Bioceramics: For Materials Science and Engineering

Related titles

Bioceramics and their clinical applications
(ISBN 9781845692049)

Hydroxyapatite (Hap) for Biomedical Applications
(ISBN 9781782420330)

Tissue Engineering Using Ceramics and Polymers
(ISBN 9780857097125)

Woodhead Publishing Series in Biomaterials

Bioceramics: For Materials Science and Engineering

Saad B. H. Farid
University of Technology
Department of Materials Engineering
Baghdad
Iraq

ELSEVIER

WP
WOODHEAD
PUBLISHING
An imprint of Elsevier

Woodhead Publishing is an imprint of Elsevier
The Officers' Mess Business Centre, Royston Road, Duxford, CB22 4QH, United Kingdom
50 Hampshire Street, 5th Floor, Cambridge, MA 02139, United States
The Boulevard, Langford Lane, Kidlington, OX5 1GB, United Kingdom

Notices

Knowledge and best practice in this field are constantly changing. As new research and experience broaden our understanding, changes in research methods, professional practices, or medical treatment may become necessary.

Practitioners and researchers must always rely on their own experience and knowledge in evaluating and using any information, methods, compounds, or experiments described herein. In using such information or methods they should be mindful of their own safety and the safety of others, including parties for whom they have a professional responsibility.

To the fullest extent of the law, neither the Publisher nor the authors, contributors, or editors, assume any liability for any injury and/or damage to persons or property as a matter of products liability, negligence or otherwise, or from any use or operation of any methods, products, instructions, or ideas contained in the material herein.

Library of Congress Cataloging-in-Publication Data
A catalog record for this book is available from the Library of Congress

British Library Cataloguing-in-Publication Data
A catalogue record for this book is available from the British Library

ISBN (Print): 978-0-08-102233-7
ISBN (Online): 978-0-08-102234-4

For information on all Woodhead Publishing publications visit our website at https://www.elsevier.com/books-and-journals

Publisher: Mathew Deans
Acquisition Editor: Laura Overend
Editorial Project Manager: Natasha Welford
Production Project Manager: Joy Christel Neumarin Honest Thangiah
Cover Designer: Christian J. Bilbow

Typeset by TNQ Technologies

To My Family
Wife Zainab
Son Zaid
Daughter Uruk

Contents

Preface

It is my privilege to write this volume in the Woodhead series in biomaterials. The plan of the book is essentially based on my lectures on bioceramics, which is part of the curriculum of "Advanced ceramics" courses for the undergraduate and postgraduate students of materials science and engineering. However, the material in this book is expanded to fully meet the requirements for the undergraduate study and most of that for the postgraduate study. The lecturer can decide student's assignments that spotlight on selected subjects.

The vision of the book is based on the issue of how to make the right introduction to the subjects of the book and how to ensure the flowability of the text in each chapter and across the book. Consequently, the book starts with a study text in character then gradually gains the flavor of review articles across the chapters. The author believes that this approach can represent a successful presentation of the book content to the students. In other words, the book supplies basic and advanced information of bioceramics following the shortest pathway. The writing style of the book contents smoothly changed from basics to higher levels. In addition, the book should help the students for understanding the subject in view of materials science and engineering. Moreover, the book should project a sufficient light on the recent concepts and state of the art of bioceramics. Undoubtedly, the fast-growing literature and innovations in bioceramics may make new concepts, appeared in the period between the writing of the book and publishing, uncovered. However, the reader is supplied with sufficient knowledge to follow recent literature.

The review questions at the end of each chapter were written for the undergraduates; although, some instructors will find they are also a challenge for a number of the postgraduates. The references of each chapter should be the first choice when an expansion of knowledge is needed.

Chapter 1 have three different goals; the first is providing a quick overview for the basics of ceramic materials science and engineering and the fundamentals of tissue–materials interaction, which should be useful to whom need to refresh his/her knowledge and filling some gaps. Second; the chapter should be useful for self-study needed by the newcomers to the subject. The third goal is to present a chapter that introduces the language of materials and medicine.

Chapter 2 provides the necessary link between the essential properties of materials (chemistry, crystalline structure, and microstructure) with the final properties such as the bioactivity, degradation, and mechanical properties. The instructor should give enough time to this chapter because it contains the basic tools for materials design that is necessary for both materials and medicine students.

Chapter 3 is aimed to fill a large gap in the knowledge of materials students who newly exposed to biomaterials field. The chapter is written in a way that introduces the new concepts gradually to dissolve any barrier and to get used to the biomaterials environment.

Chapter 4 presents a number of orthopedic and dental applications in a way that focuses on materials and processes design. Exposing to the examples of materials and processes design initiate and enhance creativity and capability for innovation. In this chapter and the next chapters, the instructor should encourage the students to point out the design elements in the presented examples and/or other examples. In addition, the instructor should always spotlight the role of characterizations throughout the materials and processes design.

Chapter 5 invested the knowledge base built through the previous chapters to start exposing to the hot disciplines of hard tissue engineering. It contains various scaffolds fabrication processes based on bioceramics and polymer–bioceramic composites. The fundamentals of the scaffold design process and the tests for bioactivity are presented to perform a wide view of the field of hard tissue engineering; however, the students can refer to the original reference article for more detailed information.

Chapter 6 illuminates the contribution of nanotechnology in tissue engineering and drug delivery. The chapter demonstrates that nanotechnology is not merely the use of nanomaterials. Various methodologies, microstructures, processes, and characterization techniques are expressed to reveal how the new and attended properties were achieved. The chapter concentrates on recent development in the field; however, the reader should gain the necessary knowledge to grasp newer achievements in the field.

I hope that the students, the instructors, and readers looking for self-contained volume will find this book useful.

Prof. Dr. Saad B.H. Farid

Overview

1

The aim of this chapter is to introduce the necessary basics of ceramics and bioceramics that are needed as a prerequisite before presenting more advanced materials. Various concepts connected to materials science and engineering are exposed. In view of this, the content of this chapter can be useful for the freshman and for those who want to refresh their basic knowledge. Depending on the level of the student, the lecturer has the option of going through the chapter, as it as a prerequisite, or bypassing it.

1.1 Ceramics and glasses [1–9]

1.1.1 Description of ceramics

Ceramic materials are chemically different from metallic and organic materials. Metallic materials are composed of metal elements such as iron (Fe), copper (Cu), nickel (Ni), and aluminum (Al). Organic materials are natural and synthetic carbon-based compounds. The important category of organic materials for engineers is polymers. Polymers are essentially very long chains of C atoms, which are connected with other atoms such as C, H, O, and N. Ceramic materials are not carbon-based materials, i.e., they are inorganic. Also, ceramic materials are compounds of two or more atoms. Most of the ceramic materials are oxides such as silica (SiO_2), alumina (Al_2O_3), zirconia (ZrO_2), and magnesia (MgO). They are also found as carbides such as SiC, nitrides such as Si_3N_4, silicates such as $ZrSiO_4$ and $MgSiO_3$, and a variety of other compounds. Ceramic materials are thus inorganic nonmetallic compounds, such as oxides, carbides, and nitrides.

The type of atomic bonding is also different between metals, polymers, and ceramics. In metals, the valence electrons are detached from the atomic nuclei and make a sort of electron cloud that bonds the positive nuclei together. This sort of bonding is called the metallic bond. On the other hand, the carbon atoms in a polymer chain are strong, directional, and covalent. Covalent bond means that there is a sharing of electrons between two atoms. In the case of ceramic materials, electrons are moved from one atom to another atom leaving anions, e.g., Si^{+4}, and cations, e.g., $2O^{-2}$. The resultant attraction is called the ionic bond. However, ceramic materials generally exhibit a combination of ionic and covalent bonds.

Consequently, the chemical, physical, and mechanical properties are expected to be distinguished between metals, polymers, and ceramics. Ceramics are hard materials; hence they are not easily scratched or dented. The high hardness of ceramics makes them resistant to mechanical wear. However, because of the ionic character of their atomic bonds, ceramics are brittle materials, i.e., they have a low resistance to impact and are easily cracked. Also, ceramics show high compression strength and low tensile

Bioceramics: For Materials Science and Engineering. https://doi.org/10.1016/B978-0-08-102233-7.00001-X

strength. However, the metallic bonds of metals give these materials different extents of ductility, and the tensile strengths exhibit values close to those of compression strengths.

As a result, ceramics being compounds are generally chemically stable, i.e., they are resistant to oxidation and acidic and alkali chemical attacks. In addition, as a whole ceramics are refractory, i.e., they maintain their strength at high temperature, which depends on the type of ceramic material. Another thermal property of ceramics is that they are thermally insulative materials. Their thermal conductivity values are greater than those of polymers and less than those of metals.

It may be useful to bring to mind that ceramic materials are usually good electrical insulators, e.g., alumina, although ceramics such as MgO are classified as semiconductors. As much as the covalent character of the atomic bonds is dominant, ceramic materials are more insulative. However, there is a class of ionically conducting ceramics that is used as solid electrolytes in high-temperature fuel cells and as chemical sensors. Generally, the electrical properties are usually described at room temperature. In fact, electrical insulation of ceramic materials is lower at higher temperatures. Ceramic materials are typically nonmagnetic. However, certain ceramic materials are strong magnets; in addition, some ceramic materials are superconductors at sufficiently low temperature, which is outside the scope of this book.

It may be noted that the average densities of ceramic materials are, roughly speaking, half of those of metallic materials. The low density, chemical stability, good mechanical strength, and other tailorable properties of ceramic materials give them great potential to produce new materials with desired properties that simplify product designs with the benefit of increased efficiency.

1.1.2 Structure and microstructure

The atoms of solid materials, including ceramics, are usually geometrically arranged in three dimensions. The geometrical arrangement is of periodical fashion. Hence they are called *crystalline materials* because they exhibit *long-range order*. X-ray diffraction patterns can tell us that the investigated solid material is crystalline when the diffraction peaks are sharp with a low background. Crystallinity is not always perfect; in other words, a combination of long-range and short-range orders may exist in the solid material. Short-range order is reflected by diffuse diffraction peaks and high background. Thus the concept of the *degree of crystallinity* is introduced to indicate the extent of the long-range order of atomic arrangement.

In the case where the short-range order is dominant, X-ray diffraction does not show diffraction peaks. Instead, the results of experiments show a wide hump that reflects the scattering phenomena of X-ray photons with randomly positioned atomic particles. In this case, the periodicity of the investigated solid material is lacking. Therefore the solid material is called *noncrystalline*, *amorphous*, or *glassy*. Here a preliminary definition of *glass* as an amorphous (noncrystalline) solid material can be introduced.

Regardless of the crystallinity of the solid material, is the solid material a sort of continuum? Using optical and electron microscopy the answer is certainly not.

The solid material is composed of building blocks called *grains*, and may contain *pores* and different kinds of materials. In addition, the solid material may have types of inhomogeneity in chemical composition, crystalline and amorphous phases, and different grain and particle sizes. These properties are called the *microstructure* of the solid material. The versatility of microstructures is the origin of the broad range of chemical, physical, and mechanical properties of the solid materials. Accordingly, the materials scientists and engineers are microstructure designers.

1.1.2.1 Structure

The repeated pattern of the atomic arrangement in three dimensions can be visualized as building blocks of solid material. The building block is called the *unit cell.* The unit cell is thus the repeated unit in three dimensions. Because of geometrical restrictions, only seven types of unit cell shapes can fill the space without vacancies. These seven unit cell shapes are called the *crystal systems*. Each crystal system can be distinguished via the lengths a, b, and c of the unit cell edges and the angles α, β, and γ between them. These lengths and angles, shown in Fig. 1.1, are called unit cell parameters.

The unit cell parameters are frequently called lattice parameters because the lattice concept is more easily represented and handled. In addition, the unit cell has a number of permutations: primitive, base centered, body centered, and face centered. However, because of geometrical considerations, there are only 14 unique permutations, called the Bravais lattices. Fig. 1.2 gives an overall appreciation of the 7 crystal systems and 14 Bravais lattices.

Ceramic materials may be found in different phases, i.e., different crystal structures. An example is that silica (SiO_2) could be in the hexagonal (quartz), cubic (cristobalite), or other phases. Each phase has its physical and mechanical properties. Another example is zirconia (ZrO_2), which exists in three phases. These phases are monoclinic at room temperature, with phase transition to tetragonal and cubic at higher temperatures. The high-temperature phases of zirconia have special mechanical properties, as will be described later.

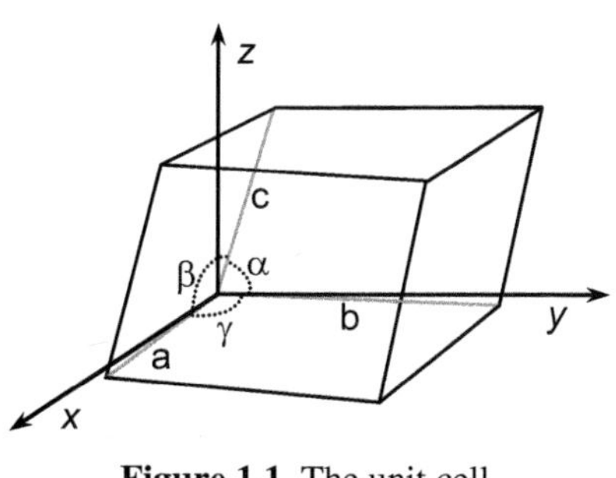

Figure 1.1 The unit cell.

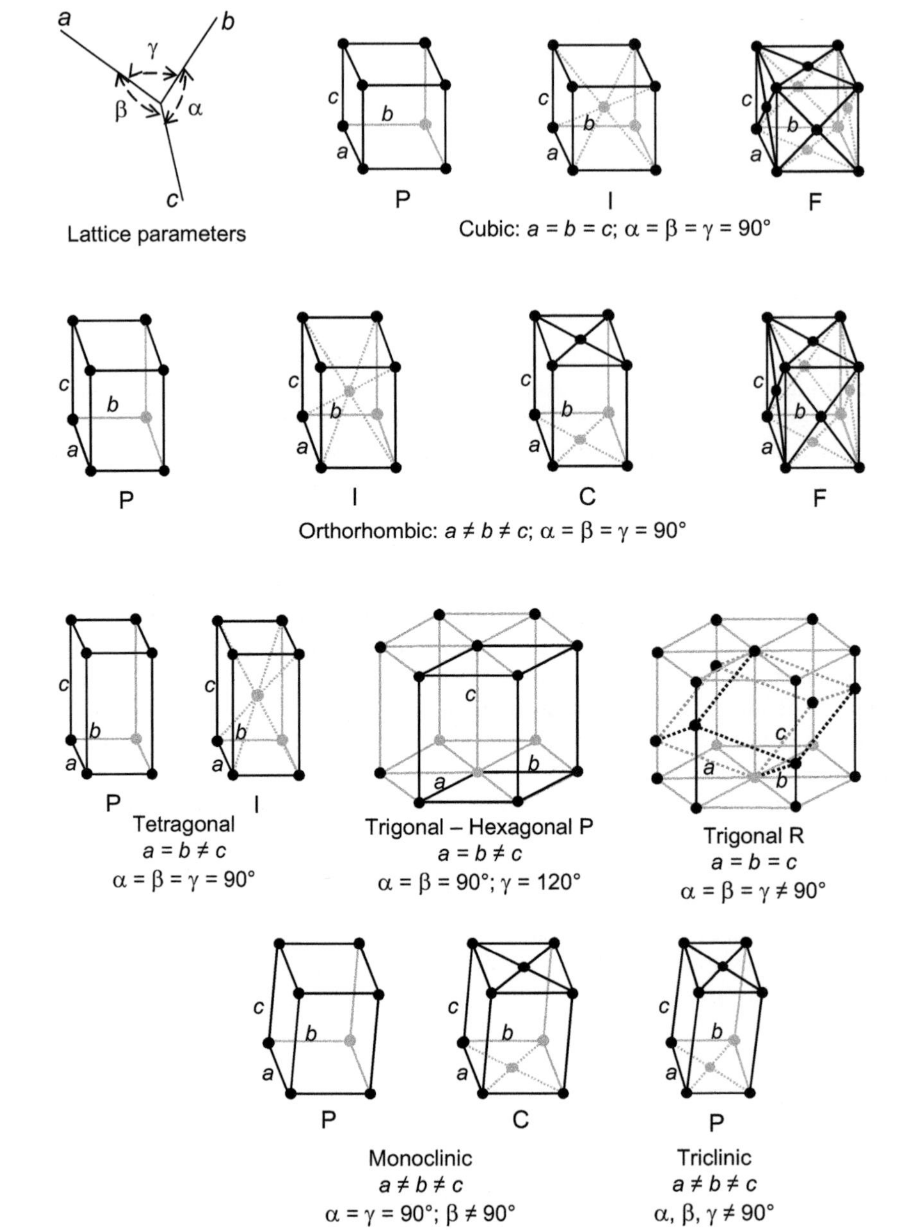

Figure 1.2 The 7 crystal systems and 14 Bravais lattices. Symbols P, C, I, F, and R refer to the different lattice types: *C*, centered in the faces perpendicular to the cell *c* axis (+1/8 of reticular point in each corner); *F*, centered in all faces of the cell (+1/8 of reticular point in each corner); *I*, centered in the body of the cell (+1/8 of reticular point in each corner); *P*, primitive (there is only one reticular point inside the cell—1 point in each of the 8 corners of the cell means 8/8 = 1 point in the cell); *R*, primitive, identical cell axes and cell angles, or hexagonal two times body centered (+1/8 of reticular point in each corner).

1.1.2.2 Microstructure

Fig. 1.3 shows a typical cross-section of a ceramic material. It is composed of an assembly of irregularly shaped grains and pores. The solid–solid interfaces are called the *grain boundaries*, and the solid–gas interfaces are called the *free surfaces*. Grain size is in the range 1–50 μm on average; hence they are visible only under a microscope. The shape and size of the grains, together with the presence of porosity, second phases, etc., and their distribution, represent the description of the microstructure.

The mechanical and physical properties of ceramics depend on their microstructure. The mechanical properties are correlated to the grain size (the diameter of the sphere of the same grain volume), which is also affected by the existence of the pore phase. On the other hand, the thermal, magnetic, and electrical properties are influenced by the existence of the interfaces (grain boundaries and free surfaces); this is why the microstructure is sometimes defined as being constituted of grain boundaries and free surfaces. In all cases, research and development in the ceramics field pays attention to grain boundary chemistry, which may be influenced by minor secondary phases but with obvious influence on the final physical and mechanical properties of the ceramic material.

It is useful to note that the ceramic material in powder form consists of an assembly of small single crystals, which is the origin of the term *polycrystalline materials*. The single crystals comprising the powder are usually called the *particles*. Particles should be differentiated from grains, which are the building blocks of the ceramic solid material.

A heat treatment process of a powder compact, termed *sintering*, converts the loose powder into a solid ceramic body. Thus the microstructure, or the microstructural features, is evolved as a result of the sintering process and its parameters (heating rate, dwell time, sintering atmosphere, etc.). The correlation between the properties of ceramics and their microstructure reflects the importance of sintering studies. Normally, these studies attempt to attain high density and controlled grain size of the product.

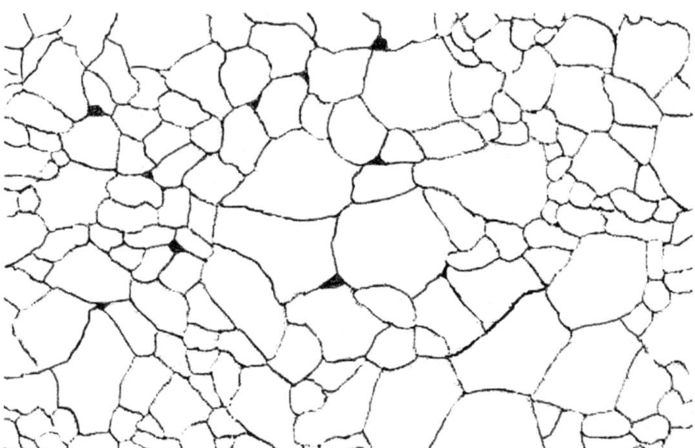

Figure 1.3 A sketch showing a cross-section of ceramic material. The *dark areas* represent the pores.

1.1.3 Sintering and microstructure of ceramics

The sintering process is described as the principal stage of the fabrication of the ceramic product. The fabrication stages are consequently the preparation of powders, shape forming, and heat treatments.

The preparation of powder includes one or more processes of extraction, purifying, grinding, milling, or chemical preparations such as the sol–gel process. The preparation step is sometimes simply the selection of materials. Shape forming includes various powder compaction processes such as die pressing, cold isostatic pressing (CIP), and hot isostatic pressing (HIP). The latter combines both the shape-forming and sintering stages. Heat treatments include one or more of drying, presintering, and sintering processes. Sintering of solid materials is a fundamental of scientific studies and continuous research and development activities in the field of ceramic materials. The preceding two stages to sintering, powder preparation and shape forming, are subjected to accumulated manufacturing experiences and innovations as well.

Usually, the sintering process is the final fabrication stage. The product may need additional processes such as rectification, decoration, surfacing coatings, or other processes. However, defects may be discovered in the product after sintering is accomplished; these defects are primarily caused by incomplete handling or manipulation in the preceding stages. As an example, the preparation of powders involves their selection or preparation according to appropriate purity, particle size and distribution, granularity of powders, sintering additives if necessary, homogeneity in the case of powder mixtures, and others.

To understand the connection between the sintering process and the final microstructure, a simple description of the sintering process may be useful. After the shaping process via casting or pressing of the loose powder, a powder compact is subjected to sintering. The compacted ceramic particle, when subjected to heat, becomes a cohesive material and subsequently begins to consolidate. In other words, the heat treatment starts an arrangement process for the compacted particle that eventually organizes a microstructure. Thus the sintering process includes several phenomena such as evolution of the size and shape of the grains (the welded particles), pore size and shape, development of new phases if any, and the possible appearance of inhomogeneities and defects. High-resolution microscopy of the fracture surface or polished and etched surface may help in the evaluation stage. The microstructure evaluation stage is important because, as stated earlier, it predicts the performance of the final product significantly.

1.1.4 Glasses and glass-ceramics

Glass is a noncrystalline solid material in which the long-range order of the constituted atoms and molecules is completely absent. The term amorphous is also used to describe glass solid material. Glass is usually prepared via melting of a mixture of precursor (starting) materials. The mixture may be composed of metal oxides, nitrates, chloride, and other salts. The mixture may also contain more complex compounds of naturally occurring ores such as kaolins and feldspars. Impurities are usually present in the glass compositions, which are not of great concern for most industrial applications. The impurities are carefully monitored and adjusted only for advanced applications of glass. When the right composition (recipe) of the precursors and melting temperature is attained, a successful preparation of the attempted glass is performed. Usually, quenching is the final step in the preparation procedure to avoid nucleation of crystalline phases within the glass. Accordingly, supercooling a viscous liquid also yields glass and the process is called vitrification.

Glass materials can be found in vast varieties of compositions according to the demanded properties. Most glasses are silica based with other components. Soda–lime glass is a good introductory example that is composed of ~72% SiO_2, 14% Na_2O, 10% CaO, and other minor additives or impurities. The prepared glass is supposed to show a unique phenomenon called glass transition or transformation behavior. Glass transition is a reversible solid–liquid transition in amorphous materials from a solid state into a molten high viscous state. Glass transition does not occur suddenly, but extends over a range of temperatures.

During glass transition, a considerable change takes place in the physical properties of the amorphous material such as density, optical, and electrical properties. In fact, any metallic, inorganic, or organic material, despite the preparation technique, that exhibits glass transition behavior is classified as glass. However, glass transition is not classified as phase transition because it does not involve the absorption or emission of thermodynamic energy, i.e., it is not accompanied by a change in molecular arrangement or crystal structure.

Glass precursor materials do not always need to be purified materials if the impurity level does not affect the desired properties of the final glass. Thus a variety may be naturally occurring and of low cost. Table 1.1 shows a few examples of cheap and abundant materials that are frequently used as glass precursor materials. The table lists the nominal compositions, but in reality the ore materials contain different levels of impurities.

In devising a glass, one of the critical design parameters is the acceptable melting temperature range. Some oxides increase the melting temperature and others decrease it. A better picture can be given if the oxides are categorized as follows:

Acidic oxides: These are the backbone of glass and mainly increase the firing temperature and improve the mechanical properties.

Formula: MO_2, e.g., SiO_2, GeO_2, ZrO_2, TiO_2, CrO_2, etc.

Table 1.1 Some popular glass precursor materials

Name	Nominal composition	Name	Nominal composition
Sand	SiO_2	Boric acid	$B_2O_3 \cdot 3H_2O$
Kaolin	$Al_2O_3 \cdot 2SiO_2 \cdot 2H_2O$	Dolomite	$CaCO_3 \cdot MgCO_3$
Albite feldspar	$Na_2O \cdot 6SiO_2$	Calcite	$CaCO_3$
Orthoclase feldspar	$K_2O \cdot Al_2O_3 \cdot 6SiO_2$	Potash	K_2CO_3
Anorthite feldspar	$CaO \cdot Al_2O_3 \cdot 2SiO_2$	Soda ash	Na_2CO_3
Petalite feldspar	$Li_2O \cdot Al_2O_3 \cdot 8SiO_2$	Caustic potash	KOH
Borax	$Na_2O \cdot 2B_2O_3 \cdot 10H_2O$	Caustic soda	NaOH

Basic oxides: These are fluxes, i.e., they reduce the firing temperature.
Formula: MO and M_2O, e.g., CaO, MgO, Na_2O, K_2O, Li_2O, etc.

Amphoteric oxides: These form bridges between acidic and basic oxides and partially substitute them.
Formula: M_2O_3 and M_2O_5, e.g., Al_2O_3, B_2O_3, Bi_2O_3, P_2O_5 PbO, Pb_3O_4, etc.

Several oxides such as SiO_2, B_2O_3, GeO_2, P_2O_5, PbO, and Pb_3O_4 are also called *glass formers* because they mainly contribute to the formation of the glass molecular network.

The most important properties that the glass designer bears in mind are the viscosity of the glass-forming melts and the thermal expansion of the prepared glass. The viscosity of the glass-forming melts, which is a measure of the resistance of a liquid to shear deformation, gives an indication of the merit of the casting process of the final product. Thermal expansion, which is the change in length of a material with increasing temperature, may contribute to the thermal behavior of the glass and the adaptation quality of a glass coat to a certain solid body. Viscosity and thermal expansion are largely dependent on glass composition.

An important application of glass is the *vitreous coating*. The vitreous coating may be classified as the coating of a ceramic body (glazing) and the coating of a metallic body (enamel). The coating includes physical and chemical adhesion of a thin layer of glass to the solid body. Applications of vitreous coatings are diverse because they add the desired chemical and physical properties to the solid part.

A key category of materials is *glass-ceramics*. Glass-ceramics consist of one or more amorphous and crystalline phases. The preparation process of a glass-ceramic includes complete melting of the batch materials. Experienced technicians prefer to quench the glass melt, crush and mix it, and then melt the batch again to attain better homogeneity. A controlled cooling process is then followed to allow for the formation and growth of crystalline nuclei (crystallization) in the glass medium. Nucleation seeds or agents are added to the glass melt, in some cases to encourage the crystallization process. The nucleation agents, such as TiO_2, assist the crystallization process and also control the speed and amount of the crystalline phase. The crystallization process is also called *controlled crystallization* and should be distinguished from *spontaneous crystallization*, which is usually avoided in glass manufacturing because it causes inhomogeneity problems. The controlled crystallization process of the glass melts is a unique ceramic fabrication process in that the final product is typically free of porosity. Unlike sintered ceramics, porosity is unavoidable unless special, expensive techniques are used such as HIP.

Several advantages are afforded by glass-ceramic materials. In addition to the preparation of zero porosity solid material, glass-ceramic material has high strength and toughness with sealing properties of glass, high chemical durability, high-temperature stability, and low thermal expansion. The glass-ceramic can also be fabricated with unique aesthetic optical properties such as fluorescence, translucency, or opacity. The fabrication process of the glass-ceramic also allows fabricating materials with favored electrical properties such as low dielectric constant and dielectric loss, high resistivity, and breakdown voltage. Machinability of ceramics can be attained with a special type of glass-ceramic called *machinable ceramics*. In addition to other advantages, the glass-ceramic is usually manufactured at relatively low cost; glass-ceramics are a favorable choice in a variety of fields.

The various applications of glass-ceramics are because of the ability to tailor the properties of the fabricated parts. Tailoring of the properties can be achieved by the design of the composition of the glass melt, type and amount of the nucleation agents, and the heat treatment crystallization program.

1.1.5 Conclusion

Materials science and engineering is exclusively discussing the interrelationships between the structure of materials, processing methodologies that result in a targeted microstructure and properties, and the study of the resultant performance of the synthetic material at the operating conditions. These research activities are always accompanied by the characterization of materials. Thus the materials scientist, after studying the required properties and performance of a product, may suggest the starting materials and the processing route that may result in a designed chemistry, crystalline structure, and microstructure. The resultant properties and performance may help in the determination of the required directions for improvement of the results. In reality, characterization of materials resembles a gauge for progress during the whole research and development process.

Bioceramics, as part of biomaterials, is an interdisciplinary field of research. The field of bioceramics comprises materials science and engineering and many aspects of biology, medicine, and clinical experience. Bioceramics have a variety of applications such as hip and knee implants and various dental implants. Bioceramics also include more sophisticated implants such as the middle ear and heart valves.

The scope of this book is to focus on materials science and engineering aspects of bioceramics needed by undergraduate and postgraduate students of materials. This scope may extend, when necessary, to other aspects of bioceramics to achieve a self-contained volume.

1.2 Types of bioceramics [10–15]

There are several classifications of biomaterials. Starting with those determined by biomaterials reaction with living tissue may be appropriate. Implant materials may be found to be toxic, inert, active, and resorbable. Metals and alloys may be toxic because of the release of toxic elements such as cadmium and vanadium. Carbides and some polymeric materials can also be toxic. Toxic effects such as the release of chemicals and promotion of a local galvanic process may lead to the rejection of toxic implants, or, in some cases, the surrounding living tissues die resulting in a complicated medical situation. On the other hand, there exist nontoxic alloys and polymers that are beyond the scope of this book. In the case of ceramic implants, they are generally nontoxic. Thus bioceramic implants fall into three main categories: bioinert, bioactive, and bioresorbable ceramics.

1.2.1 Classification of bioceramics according to the type of implant material

There are different types of bioceramics according to the type of implant ceramic material that determines the type of attachment to the host tissue. Ceramic materials can be bioinert, porous, bioactive, and resorbable. Tissue–implant interactions depend to a large extent on the similarity of implant materials to the inorganic phase of bone.

The inorganic phase of bone is called the bone apatite or the biological apatite. The composition of bone apatite is close to that of synthetic calcium hydroxyapatite ($Ca_{10}(PO_4)_6(OH)_2$), which is usually called hydroxyapatite (HA). However, the physical and mechanical properties of bone apatite are different from HA because of the deviation from stoichiometry via calcium deficiency.

1.2.1.1 Bioinert ceramics

There is no material that is completely inert when it is exposed to physiological environments. Bioinert material undergoes negligible or ineffective chemical changes when implanted in living tissue. Accordingly, bioinert material maintains its physical and mechanical properties for a long time in the host tissue.

The body's response to a bioinert implant is the formation of a fine fibrous tissue that surrounds the implant and separates it from the living tissue. Ceramic oxides are known to have strong bonds, i.e., they are chemically inert; accordingly, they show a high degree of bioinertness. Because bioinert ceramics such as aluminum oxide and zirconium oxide show higher degrees of bioinertness than alloys, the thickness of fibrous tissue is formed in the order of several molecular layers. Whereas for lesser bioinertness shown by, e.g., stainless steel, the layer thickness is several micrometers or more. Hence the fibrous tissue layer thickness can be regarded as a sort of measure of bioinertness. A morphological fixation leads to a mechanical interlocking of the bioinert ceramic to the host tissue. Porous bioinert ceramics may be used with 100–150 μm interfacial pore sizes to allow the growth of host tissue inside those pores and construct a mechanical interlocking.

An important field of application of bioinert ceramics is in frictional pairs of artificial joints. In addition to chemical inertness, bioceramics are known to show a coefficient of friction and wear rate, which are remarkably smaller than those of metals. This has resulted in the use of bioceramics, e.g., alumina extends the life of prostheses such as the knobs of hips and other parts of joints. The ceramic knob–polyethylene friction pair shows extremely fine and dispersed wear that can be discarded via kidneys. The ceramic–ceramic frictional pair also exists, but extreme care should be taken in the manufacturing process to ensure excellent interface sliding, i.e., to achieve a status of insignificant wear products.

1.2.1.2 Porous ceramics

Porous ceramics are essentially introduced as a type of bioceramics when the required function is the filling of bone defects. In fact, there are two additional functions of porous ceramics. The first is as a host for drug delivery, where microporosity is required; the second is for tissue engineering scaffold, where macroporosity (>100 μm) is needed to provide enough space for bone tissue to grow inside macropores. In all cases, porous ceramics are used as bone implants at nonload-bearing sites.

Macroporosity and interconnected porosity are required for several reasons. The first is to fulfill the morphological requirement for bone tissue integration that needs open interconnected pores to stimulate tissue ingrowth that helps in mechanical interlocking; thus loose implants are avoided. Porous implants of (HA) ceramics, with about 70% interconnected porosity, mimicking natural bone, are usually used for bioactive fixation. The coating of porous alumina or porous alloys with bioactive HA or with an HA layer that contains pores (porous coating) is also used to encourage tissue ingrowth to achieve mechanical interlocking. Hip and knee replacements are important examples of such interlocking of orthopedic implanting.

The second reason is that fluid flow is permitted via vascular growth to accomplish nutrient delivery and removal of waste, which explains why the pore network needs to be no less than 100 μm in size.

Another reason for the requirement of macroporosity is to encourage resorption of the biomaterials to promote bioactivity. Bioresorption can take place with bioactive glass because of its special formulation. It also can take place with HA and tricalcium phosphate (TCP). Accordingly, these materials found wide applications for tissue engineering scaffolds because a porous scaffold could be built outside the body, implanted in the living tissue, and a slow bioresorption process would then replace the implant with new living tissue.

1.2.1.3 Bioactive ceramics

The ability of the implant to form a bond with human bone is called bioactivity. Bioactive materials do not form fibrous tissue at the interface; instead, they form an adherent interface with extensive mechanical strength. Accordingly, a bioactive material is reliably integrated with bone and sustains its implantation for a sufficiently long time.

The interface is created via chemical reactions that lead to the formation of hydroxycarbonate apatite (HCA). The bond is stronger than the bone itself. One exception is that HA bonds directly to the bone.

Bioactive ceramics include bioactive glasses, bioactive glass-ceramics, several calcium phosphates, bioactive coatings, and bioactive composites. The difference in the solubility of the bioactive implant, which leads to a different degree of reaction, results in a range of layer thicknesses of 0.5–100 μm.

Historically, the first bioactive ceramic was the bioactive glass discovered by Hench, Splinter, Allen, and Greenlee in 1969. They found that certain compositions of glasses have the ability to form a strong adherent layer to the bone. The discovered bioglass is composed of SiO_2–CaO–Na_2O–P_2O_5. A typical composition, termed Bioglass 45S5, has the composition, in wt%, 45% SiO_2, 24.5% Na_2O, 24.5% CaO, and 6% P_2O_5. In addition, with SiO_2 content up to 52 wt%, bonding can take place to the bone and also to the soft tissue.

Another approach is the coating of alloys and ceramics with bioactive materials. To a large extent these biocomposite materials have higher strength and stiffness compared to bone. In other words, a problem of mechanical incompatibility emerges. The opposite case is that the HA is insufficiently strong, especially in porous form, for load-bearing bones. Thus research activities were focused on developing bioactive ceramics, which are designed in structures and/or microstructures to be chemically and mechanically compatible with bone.

1.2.1.4 Resorbable ceramics

A resorbable material undergoes a gradual dissolution in the living organism. The final interface is either absent or of very low thickness. Concurrently, living tissue is restored like bone regeneration and the restoration of blood vessels and nerve fibers. Resorbable ceramics include some of the bioglasses, calcium phosphate, TCP, and porous HA. These ceramics are resorbable principally because of the nature of their chemical bonds and also their ability to form microstructures. The resorption rate of the ceramics is increased with the decrease in grain and particle size. It is further increased with the decrease in crystallinity. In addition, the resorption rate is higher for a higher surface area; thus the powders show the highest resorption rate, followed by porous ceramics, and then dense ceramics.

Resorbable (or bioresorbable) ceramics integrate with tissue without toxicity or rejection and are steadily replaced by the host tissue. Bioactive ceramics may be distinguished from resorbable ceramics by the aforementioned structural and microstructural factors, e.g., HA is not resorbable in dense form and can be stable for 5–7 years in living tissue. Thus it can be concluded that bioactive ceramics lie in an intermediate location between bioinert and resorbable ceramics.

Resorption is started with the dissolving of the ceramics that creates a suitable chemical environment for tissue infiltration and substitution, i.e., tissue regeneration. The resorption rate must be controlled so that it matches the tissue repair rate to achieve a successful tissue regeneration process. The resorption rate is undoubtedly proportional to the dissolving rate of the implanted ceramics. Moreover, the dissolving rate is controlled by the structural and microstructural factors. Another requirement for the resorbable ceramic is that it can maintain a compatible mechanical performance during the tissue regeneration processes. Otherwise, the decrease in mechanical properties caused by the dissolving of the implanted ceramics can introduce difficulties in successful applications. Thus the selection and design of resorbable ceramics play a vital role in a successful repair process.

1.2.2 Classification of implants according to their tissue interactions

Tissue–implant interactions can be classified according to the type of reaction with the living tissue. The implant material determines whether the resultant reaction is toxic, compatible, bioactive, or leads to the dissolution of the implant.

1.2.2.1 Implants with toxic effect

Implanted materials may have a toxic effect on living tissue. This effect can take place when the implant releases toxic materials at risky rates. The released materials may activate the immune system. Thus material selection of the implant should take into account the risk that chemicals may be released that are harmful to the host tissue or can be transported within body fluids. In most cases, the body's response is to isolate the implant through a fibrous tissue. The fibrous tissue does not adhere to the implant and encapsulates it to separate it from the living tissue. The formation of the fibrous capsule can be understood as a protecting mechanism that develops with time. Accordingly, the fibrous capsule can be of different thicknesses; the thickness depends on the rate of the release or leaching of toxic substances. The sources of the toxic substance are metallic elements, corrosion products, wear particles, or polymer degradation. These effects are usually found when the implant materials are composed of metals or most of the polymers. The importance of ceramics as biomaterials lies in the fact that these toxic effects are rarely met.

Limited toxicity may be found with some elements such as zirconium and titanium. On the other hand, the impurities of starting materials are a potential source of toxicity. Toxicity increases with an increase in the impurity level. Another effect of impurities in the implanted materials in the physiological environment is that they gradually attack the grain boundary of implanted material, deteriorate the microstructure, especially at the surface, and increase the roughness. As a result, the wear rate is increased in the case of the frictional parts, or the strength of the load-bearing implant is reduced. Consequently, service life is reduced and the implant eventually needs to be replaced.

There are also examples of limited toxicity of ceramics such as barium sulfate. Barium is a heavy metal and its sulfate is water soluble, but it has very low solubility in body fluid. The limited solubility restricts the toxic effect of barium. Some toxic materials are introduced indirectly when implanting bioceramics, e.g., the binder introduced with bone scaffolds produced by a conventional method. Thus limited toxicity is introduced via such residuals, which can introduce thin fibrous separating tissue.

1.2.2.2 Biocompatible implants

The concept of biocompatibility is extended from inert to bioactive materials in some literature. However, biocompatibility in the context of this book denotes that the implant has no negative impact on the host tissue. The long-term contact of the implant with the living tissue requires that the implant material shows no toxic effects, good fixation to the host, and, in some cases, the mechanical properties of the implant should be attuned with that of the hard tissue.

Accordingly, the implant should be composed of biologically inert materials or, at least, the surface of the implant should show biological inertness. There are two requirements to achieve biological inertness: the first is the chemical inertness of the surface of the implant, and the second is to bring the amount of the mechanical wear products, in the case of moving parts, to an acceptable minimum. Generally, implants comply with these requirements in varying degrees.

As mentioned earlier, there is no absolutely bioinert material. Varying degrees of bioinertness are examined with the implant. The implant that induces a separating fibrous tissue layer with a lower thickness is of higher biocompatibility. In other words, the higher the biocompatibility, the lower the response of the host physiological environment and immune reactions. Thus the refractory ceramic materials are well suited for this type of application because of their unique chemical inertness. The strong chemical bonds of the ceramic materials protect them to a large extent from the effect of fermentation mechanisms in the living tissue.

The strong bonds of the ceramic materials suitable as implants also explain why there is an enhanced chemical resistance, high compression properties, and high hardness, which result in reduced wear of products at the surface of the frictional pairs of artificial joints, especially the bearing surfaces. Ceramic materials were first used in dentistry, e.g., in dental crowns, because of their aesthetic appearance and high mechanical properties; now they are being introduced into orthopedics.

1.2.2.3 Bioactive implants

Bioactive implants are distinguished from inert implants because they trigger chemical bonding with the living tissue. Numerous ceramic materials are described as bioactive because of their ability to form chemical bonds with the hard tissue. The resultant ceramic–bone interface can be stronger than the bone itself. The hard tissue is stimulated from that interface because of the composition of the bioceramics, which contains elements typically found in hard tissue such as calcium, phosphorus, and silicon. Bioceramics are occasionally described as biocompatible because they usually do not show toxic effects provided that the implant material is sufficiently pure.

The generated strong interface between the implant and the host tissue represents an adherent fixation that impedes movement of the implant or separation from the host tissue. Consequently, mechanical loads and other stresses are passed through the interface.

In fact, bioactivity is not restricted by the formation of the chemical bond with the hard tissue. Bioactivity may include fusing with the bone or soft tissue, especially with noncrystalline ceramics. This process can result in the reformation of lost bone tissue and bone reconstruction because of the existence of the necessary element at the implant interface with the proper concentration.

If total fusing of the ceramic implant takes place, then HCA replaces the implant, i.e., the implant is dissolved. Thus the bioactive ceramics can be thought of as an intermediate between inert and resorbable ceramics. The evaluation of ceramic materials as inert, bioactive, or resorbable depends on the processing routes of the implant and the site of the implantation.

1.2.2.4 Dissolved implants

If the implant–tissue interface has sufficient chemical activity, the interface location will not be fixed but will move toward the implant, i.e., there is a continuous dissolution of the implant accompanied by the formation of new surrounding tissue. This process can take place provided that the proper conditions of composition and microstructure of the implant are fulfilled. The process should end with total replacement of the implant with new tissue. The dissolved implants can be thought of as advanced bioactive materials that share load bearing with the host bone and gradually dissolve to enhance the growth of new bone cells and restore the original bone strength.

The composition of the dissolved implants should be bioactive; i.e., they contain the necessary balance of calcium, phosphorus, and silicon. Dissolution of the bioglasses is faster than calcium phosphates, and HA is the slowest. In addition, the composition should not contain toxic materials or impurities at levels that can hinder bioactivity. Dissolving is extremely slow for dense ceramics, and the implant is regarded as stable at high levels of sintered density. Thus the existence of porosity is necessary for the dissolving process to take place. An attack by body fluid to dissolve the implant is limited in the case of closed porosity. Therefore open porosity is mandatory for the process because it provides the necessary circulation of body fluid to obtain a balanced concentration of elements. Certainly, the porosity level affects the dissolution speed because of the higher surface area accompanied by higher porosity. Smaller grain sizes also increase the surface area. The fingerprints of materials science and engineering are very obvious in this type of application through experience in the development of the microstructure.

The development, or design, of the microstructure controls the dissolving rate by, e.g., the synthesis of materials with graded composition or porosity. This type of design is usually called functionally graded materials (FGMs). With such a microstructure, the dissolution and reprecipitation of calcium and phosphate ions control the formation of biological apatite. As a result, the bioactive interface is in dynamic equilibrium, and the bioceramic is gradually consumed until it diminishes without leaving a fibrous tissue behind.

1.3 Alumina and zirconia [16–27]

1.3.1 Alumina

Alumina (Al_2O_3) is a celebrated engineering material because of its diverse applications. Most of the applications of alumina rely on its strength, refractoriness, chemical stability, and electrical insulation. Alumina is only slightly soluble in strong acids and alkalis. Accordingly, alumina is usually selected for surgical devices. The application of alumina as a component of prostheses was introduced in 1970 because of its resistance to chemical attack in the living environment (in vivo) and bioinertness, which make it ideal as a material of choice for long-term stability and service in the body environment.

Alumina exists naturally as the corundum ore, which contains crystalline alumina with traces of other oxides such as iron and titanium oxides. The economic use of this ore is as an abrasive material because of its hardness, which can reach 9 on the Mohs scale for the pure phase. Alumina is usually produced commercially from more abundant ores with a chemical purification process.

The production of alumina starts with the process of extraction of its ores such as bauxite and cryolite. The ores are different in their alumina content, purity, and extraction cost. Bauxite consists of monohydrate ($Al_2O_3 \cdot H_2O$) and trihydrate ($Al_2O_3 \cdot 3H_2O$) alumina in different ratios that depend on the site of the extraction. Monohydrated alumina is called boehmite, and trihydrated alumina is called gibbsite. Other existing phases are mainly silica, in addition to various iron oxides and titanium oxides. The total alumina content in bauxite is 30%–54% depending on ore composition.

The process of extraction of alumina from bauxite was invented in 1887 by Karl Bayer and named after him as the Bayer process. The ore is first well grounded to increase the surface area of the ore powder. The higher surface area provides a more efficient and inclusive chemical reaction during the process because of increased solid–liquid contact. A solution of sodium hydroxide ($pH > 10$) is then added to dissolve the bauxite. A pressure vessel is utilized to contain the mix, and the temperature is raised. The resulting steam may boost the pressure in the vessel up to 30 atm. Boehmite dissolves at temperatures above 220°C, and gibbsite dissolves at temperatures below 150°C. These reactions yield sodium aluminates, as shown by Eqs. (1.1) and (1.2). The dissolving reaction takes around 2–3 min, which is very short compared with 4–6 h in the case of the reaction at normal pressure. The high pressure also prevents boiling of the slurry.

$$2NaOH + Al_2O_3 \cdot H_2O \rightarrow 2NaAlO_2 + 2H_2O \quad (1.1)$$

$$2NaOH + Al_2O_3 \cdot 3H_2O \rightarrow 2NaAlO_2 + 4H_2O \quad (1.2)$$

The reaction is followed by filtration to remove the solid unreacted content, which is composed mainly of silica, iron, and titanium oxides and some unreacted alumina. Then, the remaining supersaturated solution is seeded via aluminum hydroxide fine particles to initiate and accelerate the precipitation of crystalline aluminum trihydrate ($Al_2O_3 \cdot 3H_2O$), which can be easily filtered and washed. The final step is calcination of the aluminum trihydrate above 1100°C to extract the water molecules. The calcination condition determines the resultant particle size and surface area of the produced alumina. The produced crystalline phase of alumina is the thermodynamically favored form α-Al_2O_3, but other phases can exist indicating the need for further calcination.

For the synthesis of alumina medical parts, the use of high-purity alumina is essential to secure the implant from attack from body fluid. The standard specification ASTM F603-00 requires that the alumina content is not less than 99.5%, with MgO not exceeding 0.5%, and other oxides not exceeding 0.1%. The cold isostatic press is usually used for the formation of implant shapes (shape forming) to achieve high green density, reproducible results, and to avoid the inclusion of impurities. In some cases, the green part, or compact, needs machining to obtain the desired details.

Sintering of alumina is performed at 1600–1800°C depending on the particle size and distribution of the starting powder, compact density, sintering additive, and the desired final density. These parameters are very important to produce the required final dimensions of the sintered part, especially for medical applications. Sintering additives, such as MgO or CaO (usually called fluxes), may be included in the starting powder to adjust the sintering temperature. A quantity of MgO less than 0.5% may be added to inhibit abnormal grain growth that may degrade the mechanical properties of the final product. Doping (addition of less than 100 ppm) of rare earth oxides may alter the grain boundary lattice and inhibit grain growth. The addition of small amounts (≤0.5) of CaO may be used to decrease the sintering temperature. The addition of CaO to alumina produces a liquid phase that facilitates mass transport during sintering, but the liquid phase will exist at the grain boundaries after cooling. The residual liquid (glassy) phase may reduce the chemical stability that can negatively affect the mechanical properties of the product. The existence of SiO_2 impurity usually promotes grain growth and decelerates the densification mechanisms, and the sintering process ends with lower sintered density.

As mentioned in Section 1.2, the bioinertness of alumina stimulates the body to isolate it via a thin fibrous capsule. The sintered alumina encounters minimal response at the body environment because of its chemical stability. On the other hand, if wear products are produced in a site of moving parts, the isolation fibrous capsule becomes thicker. For this reason, a postsintering finishing process attempts to reduce the surface roughness of the sintered alumina implant to less than 0.02 μm. The surface of the alumina can also be modified in terms of chemistry and microstructure via the art of surface engineering such as coating.

Since the 1970s, alumina implants with smooth polished surfaces were used in joint replacement prostheses because of their high-quality chemical and wear properties. Alumina femoral heads are regularly used for hip replacement implants, as seen in Fig. 1.4. Initially, an acetabular cup (the hip socket, a cup-shaped part for the opposing articulating surface to assemble with the femoral head) is made from ultrahigh molecular weight polyethylene (UHMWPE). Then, alumina is introduced for the production of the acetabular cup, usually called ceramic-on-ceramic (COC) hip replacement or arthroplasty. The COC or alumina–alumina ceramic bearing couple has the advantage of better wear resistance compared with cases where UHMWPE or metal is included. The ceramic wear debris is also less inflammatory than that of UHMWPE and far less than that of metal. The ceramic bearing couple also gives the surgeon the freedom to use a larger femoral head in an attempt to reduce the probability or risk of dislocation of the implant from its site.

Fracture of the alumina femoral head was an important concern in early applications. Materials scientists have directed the focus of their research on the origin of such a negative aspect and attempted to solve the problem. The early production of the alumina femoral head was not free of porosity, and it is concluded that the residual porosity and the inhomogeneous microstructure resemble the origin of a slow retard of the microstructure and associated mechanical properties. Accordingly, a lot of work has been carried out to improve the properties of the starting materials and fabrication techniques, including the sintering techniques. CIP of nanoalumina powder with subsequent sintering and polishing represents the general practice. On the other hand, techniques such as HIP are also part of the practice. In all cases, a homogeneous, fine-grained microstructure is attained with average grain size not exceeding 4 μm. Accordingly, a fracture rate of 0.004% is achieved for the femoral head.

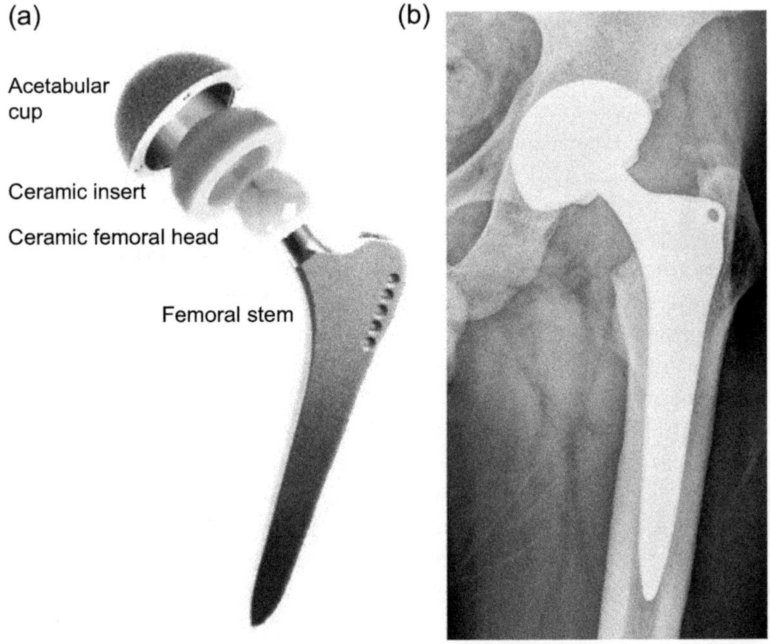

Figure 1.4 (a) A hip prosthesis implant design, (b) a radiograph of a successfully implanted hip prosthesis after 3 years.
Reused from T.V. Swanson, D.J. Peterson, R. Seethala, R.L. Bliss, C.A. Spellmon, Influence of prosthetic design on squeaking after ceramic-on-ceramic total hip arthroplasty, The Journal of Arthroplasty 25 (2010) 36–42. https://doi.org/10.1016/j.arth.2010.04.032; B.-J. Kang, Y.-C. Ha, S.-C. Hwang, Y.-K. Lee, K.-H. Koo, Midterm results of large diameter biolox forte ceramic head on delta ceramic liner articulation in total hip arthroplasty, The Journal of Arthroplasty 29 (2014) 2412–2414. https://doi.org/10.1016/j.arth.2014.03.003 after license via (copyright.com) number 4082891318449 and 4082920848195, respectively.

Alumina–zirconia composite ceramics are also used in total knee replacement (Fig. 1.5). In this figure, the upper part, the femoral component, which articulates with the lower part, a tibial component, are both made of ceramics. A plastic spacer between them is usually made of UHMWPE. As the femoral component slides on the spacer, also called the wear plate, the formation of debris is unavoidable because of the wear of UHMWPE. Fortunately, the wear plate can be replaced in a quick and simple operation, and recovery is relatively rapid. Anyway, the ceramic femoral component is superior to that of metal because of the reduced amount of polyethylene wear debris as a result of the smooth and hard surface of the alumina. In addition, the release of ions in the case of the metallic femoral component produces more serious wear debris because of their chemical activity and solubility, which causes an inflammatory response.

An important point with the ceramic implant is the mismatch of Young's modulus of the ceramic and bone. The Young's modulus of alumina (380–420 GPa) is far more than that of cancellous bone (0.05–0.5 GPa) and cortical bone (7–25 GPa). This

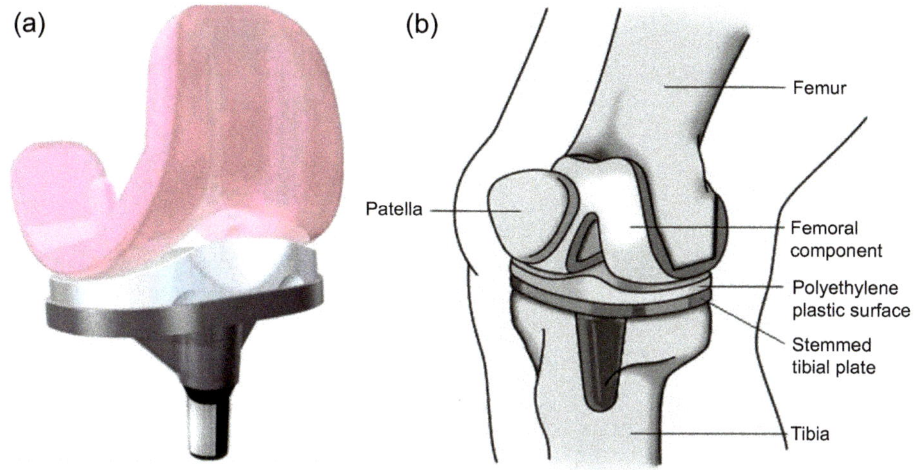

Figure 1.5 (a) Knee with ceramic (BIOLOX delta) femoral component, (b) a sketch showing a knee implant in vivo.
Reused from P. Bergschmidt, R. Bader, D. Ganzer, C. Hauzeur, C.H. Lohmann, A. Krüger, W. Rüther, D. Tigani, N. Rani, J.L. Esteve, F.L. Prats, C. Zorzi, V. Madonna, S. Rigotti, F. Benazzo, S.M.P. Rossi, W. Mittelmeier, Prospective multi-centre study on a composite ceramic femoral component in total knee arthroplasty: five-year clinical and radiological outcomes, The Knee 22 (2015) 186–191. https://doi.org/10.1016/j.knee.2015.02.003; B.C. Carr, T. Goswami, Knee implants – review of models and biomechanics, Materials and Design 30 (2009) 398–413. https://doi.org/10.1016/j.matdes.2008.03.032 after license via (copyright.com) number 4082921368191 and 4082930375115, respectively.

situation impedes the transfer of stress from the ceramic implant to the bone, i.e., a mechanical shielding by the ceramic prevents the distribution of stress along the implant and the bone. Thus the stresses will be concentrated as net compressive stress by the implant on the bone. As a result, the bone starts deteriorating, which leads to its resorption, and the entire implant site fails.

Porous alumina found application as bone spacers. Sections of the bone may be surgically removed to, e.g., eliminate cancer. The bone spacer is used to replace lost bone sections. The porous alumina should have interconnected porosity with pore size >100 μm and total porosity >30%. This type of porosity allows bone ingrowth and formations of new blood vessels through the interconnected pore structure, i.e., the bone spacers represent scaffolds for the formation of new bone tissue. Sol–gel processing and additive manufacturing (3D printing) are among the fabrication techniques for porous ceramics. However, a balance between the mechanical properties, the required porosity, and manufacturing techniques is an active field of research.

Alumina is also present in dental implantation. A permanent ceramic implant as part of an artificial tooth may be composed of monolithic alumina as a basic practice, or alumina–zirconia composite and zirconia-toughened alumina (ZTA) as advanced implantology. More information is available in the description of zirconia.

1.3.2 Zirconia

Zirconia (ZrO_2) has three polymorphic forms: monoclinic, tetragonal, and cubic. The monoclinic phase is stable at room temperature; the tetragonal phase is a metastable phase that forms at 1170–2370°C; and the cubic phase starts evolving above 2670°C. On cooling from high temperature, the cubic–tetragonal transformation takes place with a slight expansion of the unit cell volume. On the other hand, the tetragonal–monoclinic and cubic–monoclinic transformations are accompanied by high-volume expansions (3%–5%). Hence the sintered pure zirconia undergoes the formation of cracks caused by large stresses during the cooling period. To overcome this difficulty, oxide additives, e.g., CaO, MgO, and Y_2O_3, are used to stabilize the cubic or tetragonal phase of zirconia when cooled from the sintering temperature to room temperature. The zirconia powder is thus called stabilized zirconia.

The addition of about 8 mol% CaO or MgO produces partially stabilized zirconia (PSZ), i.e., the cubic or tetragonal transformation to monoclinic phase is bounded during cooling, and accordingly the formation of cracks does not occur. Roughly speaking, the mount of monoclinic phase is around 10%–20% and can be reduced to less than 5% via thermal aging. Improved mechanical properties are achieved with PSZ because of the phenomenon of transformation toughening (TT). TT is an induced transformation of the tetragonal phase into the monoclinic phase caused by the exposure to crack stress energy. The grains that constitute the microstructure turn into monoclinic within several microns of the crack tip. Volume expansion is accompanied by a compressive stress that stops crack propagation.

Fully yttria-stabilized zirconia (Y-TZP) can be achieved with about 8 mol% Y_2O_3. With the development of powder technology, 5 and 3 mol% of Y_2O_3 are enough for full stabilization because of the improved homogeneity of the powders and the smaller particle size of the zirconia and Y_2O_3 additive. At present, 3 mol% addition of Y_2O_3 to produce stabilized tetragonal zirconia powder, or polycrystals (3Y-TZP), is commercially available as a nanopowder and often used to produce sintered zirconia products.

Zirconia is often produced via the decomposition of zircon ($ZrSiO_4$) with the aid of decomposition agents and followed by a purification stage. Details of the process depend on the nature of the raw materials and the targeted properties. Low-temperature high-purity tetragonal zirconia can be produced by means of a special technique called the sol–gel process. Generally, the sol–gel process includes acid dissolving a zirconium salt followed by nucleation and growth of zirconia. Thus the sol–gel technique is used to produce nanosized zirconia via controlling particle growth. Other chemical techniques for the preparation of zirconia are available, but are not covered in this book. One of the advantages of the sol–gel process is that the additives, such as Y_2O_3, can be incorporated during the process. Accordingly, a high degree of homogeneity and particle size control that aids the stabilization of tetragonal zirconia is achieved.

MgO-PSZ was introduced in the mid-1980s as a bioceramic for the production of ball heads for total hip replacements. Better wear resistance, bending strength, and fracture toughness compared with alumina were obtained. On the other hand, the large grain size of the sintered product (40–50 μm) increases the wear rate of the polyethylene acetabular component. Thus yttria-stabilized tetragonal zirconia ball heads were introduced because the submicron grain size of the sintered product significantly improves the wear properties.

The process of manufacturing yttria-stabilized tetragonal zirconia involves a precise and complicated heat treatment program that ensures the precipitation of the tetragonal acicular phase at the grain boundaries of the cubic phase. It was found that the stability of zirconia strongly depends on such processing conditions. In addition, the environmental conditions faced by the implant also affect the stability of zirconia. Explicitly, the surface of the zirconia implant is exposed to the body (synovial) fluid that causes low-temperature degradation (LTD) of the implant. LTD is the increase in the monoclinic phase that significantly leads to the increase in roughness. Overstabilization of the tetragonal phase by a minor increase in the stabilizer may reduce the LTD effect. On the other hand, the enhanced stabilization should not hinder the TT and accordingly should reduce the mechanical properties. These complications put the process at a slight disadvantage. Accordingly, the production of zirconia balls has been gradually reduced. Alternatively, research activities attempt to include zirconia in alumina composite, as shown next.

Alumina reinforced with tetragonal zirconia has been used successfully for total hip arthroplasty (THA) because of the improved hardness, strength, toughness, and thermal conductivity of that composite. The TT of zirconia in ZTA is the origin of the improved mechanical properties. The improved mechanical properties reduce the design limitations of the implant components. Another advantage of ZTA is that the LTD, also called aging of the zirconia phase, is considerably slower compared with the zirconia matrix. The homogeneous distribution of the zirconia reinforcement should be ensured to accomplish that advantage. The alumina matrix appears to hinder the transformation of zirconia to the monoclinic phase; thus the surface of the implant is free from large grains that negatively affect the wear properties of the couple-bearing implant.

Alumina and zirconia also contribute to dental restorations. Dental restorations started in the 1960s with metal–ceramic systems. The metal–ceramic system is composed of a metal substructure coated with two or three layers of feldspathic porcelain (a leucite-based glass-ceramic). The first layer, the opaquer, acts to ensure mechanical interlocking to the metal base to provide the desired opacity to conceal the metal color, and to give the desired color with the aid of coloring agents. The second layer, the dentine, is desired to provide the required translucency necessary for the aesthetic look of the tooth. The third layer, the glaze, is added in some cases to further improve the aesthetic properties because of its higher light refraction, which improves the luminosity. Every coat should have thermal expansion larger than that of its base by not more than $0.3\times10^{-6}K^{-1}$, and a lower melting point not more than 30K. These prerequisites make achieving a successful coating a real challenge, and it was the objective of vast research studies. Alternatively, metal-free systems have evolved for dental restorations.

PSZ was used in the early 1990s as a dental implant and was gradually adopted by the all-ceramic restoration systems utilizing various ceramic fabrication processes. The crystalline nature of ceramic restoration offers greater durability and mechanical properties. ZTA and silicon nitride (Si_3N_4) are also used after some surface modifications.

Y-TZP ceramics have been commercially utilized to produce all-ceramic restoration systems for their unique mechanical properties. CIP is utilized to produce cylindrical blanks of Y-TZP ready for machining. The emergence of computerized digital dental photography and CAD–CAM milling machines facilitates the synthesis of veneers, crowns, bridges, etc. These machines provide the demanded dimensional accuracy of the product and noticeably decrease the production time. A final step of sintering is performed via a sintering program usually provided by the manufacturer of CAD–CAM blanks.

1.4 Glasses and glass-ceramics [28–35]

Working with glasses and glass-ceramics is attractive because of the relatively low temperature of preparation and the ability to design their final properties via their compositions. Glass-ceramics also introduce the flexibility of machinability of the cast that greatly facilitates the desired shaping of the final product. Bioactive glasses or glass-ceramics are capable of bonding to living bone. Bioactive glass and glass-ceramic implants are found in a variety of forms, and their bone-bonding properties are controlled mainly by their chemical composition and the final constituent phases. The bioactivity of glasses and glass-ceramics is evaluated as a function of the bone formation rate on the implant.

1.4.1 Glasses

The most important material properties of glasses that can be controlled via their compositions are the coefficient of thermal expansion and the melt viscosity at a given temperature. In the late 1960s, Hench was able to discover that glass composition affects its bioactivity. The 45S5 bioactive glass designed by Hench is composed of 45% SiO_2, 6% P_2O_5, 24.5% CaO, and 24.5% Na_2O (termed Bioglass as a trademarked name). The stronger 52S4.6 bioactive glass is composed of 52% SiO_2, 6% P_2O_5, 21% CaO, and 21% Na_2O. As is obvious, these bioactive glasses are silicate-based glasses with different alkali contents and fixed P_2O_5 at 6%.

The bone-bonding mechanism is the formation of a carbonated hydroxyapatite (HCA) layer on the glass surface as a result of exposure to body fluid. The HCA layer stimulates the formation of the bond to bone because of the chemical similarity. The formation of the bond is found to be more rapid with the bioactive glass implant compared with the synthetic hydroxyapatite (sHA) because of the higher dissolution rate of vitreous materials compared with those of crystalline materials. In addition, bioactive glass stimulates bone growth past the bone–implant interface (osteoinductive), whereas bone growth is limited at the bone–implant interface in the case of sHA (osteoconductive).

In vitro, or outside the living body, investigation of bioactivity has become possible since the invention of simulated body fluid (SBF). It is a highly saturated solution of salts that simulate the blood content of inorganic materials and is adjusted to a pH 7.25–7.4 at 37°C. The glass is found bioactive via an in vitro test when immersion in

SBF results in a change in pH of the solution and weight loss, and the surface morphology of the glass is affected. Research activities attempt to increase the durability of the bioactive glass by introducing other constituents, but the bioactivity should be monitored; for example, it is found that including Al_2O_3 by only 1%–1.5% severely reduces bioactivity.

Bioactive glass and glass-ceramic compositions are illustrated in Fig. 1.6. The P_2O_5 is fixed at 6% of Na_2O–CaO–SiO_2 in the diagram. It is obvious that each region, A, B, C, and D, has different bioactivity. The bioactive glasses are bonded to both bone and soft tissues at the subregion S of region A. Another condition for the bonding of bioactive glass to soft tissue is that the interfaces are immobile. The subregion E is the Bioglass introduced by Hench, which is in the vicinity of the ternary eutectic of Na_2O–CaO–SiO_2 that facilitates melting.

A notable advance in the field of bioactivity is the research and development field of regeneration of tissue. The concept is to control ion release from the bioactive and biodegradable glass via a prior design of the glass composition and microstructure. This strategy allows the bioactivity and dissolution process to be adapted to the normal process of tissue regeneration and enhances it. The designed glasses for this purpose are called bioactive bone grafts. The bioactive bone grafts are thus designed for in situ regeneration of bone in a manner that restores bone structure and architecture. Accordingly, the resultant mechanical strength is equivalent to the original as shown for successful cases with cortical and cancellous bone.

Alternatively, utilization of biodegradable glasses in the form of powders or solution for application on the defected tissues is called in situ tissue regeneration. Local tissue repair is stimulated in this process via special formulations of glasses that allow controlled rate of dissolution. The design principles of these materials are obtained from the prior understanding of the requirements of ion supply and are rated to encourage local generation of new cells, i.e., osteoconduction is developed into osteoinduction

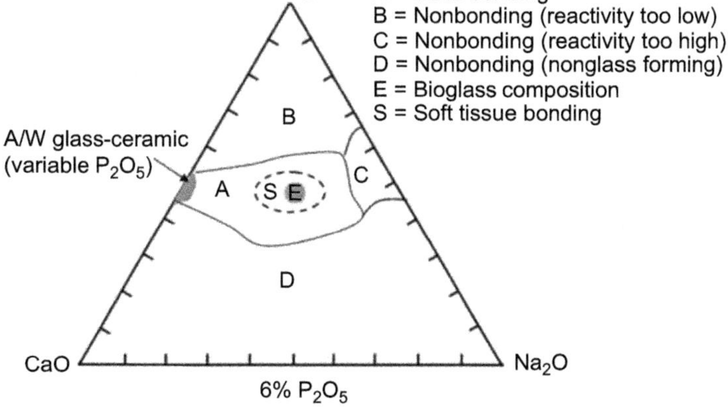

Figure 1.6 Compositional diagram of bioactive glasses and glass-ceramics.
Reused from T. Kokubo, Bioceramics and Their Clinical Applications, Elsevier, 2008 after license via (copyright.com) number 4115250000868.

(also called osteostimulation or osteoproduction) At these conditions, the new cells are allowed to self-assemble with proper chemical and structural gradients that result in appropriate architecture and mechanical properties of the repaired tissue.

The synthesis of the bioactive glass can be performed either by the conventional method or the sol–gel method. Originally, Bioglass was made via the conventional method. In this method, a mixture of the starting raw powders is prepared via weighing according to a prescribed recipe, followed by good mixing to attain homogeneity. The typical starting raw powders are high-purity oxides and carbonates (SiO_2, Na_2CO_3, $CaCO_3$, and P_2O_5). Other components can be added if required provided that their effect on melt viscosity is noted. The mixture is then melted in a platinum crucible in a furnace. The melting temperatures are ranged between 1300 and 1450°C according to the composition; it was 1370°C for Bioglass. Quenching in water or a suitable liquid is carried out to avoid partial crystallization of the melt. The produced frit is then dried and milled to attain homogeneity and to obtain the desired particle size of the glass powder. The glass melt can also be cast as rods or other desired shapes using preheated graphite or other appropriate molds at 350°C. The preparation steps should be done with great care to avoid introducing impurities or partial volatilization of sodium and phosphorous components. The sodium component is not required for bioactivity, but is introduced to lower the melting temperature to a practical range. Also, sodium is introduced as carbonate as a starting material because sodium oxide is extremely volatile and does not exist in nature. Calcium is also introduced as carbonate to avoid segregation of the calcium components and to obtain better homogeneity.

The sol–gel method for synthesis of a bioactive glass provides exceptionally high surface area as a result of an interconnected nanopore network of the resultant microstructure. The high surface area enhances the rates of dissolution and resorbability. Thus the 60 mol% limit of silica content for bioactivity of the dense glass is now extended to 80 mol% with sol–gel–derived bioactive glasses. In other words, the formation of an HCA layer is more rapid with sol–gel–derived bioactive glasses because of the inherent nanoporosity compared with the melt-derived bioactive glass.

The sol–gel technique for the fabrication of ceramic materials (including glass) is a wet chemical process based on metal alkoxides, chlorides, nitrites, or any salt that can be dissolved in water (hydrolysis) and suspended because of Brownian motion (sol), i.e., forms a colloid. The sol molecules gradually evolve into or form an inorganic network of the solid phase (polycondensation) that contains a liquid phase (gel). The speed of gel formation, and the accompanying increase of viscosity, may be affected by the temperature and pH of the sol. Then, the liquid is removed from the gel via a drying process. The concentration of the gel, the drying procedure, and other conditions control the size of the final powder. The sol–gel process is also called the bottom-up procedure to fabricate nanosized ceramics.

The sol–gel process for the synthesis of bioactive glass is outlined in Fig. 1.7. The precursors are a silicon alkoxide-like tetraethyl orthosilicate (TEOS), triethyl phosphate, and calcium nitrate tetrahydrate as a source of silicon, phosphorus, and calcium oxide. Nitric acid is added as an acidic catalyst to facilitate the hydrolysis of the TEOS. Formation of the gel is rather slow and may take up to 3 days. Aging at 60°C also takes 3 days to enhance the networking. Carefully controlled drying is performed (at 60°C

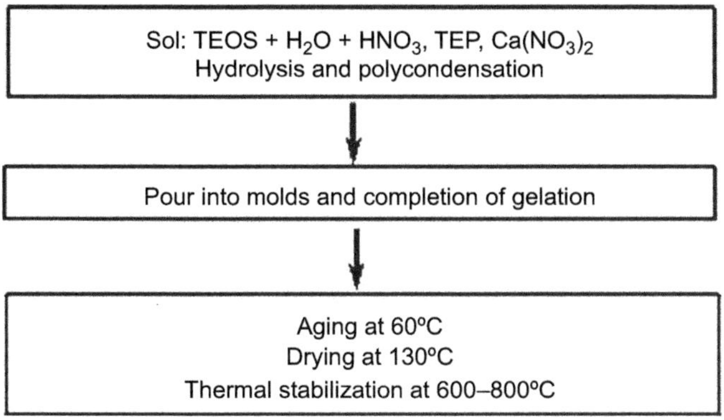

Figure 1.7 The synthesis steps of sol–gel bioactive glass. *TEOS*, tetraethyl orthosilicate; *TEP*, triethyl phosphate.

for 1 day, 90°C for 1 day, and 130°C for 2 days) to avoid the formation of coarse particles. A final burning step is performed to remove organic by-products and nitrates.

1.4.2 Glass-ceramics

As mentioned in Section 1.1.4, crystalline phases can be nucleated and grow on controlled heat treatment of glass. This process produces a composite of glass matrix that contains one or more crystalline phases. The volume fractions and grain (crystal) sizes depend on the starting composition coupled with the heat treatment program. The efforts made for the syntheses of bioactive glass-ceramics are aimed at preparing bioactive materials with better mechanical properties than apatite and bioglass. The apatite phase is a prerequisite because one of the crystalline phases of glass-ceramics is its role in bioactivity. The apatite has the general chemical formula $Ca_{10}(PO_4)_6(OH,F,Cl)_2$ signifying HA, fluorapatite, and chlorapatite. In fact, HA exists in the bone as an assembly of crystalline particles reinforced by the organic collagen fibers. In addition, including β-wollastonite ($CaO{\cdot}SiO_2$) is attractive because it crystallizes as a silicate chain structure, which is known as a strong fibrous phase. Thus apatite–wollastonite (A–W) glass-ceramics are suggested as an alternative bioactive material.

In this section, (A–W) glass-ceramics are introduced because of their importance as bioactive materials. The A–W glass-ceramic implant forms an HCA layer on the interface in a similar bioactivity mechanism found with Bioglass. On the other hand, Bioglass forms a silica gel layer on its surface, and the HCA layer covers the gel layer. The gel layer is a source of mechanical weakness that makes the mechanical properties lower than those of human cortical bone. The formation of the gel layer did not occur in the case of A–W glass-ceramics, which provides higher mechanical properties. A–W glass-ceramics have thus found wider clinical use than Bioglass. Among the advantages of glass-ceramics is their machinability, so they can be shaped via machining to the desired shapes of the bone substitutes.

The fabrication of A–W glass-ceramics includes the addition of MgO in small amounts (not exceeding 0.5%) to reduce the liquidus temperature of the pseudobinary system ($3CaO{\cdot}P_2O_5$–$CaO{\cdot}SiO_2$), which is 1420°C at 36 wt% ($3CaO{\cdot}P_2O_5$)—64 wt% ($CaO{\cdot}SiO_2$). High-purity MgO, $CaCO_3$, SiO_2, and $CaHPO_5{\cdot}2H_2O$ are used as starting materials. The batch is usually melted in a Pt-10% Rh crucible at 1450°C for 2 h to ensure complete melting and best homogeneity. The glass is then cast and pressed in stainless steel to produce a glass plate thickness of about 2 mm. At this stage the glass can be represented as a pseudoternary system ($3CaO{\cdot}P_2O_5$–$CaO{\cdot}SiO_2$–$MgO{\cdot}CaO{\cdot}2SiO_2$). The crystalline phases of glass-ceramics are then encouraged to nucleate via heat treatment at a heating rate of 5°C/min up to 1050°C.

The crystalline phases of the produced A–W glass-ceramics are nanometer-sized apatite crystals and wollastonite fibers. However, the preferred orientation of the wollastonite fibers is perpendicular to the surface of the glass. Explicitly, thermal contraction is not isotropic, which leads to large internal stresses and the formation of macrocracks. To avoid this situation, the glass is crushed into a fine powder. Then, the powder is pressed into discs via CIP and heat treated again with the same procedure mentioned earlier. The result is a glass-ceramic with a homogeneous distribution of crystalline phases that overcomes the problem of crack formation. As expected, the pressed and heat-treated powder does not have zero porosity like the cast glass melt. About 3.5% of porosity thus remains in the bulk glass. To avoid the remaining porosity, CaF_2, which acts as a flux, may be added to the parent glass in small amounts (~0.5%) to decrease the softening temperature of the glass and encourage pore diffusion outside the bulk. The glass is fully densified at 830°C, oxyfluoroapatite ($Ca_{10}(PO_4)_6(O,F_2)$) crystals appear at 870°C, and wollastonite at 900°C. The resultant glass is homogeneous, crack free, and has zero porosity.

The density of A–W glass-ceramics is typically slightly above 3 g/cm^3. The approximate value of the bending strength of A–W glass-ceramics is 220 MPa and fracture toughness is 2.0 MPa·m$^{1/2}$. These values are fairly close to those of human cortical bone, which is 160 MPa and 2–6 MPa·m$^{1/2}$, respectively. In general, the mechanical properties of A–W glass-ceramics are better than those of bioglass and apatite as will be detailed later in this book.

1.5 Hydroxyapatite [36–39]

HA is a crystalline material with the chemical formula $Ca_{10}(PO_4)_6(OH)_2$. The crystal structure is hexagonal close-packed with a=9.42 Å and c=6.88 Å. F and Cl can partially substitute for OH, and CO_3 for PO_4. Carbon is also found to partially substitute for Ca. The unit cell and Ca/P ratios are thus subjected to change according to these substitutions. Bone is composed of 33 wt% organic matrix and 67 wt% HCA and calcium phosphate. HA is a bioactive material that forms a strong bone–implant interface, and it is also osteoconductive, i.e., it encourages bone growth outside the interface region. sHA is produced in powder form in addition to various shapes of solid forms, both densified and porous according to the demanded application.

1.5.1 Preparation of hydroxyapatite

There are several methods for the preparation of HA. Among these methods are the following:

- Precipitation method
  There are two precipitation methods of HA: the first is the Rathje method and the second is the Hayek and Newesely method. In the first method, $Ca(OH)_2$ suspension in water is continuously stirred while drops of phosphoric acid (H_3PO_4) are added. The apatite powder is precipitated according to the following reaction:

$$10Ca(OH)_2 + 3H_3(PO_4)_2 \rightarrow Ca_{10}(PO_4)_6(OH)_2 \qquad (1.3)$$

  The pH of the solution is kept highly alkaline via the addition of ammonia (NH_4OH) to encourage the formation of stoichiometric HA after sintering of the powder precipitate.
  In the second method, the formation of the apatite powder is via the reaction of calcium nitrate ($Ca(NO_3)_2$), ammonium phosphate ($(NH4)_2HPO_4$), and ammonia:

$$10Ca(NO_3)_2 + 6(NH_4)_2HPO_4 + 2NH_4OH \rightarrow Ca_{10}(PO_4)_6(OH)_2 \qquad (1.4)$$

  Again, the pH of the solution influences the formation of HA after powder sintering. Calcium nitrate may be substituted by calcium acetate ($Ca(CH_3COO)_2$) to avoid the existence of trace nitrates in the final powder.
  In either method, precipitation is rather slow; thus stirring is accompanied by heating of the solution to about 70–80°C.
- Hydrolysis method
  The hydrolysis method comprises the decomposition of acidic calcium phosphates in basic solutions. The calcium phosphates include dicalcium phosphate dihydrate ($CaHPO_4{\cdot}2H_2O$), octacalcium phosphate ($Ca_8H_2(PO_4)_6{\cdot}5H_2O$), and dicalcium phosphate anhydrous ($CaHPO_4$). The basic solutions include ammonium, sodium, or potassium hydroxide. The hydroxide can be replaced by carbonate, fluoride, or chloride according to the targeted type of the apatite. Other starting materials for hydrolysis are calcium carbonate ($CaCO_3$) in ammonium or sodium phosphate solutions. These are examples of many chemical routes for the hydrolysis method.
- Hydrothermal method
  The hydrothermal method also includes various chemical routes. Among these are the following reactions:

$$6CaHPO_4 + 4Ca(OH)_2 \rightarrow Ca_{10}(PO_4)6(OH)_2 + 6\ H_2O \qquad (1.5)$$

$$3Ca_3(PO_4)_2 + Ca(OH)_2 \rightarrow Ca_{10}(PO_4)6(OH)_2 + H_2O \qquad (1.6)$$

$$4CaCO_3 + 6CaHPO_4 \rightarrow Ca_{10}(PO_4)6(OH)_2 + 6H_2O + 4CO_2 \qquad (1.7)$$

$$10CaCO_3 + 6(NH_4)_2 \rightarrow Ca_{10}(PO_4)6(OH)_2 + H_2O + CO_2 \qquad (1.8)$$

  The hydrothermal reaction is carried out in steam at a temperature of 275°C and pressure of 12,000 psi.

- Solid-state reactions method
  The reactions, shown in Eqs. (1.5) and (1.6), can be carried out in a solid-state homogeneous and stoichiometric mix of powders. The powder mix is compacted and then heat treated at 950°C. Technically, the prepared apatite powder by any of the foregoing methods can be compacted and sintered to have a solid body.

  The process of sintering of HA produces solid bodies with inherent porosity. By convention, the dense HA has porosity and pore size that do not exceed 5% and 1 μm, respectively. The porosity and pore size depend on the sintering conditions. Usually, the sintering temperature lies between 950 and 1300°C for 2–8 h. The sintering duration is usually decreased with the decrease in the average particle size of the starting powder. On the other hand, macroporosity may be required and can be introduced via the addition of volatile materials such as naphthalene, paraffin oil, polyvinyl butyral, or hydrogen peroxide to the apatite powder before compaction. HIP can also be used with the advantages of lower sintering temperature (~900°C) and the prevention of the formation of other calcium phosphate phases in the HA matrix.

1.6 Different forms of tricalcium phosphate [40,41]

The chemical formula of TCP ($Ca_3(PO_4)_2$) is close to that of HA ($Ca_{10}(PO_4)_6(OH)_2$) and can be easily hydrolyzed and converted to it at proper conditions. TCP is bioactive and resorbable. There are four different forms of TCP, which are more soluble than stoichiometric HA. The first two forms of TCP are the low-temperature and unstable phases, which are amorphous (am-TCP) and apatitic (ap-TCP). The last two forms are high-temperature and crystalline phases, known as α-TCP and β-TCP. The crystalline phases of TCP are not fully crystalline, and their degree of crystallinity and composition is close to that which exists as the inorganic component of bone.

The dissolution rate of TCP is higher than that of HA. They hydrolyze in vivo to the bone-like HA. am-TCP and α-TCP have the highest dissolution rates among the TCP family. ap-TC has a lower dissolution rate, and β-TCP has the lowest dissolution rate compared with other forms of TCP. Accordingly, TCP has been used for bone filling for orthopedic and dental purposes. The bone-filling process can be controlled and enhanced to osteoconduction quality via utilization of TCP with smaller particle size and increased microporosity. Both the osteoclastic activity and in vivo resorption rate of TCP control bone filling and remodeling.

There are two main preparation methods for TCP. The first is the low-temperature precipitation of TCP from a solution. am-TCP and ap-TCP are produced by this method. The important process parameters are usually concentration, pH, and temperature of the solutions. The second method is the high-temperature solid–solid reaction method. Crystalline TCP (α and β) is produced, and the result depends on the properties of the starting powders, stoichiometry, and the time–temperature schedule.

The reaction between a solution of a calcium salt and phosphoric acid at room temperature and a pH of 10 produces am-TCP. Introducing ethanol into the aqueous medium improves dispersion, amorphous phase, and stoichiometry of the product. am-TCP should be freeze-dried and stored in a dry environment because of its high reactivity. If the drying stage is performed in an oven at 80°C, internal hydrolysis takes place that produces ap-TCP, which has a Ca/P ratio close to 1.5.

Solid-state reaction at around 1200°C of any of the Ca and P salts, with the correct Ca/P ratio, produces α-TCP. In addition, prolonged heat treatment of α-TCP at 900°C leads to the formation of β-TCP. In fact, the same heat treatment for am-TCP and ap-TCP results in β-TCP provided that the Ca/P ratio is corrected by the addition of the proper salt in the right amount. An inappropriate Ca/P ratio leads to the formation of other phases, and the produced β-TCP is regarded as impure. Heat treatment of β-TCP above the $\beta \rightarrow \alpha$ transition temperature (1125°C) results in the formation of α-TCP.

There are other forms of TCP, which are not mentioned in this overview. The synthesis, structure, properties, and uses of the different types of TCP will be presented later in this book.

1.7 Pyrolytic carbon [16,36]

Carbon as bioceramics is currently known as turbostratic carbon, graphite, or graphene. Generally, it is described as having a disordered lattice structure and a slipped basal plane or rotationally disordered layers. It is obvious that the term "turbostratic" indicates a structural feature. Originally, carbon as bioceramics is called low-temperature isotropic (LTI) carbon and ultralow temperature isotropic (ULTI) carbon, indicating the processing routes, which are variants of chemical vapor deposition (CVD). In addition, the term "pyrolytic" is related to its original development for elevated temperature applications.

The pyrolytic carbon shows hemocompatibility, i.e., compatible with blood, compatibility with soft tissue, and high resistance to blood clotting (thromboresistant). The pyrolytic carbons also show high strength, excellent durability, and wear and fatigue resistance. Although medical devices completely made of pyrolytic carbons may be found when its mechanical properties are sufficient for the purpose, the major utilization of the pyrolytic carbons is as a coating, e.g., on heart valve prostheses. Accordingly, the mechanical properties of the prostheses are related to the substrate. However, the stiffness, hardness, and wear resistance of the coat may be improved by the addition of up to 20% silicon to the carbon.

A general description of the CVD process to produce pyrolytic carbon mixed with silicon is the utilization of a hydrocarbon gas as a source of carbon and an organosilicon compound. Decomposition of the starting materials is performed at a temperature of 1000–1500°C. The following set of equations is an example of the decomposition and the products:

$$C_3H_8 \rightarrow 3C + 4H_2 \tag{1.9}$$

$$CH_3Cl_3Si \rightarrow SiC + 3HCl \tag{1.10}$$

The products are pyrolytic carbon and β-SiC, in addition to by-products of hydrogen and hydrogen chloride vapors. The solid products are deposited on a substrate, often graphite. The silicon content depends on process parameters, and it is usually around 10%. The carbon has a turbostratic structure with nanometer particle sizes. The mechanical properties of the resultant coat together with the associated applications will be detailed in the next chapter.

1.8 Composites [11–13,18]

Composite is an important class of materials that combines the properties of two or more different materials. In materials science and engineering, the composite material consists of a matrix and one or more fillers. The filler is also called a reinforcement because it is added to the matrix to improve a targeted property. Usually, the matrix has the largest volume fraction because it completely surrounds the fillers, but there are many examples where the volume fraction is smaller than that of the fillers. In all cases, the matrix contains the fillers with a distinct matrix–filler interface.

A well-known example of composite materials is the polymer matrix glass fiber-reinforced composite, frequently called glass fiber-reinforced plastic. Here, the glass fibers are added and aligned in one direction to improve the tensile property in the direction of the filler. The composite material is anisotropic in this case. In addition, the bending strength is improved in perpendicular directions to the fillers. In many cases, the fillers are aligned in more than one direction to improve the tensile property in the directions of the fibers. Another example is when a polymer is reinforced with ceramic particulates. In this case, the improved property is the compression strength. If the particulates filler is uniformly distributed in the polymer matrix, the composite material is isotropic. A final example is laminate composite material, in which laminates of two or more materials are sequentially distributed one after another. Other models of distributions certainly exist. The laminate thicknesses are predesigned to optimize the targeted property. Thermal, mechanical (such as the impact strength), and other properties can be optimized with the laminate composite design of materials.

The filler–matrix interface plays a major role in the final property of the composite material. Filler adhesion to the matrix, the interface chemistry, etc., can dramatically modify the macroscopic property of the composite material. Any two or more of the major classes of materials (metals, ceramics, including the glass, and polymers) can exist in the composition of the composite materials. The composite materials find application in all fields of science and engineering with tailored properties such as electrical, magnetic, thermal, mechanical, and other properties. Bone is an elaborated composite of a natural polymer matrix (aligned bundles of collagen fibers) reinforced with ceramic particulates (apatite). The apatite particles are not evenly distributed, which makes the bone anisotropic and graded, i.e., a compositional gradient characterizes the bone that is reflected in the bone mechanical properties, especially the stiffness.

Usually, two or more properties are desired in the synthetic composite material. An example is the HA–polyethylene composite. This composite is used as the sockets of the joint prostheses. In this case, the toughness and ductility of the polyethylene matrix are close to that of the bone, and the apatite particulates (>20 vol%) are biocompatible. This composite is machinable, which is an added advantage because it gives it the ability to refine the shape at the time of the surgical operation. It is normal to try fillers other than HA with the polyethylene matrix. Bioglass and A–W glass-ceramics are also studied as fillers for polyethylene.

Another matrix used with HA particulates is the biodegradable poly(L-lactide) (PLLA) polymer. This composite is fabricated via a different route. The utilization of noncalcined nonsintered HA enhances the formation of a bone-like apatite layer on its surface. Afterward, the biodegradable composite is gradually substituted by bone tissue. Accordingly, fixation of bone fractures takes place. A range of clinical applications, including orthopedic, reconstructive, oral, facial, etc., makes use of the biodegradability of this composite.

Another widely used composite is that composed of a matrix of type I collagen (an abundant type of collagen in the human body that forms the collagen fibers). The filler is a combination of HA (65%) and TCP (35%). This composite is registered as Collagraft. The composition is very similar to that of bone and has proved useful, when used with bone marrow, for bone reconstructions. Thus problematic surgeries of autografting or allografting, usually used for the treatment of long-bone fractures and traumatic defects, are avoided.

Nanomaterials, the sol–gel preparation process, and other improved preparation techniques will be discussed in another chapter.

Review questions

Note: Use available literature, matweb.com, azom.com, or any suitable source to find material properties data if required.

1.1 Ceramics and glasses

1. Make a table that compares the composition and properties of ceramic, metallic, and polymeric materials.
2. What type of bonds are usually found in ceramic materials? What are their consequences on the mechanical and thermal properties of ceramic materials?
3. Ceramic materials may be insulators, semiconductors, ionic conductors, and semiconductors. Find three examples of each type.
4. Define crystalline materials, amorphous materials, and the degree of crystallinity.
5. What is the information that can be extracted from an electron microscope micrograph? What kind of indications can be given when carefully examining such a micrograph?
6. Introduce the term "structure" of a material. Compare it with "microstructure."
7. How can the structure of materials give an indication of its macro properties? How do microstructural features influence these properties?
8. How are the mechanical, thermal, magnetic, and electrical properties of materials influenced by their microstructure?
9. How do the process parameters of sintering affect the final material properties?
10. Draw a flowchart that describes the principal stages of the fabrication of a ceramic product.
11. The sintering process includes several phenomena; briefly describe them.
12. Describe glass and its preparation from the starting materials.

13. Define the phenomenon of glass transition and its macroscopic effects. Does the glass transition or transformation is a phase transition? Why?
14. Why are most glass productions of relatively low cost?
15. Classify oxides relative to their effect on the glass melting temperature.
16. What is the most important properties in glass design? Explain.
17. Briefly introduce vitreous coating.
18. Describe glass-ceramics and their preparation process.
19. Explain the term "controlled crystallization" and the importance of this process.
20. State the advantages of glass-ceramics materials.
21. What are the process parameters that allow the tailoring of glass-ceramics' final properties?
22. Write a short essay that introduces the structure–microstructure–processing relation to the final properties of materials.

1.2 Types of bioceramics

23. What is the main reason behind the toxicity of incompatible implant materials?
24. Explain why ceramic biomaterials are generally nontoxic?
25. On what parameter do tissue–implant interactions mainly depend?
26. Explain why the physical and mechanical properties of bone apatite are different from synthetic HA.
27. Construct a table that classifies bioceramics according to the type of implant material.
28. Why does the thicknesses of fibrous tissue formed by living tissue to encapsulate the implant differ in different cases?
29. Explain mechanical interlocking of an implant to the host tissue.
30. Explain why the synthesis of the frictional pairs of artificial joints is an important field of application of bioinert ceramics.
31. What are the main functions intended from porous bioceramics?
32. Macroporosity and interconnected porosity are required for several reasons. Explain.
33. What type of interface is formed for the bioactive ceramic and host tissue? Does that interface also form with HA?
34. State a typical composition for Bioglass 45S5. What component is typically of fixed wt% in variations of bioactive glass?
35. What are the effects of variant SiO_2 content in bioactive glass?
36. Is chemical compatibility enough for implantation? Explain.
37. Why are structure and microstructure important design parameters for bioactive implants?
38. What are the main purposes of resorbable bioceramics?
39. What are the factors that affect the resorption rate of bioceramics?
40. Explain dissolving rate–resorption rate–tissue repair interrelations.
41. Construct a table that classifies implants according to their tissue interactions.
42. Explain the protecting mechanism of the host body when a toxic material is implanted.
43. Describe the multiple effects of impurities of implanted materials.
44. Give examples of limited toxicity that takes place after implantation.
45. What are the two requirements to achieve biological inertness?
46. What are the benefits of strong bonds of ceramics as biomaterials?
47. What bioactivities are there other than chemical bonding?
48. What are the parameters that determine whether the ceramic implant is inert, bioactive, or resorbable other than chemical composition?
49. What is the role of dissolved implants during tissue repair? What are the conditions that should be fulfilled that allow the process to continue?

50. Sort HA, bioglasses, and calcium phosphates according to their dissolution rate. What are the factors that affect the dissolution rate?
51. Why are open porosity and porosity level so important for dissolved implants?
52. Explain why the FGM design is better for dissolved implants?

1.3 Alumina and zirconia

53. What are the properties of alumina that make it ideal for surgical devices?
54. Draw a flow diagram for the extraction of alumina via the Bayer process.
55. What is the role of the calcination condition in the properties of the final alumina powder produced via the Bayer process?
56. What is the accepted purity of alumina and impurity levels for the production of medical parts?
57. What is the accepted shape-forming process for alumina medical parts?
58. Explain the role of additives and impurities in the sintering of alumina.
59. Explain the role of the postsintering process of alumina for the production of medical parts.
60. What are the advantages of COC hip replacement or arthroplasty?
61. What is the origin of the fracture of the alumina femoral head at the early application experience? What are the attempted solutions?
62. Discuss the use of UHMWPE as part of total knee replacement.
63. Discuss "mechanical shielding" caused by a ceramic implant.
64. Explain the use of porous alumina implants.
65. Explain the term "stabilized zirconia."
66. Define the term "transformation toughening" and show how it is employed.
67. Why is 3 mol% Y_2O_3 currently enough to stabilize zirconia while 8 mol% Y_2O_3 was needed previously?
68. What are the advantages of the sol–gel process to produce toughened zirconia?
69. Why are yttria-stabilized tetragonal zirconia ball heads superior to MgO-PSZ?
70. Explain LTD for a zirconia implant.
71. What are the motivations behind replacing the stabilized zirconia balls with tetragonal zirconia-reinforced alumina?
72. What are the advantages of the use of tetragonal zirconia-reinforced alumina in THA?
73. Explain the metal–ceramic systems for dental restorations and state why achieving a successful coating is a difficult task?
74. Describe the CAD–CAM blanks, their synthesis, and uses.

1.4 Glass and glass-ceramics

75. What are the parameters that control the bone-bonding properties of glasses and glass-ceramics?
76. What are the most important material properties of glasses that can be controlled via their compositions?
77. State the chemical composition of the 45S5 bioactive glass and the 52S4.6 bioactive glass.
78. State the mechanism of bone bonding to the surfaces of glass and the reason why it is more rapid than the case of sHA.
79. What is the difference between bone growth stimulated by bioactive glass and that stimulated by sHA?

80. Define SBF and describe the in vitro test for bioactivity of a glass.
81. Sketch the compositional diagram of bioactive glasses and glass-ceramics and describe its subregions.
82. Explain bioactive bone grafts, their design, and merits.
83. Explain in situ tissue regeneration, materials, applications, and design principles.
84. Draw a flow diagram that illustrates the conventional method of the synthesis of bioactive glass.
85. State the role of sodium in a bioactive glass recipe. Why is it included as carbonate?
86. State the role of calcium in a bioactive glass recipe. Why is it included as carbonate?
87. State the advantages of the sol–gel method for the synthesis of a bioactive glass.
88. Explain the sol–gel technique for the fabrication of ceramic and glass materials. Why is the drying step so important?
89. Draw a diagram that illustrates the synthesis steps of sol–gel bioactive glass. Explain the abbreviations if any.
90. Briefly describe the synthesis of glass-ceramics.
91. Why are bioactive glass-ceramics favorable to apatite and bioglass? Why is the apatite phase a must in bioactive glass-ceramics?
92. What is the advantage of the β-wollastonite phase in glass-ceramics that qualify A–W glass-ceramics?
93. Explain the A–W glass-ceramics implant that provides higher mechanical properties compared with bioglass.
94. What are the advantages of A–W glass-ceramics other than bioactivity?
95. Draw a detailed flow diagram that illustrates the fabrication of A–W glass-ceramics.
96. Describe the crystalline phases of the just-produced A–W glass-ceramics and mention the problem of the formation of macrocracks.
97. Describe the extra process applied to the produced A–W glass-ceramics to avoid the formation of macrocracks and for it to have zero porosity.
98. State some of the physical and mechanical properties of A–W glass-ceramics and state why it is more favorable than apatite and bioglass.

1.5 Hydroxyapatite

99. Explain the preparation of HA according to the following methods:
  a. The precipitation method
  b. The hydrolysis method
  c. The hydrothermal method
  d. The solid-state reactions method
100. Discuss the presence of inherent porosity in sintered HA, the effect of the addition of volatile materials before sintering, and the advantages of using HIP as the sintering process.

1.6 Tricalcium phosphates

101. State the different forms of TCP and compare their crystallinity and stability.
102. Compare the dissolution rate between different forms of TCP.
103. What are the main uses of the different types of TCP as biomaterials? What are the advantages?
104. Explain the preparation of the different types of TCPs by the low-temperature method and the process parameters.
105. Explain the preparation of the different types of TCP by the high-temperature solid–solid reaction method and the process parameters.

1.7 Pyrolytic carbon

106. What is the origin of the term "pyrolytic carbon"? What is meant by the term "turbostratic carbon"? Also explain the abbreviations LTI and UTLI.
107. Explain the terms "hemocompatibility" and "thromboresistant." State the properties of pyrolytic carbon as a medical device.
108. What is the role of silicon addition to pyrolytic carbon?
109. State a general description of the CVD process that is used to produce pyrolytic carbon mixed with silicon. And describe the resultant product.

1.8 Composites

110. Describe composite materials as a class of materials.
111. What is the role of the filler type on the properties of the final composite?
112. Explain the role of the filler–matrix interface in the final properties of the composite.
113. Describe natural bone as a composite.
114. Explain the properties of HA–polyethylene composite and its advantage.
115. Explain the composite of an HA particulate-reinforced PLLA polymer, its bioactivity, and clinical applications.
116. Explain the uses of type I collagen as a matrix, its fillers, clinical applications, and advantages.

References

[1] M. Barsoum, M.W. Barsoum, Fundamentals of Ceramics, CRC Press, 2002.
[2] G. Phillips, A Concise Introduction to Ceramics, Springer Science & Business Media, 2012.
[3] P. Boch, J.-C. Nièpce, Ceramic Materials: Processes, Properties, and Applications, John Wiley & Sons, 2010.
[4] A. Koller, Structure and Properties of Ceramics, Elsevier, 1994.
[5] R.A. Terpstra, P. Pex, A. de Vries, Ceramic Processing, Springer Science & Business Media, 1995.
[6] G. Elssner, H. Hoven, G. Kiessler, P. Wellner, Ceramics and Ceramic Composites: Materialographic Preparation, Elsevier, 1999.
[7] J.E. Shelby, Introduction to Glass Science and Technology, Royal Society of Chemistry, 2005.
[8] N.P. Bansal, R.H. Doremus, Handbook of Glass Properties, Elsevier, 2013.
[9] R.A. Eppler, D.R. Eppler, Glazes and Glass Coatings, American Ceramic Society, 2000.
[10] K.C. Dee, D.A. Puleo, R. Bizios, An Introduction to Tissue-Biomaterial Interactions, John Wiley & Sons, 2003.
[11] W. Höland, A.R. Boccaccini, Inorganic Biomaterials, Frontiers Media, SA, 2016.
[12] D. Shi, Introduction to Biomaterials, Tsinghua University Press and World Scientific Publishing Co. Pte. Ltd., 2006.
[13] L.L. Hench, J.R. Jones, Bioactive glasses: frontiers and challenges, Frontiers in Bioengineering and Biotechnology 3 (2015) https://doi.org/10.3389/fbioe.2015.00194.
[14] V.A. Dubok, Bioceramics — yesterday, today, tomorrow, Powder Metallurgy and Metal Ceramics 39 (2000) 381–394, https://doi.org/10.1023/A:1026617607548.

[15] P.N. de Aza, A.H. de Aza Moya, S. de Aza, Crystalline bioceramic materials, Boletín de La Sociedad Española de Cerámica y Vidrio 44 (2005) 135–145.
[16] J. Park, R.S. Lakes, Biomaterials: An Introduction, Springer Science & Business Media, 2007.
[17] I.V. Antoniac, Handbook of Bioceramics and Biocomposites, Springer International Publishing, 2016.
[18] C.M. Agrawal, J.L. Ong, M.R. Appleford, G. Mani, Introduction to Biomaterials: Basic Theory with Engineering Applications, Cambridge University Press, 2014.
[19] F. Mussano, T. Genova, L. Munaron, M.G. Faga, S. Carossa, Ceramic Biomaterials for Dental Implants: Current Use and Future Perspectives, 2016https://doi.org/10.5772/62701.
[20] W. Höland, M. Schweiger, R. Watzke, A. Peschke, H. Kappert, Ceramics as biomaterials for dental restoration, Expert Review of Medical Devices 5 (2008) 729–745, https://doi.org/10.1586/17434440.5.6.729.
[21] I. Denry, J.A. Holloway, Ceramics for dental applications: a review, Materials 3 (2010) 351–368, https://doi.org/10.3390/ma3010351.
[22] W. Höland, V. Rheinberger, E. Apel, C. Ritzberger, F. Rothbrust, H. Kappert, F. Krumeich, R. Nesper, Future perspectives of biomaterials for dental restoration, Journal of the European Ceramic Society 29 (2009) 1291–1297, https://doi.org/10.1016/j.jeurceramsoc.2008.08.023.
[23] M.J. Nine, D. Choudhury, A.C. Hee, R. Mootanah, N.A.A. Osman, Wear debris characterization and corresponding biological response: artificial hip and knee joints, Materials 7 (2014) 980–1016, https://doi.org/10.3390/ma7020980.
[24] T.V. Swanson, D.J. Peterson, R. Seethala, R.L. Bliss, C.A. Spellmon, Influence of prosthetic design on squeaking after ceramic-on-ceramic total hip arthroplasty, The Journal of Arthroplasty 25 (2010) 36–42, https://doi.org/10.1016/j.arth.2010.04.032.
[25] B.-J. Kang, Y.-C. Ha, S.-C. Hwang, Y.-K. Lee, K.-H. Koo, Midterm results of large diameter biolox forte ceramic head on delta ceramic liner articulation in total hip arthroplasty, The Journal of Arthroplasty 29 (2014) 2412–2414, https://doi.org/10.1016/j.arth.2014.03.003.
[26] P. Bergschmidt, R. Bader, D. Ganzer, C. Hauzeur, C.H. Lohmann, A. Krüger, W. Rüther, D. Tigani, N. Rani, J.L. Esteve, F.L. Prats, C. Zorzi, V. Madonna, S. Rigotti, F. Benazzo, S.M.P. Rossi, W. Mittelmeier, Prospective multi-centre study on a composite ceramic femoral component in total knee arthroplasty: five-year clinical and radiological outcomes, The Knee 22 (2015) 186–191, https://doi.org/10.1016/j.knee.2015.02.003.
[27] B.C. Carr, T. Goswami, Knee implants – review of models and biomechanics, Materials and Design 30 (2009) 398–413, https://doi.org/10.1016/j.matdes.2008.03.032.
[28] T. Kokubo, Bioceramics and Their Clinical Applications, Elsevier, 2008.
[29] E. El-Meliegy, R. van Noort, Glasses and Glass Ceramics for Medical Applications, Springer Science & Business Media, 2011.
[30] H. Bach, D. Krause, Analysis of the Composition and Structure of Glass and Glass Ceramics, Springer Science & Business Media, 2013.
[31] A.R. Boccaccini, D.S. Brauer, L. Hupa, Bioactive Glasses: Fundamentals, Technology and Applications, Royal Society of Chemistry, 2016.
[32] M. Magallanes-Perdomo, Z.B. Luklinska, A.H. De Aza, R.G. Carrodeguas, S. De Aza, P. Pena, Bone-like forming ability of apatite–wollastonite glass ceramic, Journal of the European Ceramic Society 31 (2011) 1549–1561, https://doi.org/10.1016/j.jeurceramsoc.2011.03.007.
[33] M. Diba, O.-M. Goudouri, F. Tapia, A.R. Boccaccini, Magnesium-containing bioactive polycrystalline silicate-based ceramics and glass-ceramics for biomedical applications, Current Opinion in Solid State and Materials Science 18 (2014) 147–167, https://doi.org/10.1016/j.cossms.2014.02.004.

[34] M. Magallanes-Perdomo, A.H. De Aza, I. Sobrados, J. Sanz, P. Pena, Structure and properties of bioactive eutectic glasses based on the Ca3(PO4)2–CaSiO3–CaMg(SiO3)2 system, Acta Biomaterialia 8 (2012) 820–829, https://doi.org/10.1016/j.actbio.2011.10.017.

[35] R.G. Hill, M.D. O'Donnell, R.V. Law, N. Karpukhina, B. Cochrane, D.U. Tulyaganov, The early stages of nucleation and crystallisation of an apatite glass-ceramic: evidence for nano-scale crystallisation, Journal of Non-Crystalline Solids 356 (2010) 2935–2941, https://doi.org/10.1016/j.jnoncrysol.2010.05.102.

[36] A. El-Ghannam, P. Ducheyne, 1.109-Bioactive ceramics, in: Comprehensive Biomaterials, Elsevier, Oxford, 2011, pp. 157–179, https://doi.org/10.1016/B978-0-08-055294-1.00021-0.

[37] M. Mucalo, Hydroxyapatite (HAp) for Biomedical Applications, Elsevier, 2015.

[38] V.S. Gshalaev, A.C. Demirchan, Hydroxyapatite: Synthesis, Properties, and Applications, Nova Science Publishers, 2012.

[39] M.P. Ferraz, F.J. Monteiro, C.M. Manuel, Hydroxyapatite nanoparticles: a review of preparation methodologies, Journal of Applied Biomaterials and Biomechanics 2 (2004) 74–80, https://doi.org/10.1177/228080000400200202.

[40] S.V. Dorozhkin, Calcium Orthophosphate-Based Bioceramics and Biocomposites, John Wiley & Sons, 2016.

[41] N. Eliaz, N. Metoki, Calcium phosphate bioceramics: a review of their history, structure, properties, coating technologies and biomedical applications, Materials 10 (2017) 334, https://doi.org/10.3390/ma10040334.

Structure, microstructure, and properties of bioceramics

2

2.1 Oxide ceramics

2.1.1 Alumina

Alumina (Al_2O_3) may be found in many metastable phases (γ, η, θ, ϱ, and χ) other than the thermodynamically stable phase α-alumina. The metastable phases transform into the α-phase upon heat treatment above 1200°C. The oxygen atoms of α-alumina are arranged in hexagonal close-packed planes, which are intercalated with aluminum planes. The crystal structure of α-alumina is hexagonal and can also be expressed as rhombohedral with a space group of R3c. Fig. 2.1 shows the hexagonal close-packed structure of oxygen (O^-) ions. Aluminum (Al^+) ions occupy two-thirds of the octahedral sites. Each octahedron touches an upper and lower octahedron via common faces. The octahedrons are slightly distorted as a result of the repulsion between aluminum ions.

The strong chemical bonds between oxygen and aluminum ions (both ionic and covalent) are the origin of the superior properties of α-alumina, such as thermodynamic stability and resistance to chemical attacks like that of strong inorganic acids such as orthophosphoric and hydrofluoric acids. In living environments, α-alumina has excellent corrosion resistance against body fluids. Also, the surface of the alumina is ready for chemisorption of hydroxyl groups by oxygen anions, which give rise to wettability or bonding to proteins. Consequently, α-alumina is suitable for use as a biomaterial. Alumina in α-phase also has good mechanical and thermal properties because of its close-packed structure of oxygen and aluminum. Such strong bonding also results in low electric and thermal conductivity and a high melting point.

2.1.2 Properties of alumina

The most important factors that influence the physical and mechanical properties of ceramics are grain size, porosity, and purity of the ceramics. The properties of 99.5% pure α-alumina are listed in Table 2.1. The particle size of the alumina starting powder has a prime importance. The finer the particle size of the starting powder, the better the sintering process because of the higher surface area of the finer particles. The sintered particles are called grains, and the finer particles should result in finer grains in a controlled sintering process. Accordingly, a better microstructure is developed. As a result, better mechanical properties of the final product are achieved. ASTM F603 indicates that excellent compressive and flexural strength can be achieved with an alumina starting powder of purity higher than 99.7% and average grain size of less than 4 μm.

In addition to the purity and grain size of the sintered alumina, porosity plays an important role in microstructure development. A rigid microstructure results from

Bioceramics: For Materials Science and Engineering. https://doi.org/10.1016/B978-0-08-102233-7.00002-1

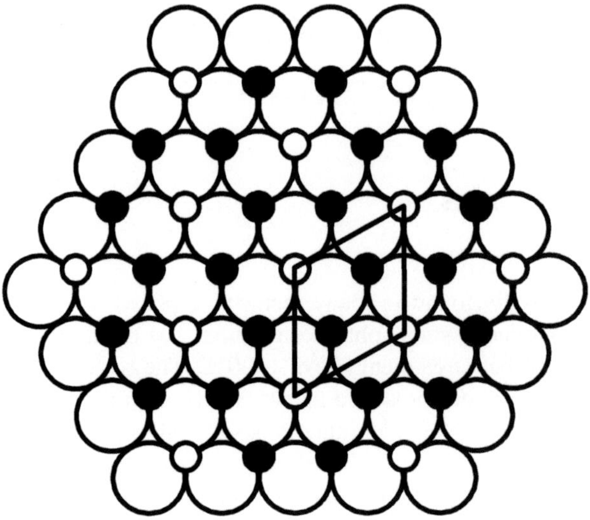

Figure 2.1 Crystal structure of alumina. The *empty circles* represent aluminum and the *filled circles* represent oxygen.
Reused from K.C. Popat, T.A. Desai, B - alumina, in: B.D. Ratner, A.S. Hoffman, F.J. Schoen, J.E. Lemons (Eds.), Biomaterials Science, third ed., Academic Press, 2013, pp. 162–166. https://doi/10.1016/B978-0-08-087780-8.00018-8 after license via (copyright.com) number 4178980884485.

Table 2.1 Mechanical properties of 99.5% pure alumina

Density	3.97 g/cm^3
Flexural strength	345 MPa
Elastic modulus	300 GPa
Shear modulus	124 GPa
Bulk modulus	172 GPa
Poisson's ratio	0.21
Compressive strength	2100 MPa
Hardness	1000 kg/mm^2
Fracture toughness	3.5 $MPa{\cdot}m^{1/2}$

Reused from K.C. Popat, T.A. Desai, B - alumina, in: B.D. Ratner, A.S. Hoffman, F.J. Schoen, J.E. Lemons (Eds.), Biomaterials Science, third ed., Academic Press, 2013, pp. 162–166. https://doi/10.1016/B978-0-08-087780-8.00018-8 after license via (copyright.com) number 4178980884485.

smaller porosity fraction, evenly distributed porosity, and closed porosity. The open pores represent weak points in the microstructure that allow penetrations of liquids and gases and provide higher contact areas for chemical attack. Thus open porosity should be minimized, or diminished, at the surface of the ceramic implant and a few micrometers behind the surface. Fig. 2.2 shows a typical microstructure for alumina intended for bioapplications. The features of this microstructure clearly indicate grain sizes in the intended range, almost zero porosity, and clean grain boundaries with no indication of inclusion of foreign materials that can distort the grain–grain contacts.

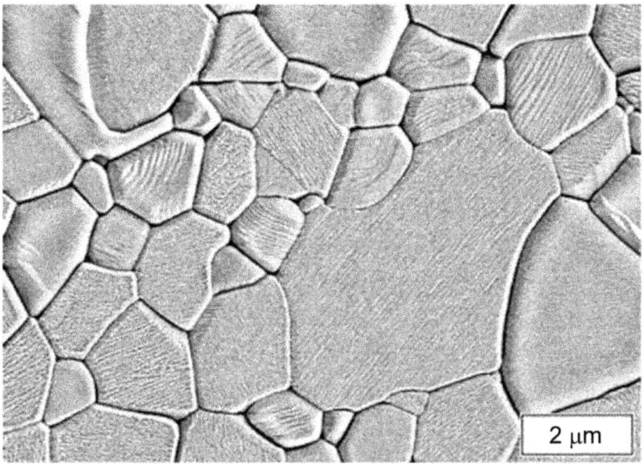

Figure 2.2 Microstructure of the monolithic alumina BIOLOX Forte.
Reused from C. Piconi, A.A. Porporati, Bioinert ceramics: zirconia and alumina, in: Handbook of Bioceramics and Biocomposites, Springer, Cham, 2016, pp. 59–89. https://doi/org/10.1007/978-3-319-12460-5_4 after license via (copyright.com) number 4175321377496.

The surface wettability of α-alumina is attributed to the formation of an absorbed surface layer of water and biological molecules that reduce direct contact with the solid alumina surface, and accordingly the coefficient of friction is reduced. The reduced coefficient of friction, combined with the high hardness, results in low wear rates of the articulating solid surfaces. Thus α-alumina represents a typical implant material for wear applications. The low wear rates of α-alumina can only be found when the surface roughness is less than 0.02 μm, which can be attained after costly machining of the hard sintered parts of alumina with a grain size smaller than 4 μm and a very narrow grain-size distribution. When the condition of low wear rates is fulfilled, the α-alumina can be used in joint replacement bearings.

As mentioned in Chapter 1, alumina is usually extracted by the Bayer process from bauxite. This extraction process has a major environmental impact on the use of alumina. Another major environmental impact comes from the shape-forming processes that may include plasticizers and binders that are burned during the sintering process. The use of plasticizers and binders may be minimized when utilizing nanosized alumina powders, but the sol–gel process utilized to produce nanoalumina consumes chemicals that in turn make a negative environmental impact. However, sintered alumina products have negligible environmental impacts.

Alumina is known to be chemically stable and corrosion resistant, insoluble in water, and shows slight solubility in strong acids and alkalis. Thus ion release is negligible in the physiological environment. However, this is true for zero-porosity sintered alumina parts. When open porosity exists, the liquids in the living environment can penetrate the solid part through the available pore channels. Taking into consideration that the defects exist inherently in the microstructure of sintered ceramics, the open porosity helps the liquid to reach and react with the intrinsic defects in the alumina microstructure. Impurities such as silica, calcia, alkalis, and high concentrations of defects may all contribute to the permeation of water molecules and lead to strength degradation. The ISO 6474 standard specifies the purity requirements of alumina for surgical implants.

2.1.3 Zirconia

Zirconia (ZrO_2) is also found in many phases: monoclinic, tetragonal, and cubic phases. Up to 1170°C, zirconia is monoclinic. Then, it converts to tetragonal until the temperature reaches 2370°C. Zirconia is cubic at this temperature until the melting point at 2680°C. Fig. 2.3 shows these major polymorphs of zirconia. Zirconia phase transformations are reversed on cooling and accompanied by volume expansions. Below 2370°C, cubic zirconia transforms into tetragonal with a change in theoretical density from 6.06 to 6.1. At around 1170°C, the tetragonal phase transforms to monoclinic, and the density decreases from 6.1 to 5.83. Obviously, the transformations into the monoclinic phase are accompanied by volume expansions of about 4%. The transformed grains undergo volume expansion-induced strains and phase transformation-induced shape changes, accompanied by shear strains. These strains apply stresses to the adjacent grains. Thus sintered pure zirconia suffers a microscopic cracking, which limits its application as refractory ceramics or pigments. This situation changed when the stabilization of zirconia was first achieved in 1929.

Additives to zirconia such as calcium oxide, magnesium oxide, cerium oxide, and yttrium oxide are utilized to stabilize high-temperature phases and are given the name "partially stabilized zirconia (PSZ)." At room temperature, PSZ as a biomaterial contains the cubic phase as the major phase and the monoclinic phase as the minor phase. Another minor phase in PSZ is the metastable tetragonal phase, which exists by an amount that depends on many "material design parameters" such as amount of stabilizer, particle sizes of zirconia and stabilizer, chemical history, and processing method. The processing method affects the homogeneity of the final powder mix and the final particle shape, which influence the surface area. For the sintered product, the residual stresses in the bulk depend on the cooling procedure and by decreasing it, the more likely will the demanded phase transformation take place.

The tetragonal metastable phase helps to enhance the fracture toughness via a mechanism known as transformation toughening. When a stress is applied, it is

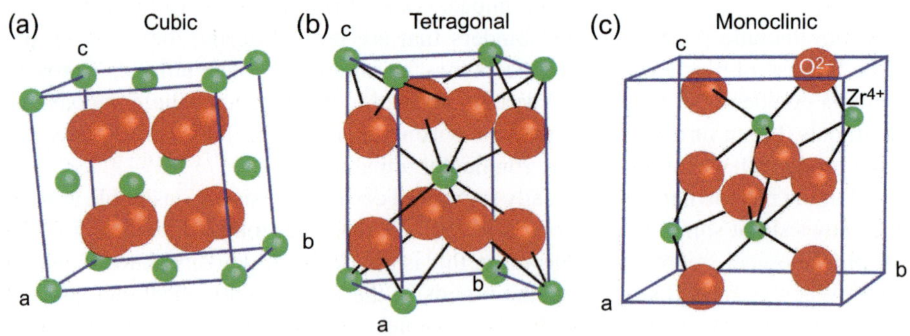

Figure 2.3 The unit cell of (a) cubic, (b) tetragonal, and (c) monoclinic zirconia. Reused from J. Chevalier, L. Gremillard, 1.106-Zirconia as a biomaterial, in: P. Ducheyne (Ed.), Comprehensive Biomaterials, Elsevier, Oxford, 2011, pp. 95–108. https://doi.org/10.1016/B978-0-08-055294-1.00017-9 after license via (copyright.com) number 4178960012771.

magnified at the crack tip and called stress concentration. The magnified stress may reach a value that is sufficient to develop tetragonal–monoclinic phase transformation. This is associated with a volume expansion, which applies a compression on the crack tip. Consequently, crack growth is retarded and fracture toughness is enhanced. The absorption of the some of the crack energy caused by phase transformation also contributes to the retardation of the crack and the enhancement of the fracture toughness. Evidently, the enhanced fracture toughness improves the reliability of the product and increases its lifetime.

When yttria (Y_2O_3) is used as a stabilizer, full stabilization may be achieved with yttria tetragonal zirconia particles (Y-TZP). The amount of stabilization depends on the materials' design parameters mentioned earlier. Thus 8 mol%, 5% mol%, 3 mol%, and recently 2 mol% yttria fully stabilized zirconia are found in various applications. Here, the term "fully stabilized zirconia" is used for almost fully stabilized zirconia because the cubic and monoclinic phases still exist as minor phases. The particle sizes of the yttria stabilizer may range from 0.5 μm to around 0.1 μm.

2.1.4 Properties of zirconia

A summary of the mechanical properties of zirconia is shown in Table 2.2. The encouraging mechanical properties of zirconia are flexural strength and fracture toughness. In addition, the elastic modulus of zirconia is close to that of titanium alloys (≈200 GPa), which minimizes strains at the metal–ceramic joints that form under load. The mechanical properties of zirconia can only be attained with a successful sintering process that leads to an evenly distributed fine-grained microstructure with minimum porosity. Fig. 2.4 shows a typical microstructure of stabilized zirconia.

On the other hand, zirconia has low thermal conductivity. Thus care should be taken to avoid thermal inhomogeneities or thermal spikes during machining or grinding of the restorative dental part. This is also the case with implanted hip replacements because they experience low lubrication. This effect may trigger a progressive degradation called low-temperature degradation (LTD) of the mechanical properties of zirconia. The other drawback of zirconia is that it has low hardness (12–23 GPa) compared with that of alumina (20–21 GPa). Thus research activities, such as coating of zirconia surfaces, may be used that aim to improve the hardness and wear resistance of zirconia.

LTD, also called aging, is a hydrothermal transformation, mostly at the temperature range of 200–300°C, in which the metastable tetragonal phase of zirconia spontaneously transforms into monoclinic. The effect starts at the surface of the solid zirconia part and then progressively penetrates the bulk. Tetragonal–monoclinic transformation is initiated first at the grain boundaries and then proceeds. The process initiates microcracking, which gradually develops into macrocracks. Eventually, the density of the solid zirconia starts to decrease and the mechanical properties degrade.

The rate of tetragonal–monoclinic transformation can be reduced with smaller and more evenly distributed zirconia particle sizes, lower porosity, and higher yttria stabilizer content and/or higher yttria content at the surface. In fact, LTD is observed with Y-TZP and is not detected with other kinds of stabilized zirconia such as Mg-PSZ or

Table 2.2 Properties of alumina, stabilized zirconia, and zirconia-toughened alumina (ZTA)

Property	Unit	Alumina	Mg-PSZ	Y-TZP	ZTA
Chemical composition		99.9% Al_2O_3+0–0.25 mol% MgO	ZrO_2+8–10 mol% MgO	ZrO_2+3 mol% Y_2O_3	Al_2O_3+5–20 mol% ZrO_2+Y_2O_3
Density	g/cm^3	3.97	5.74–6	>6	4.1
Porosity	%	<0.1		<0.1	<0.1
Average grain size	μm	2–4	20–40	<0.5	<1
Bending strength	MPa	>500	450–700	900–1200	800–1200
Compression strength	MPa	4100	2000	2000	2000
Young's modulus	GPa	380	200	210	380
Fracture toughness (K_{IC})	MPa/m	4	7–15	7–10	4–8
Hardness	HV 0.1	2200	1200	1200	1500–1800

PSZ, partially stabilized zirconia; *Y-TZP*, yttria tetragonal zirconia particles.
Reused from C. Piconi, Oxide ceramics for biomedical applications, in: K.H.J. Buschow, R.W. Cahn, M.C. Flemings, B. Ilschner, E.J. Kramer, S. Mahajan, P. Veyssière (Eds.), Encyclopedia of Materials: Science and Technology, second ed., Elsevier, Oxford, 2001, pp. 6595–6601. doi:10.1016/B0-08-043152-6/01165-7 after license via (copyright.com) number 4184121220528.

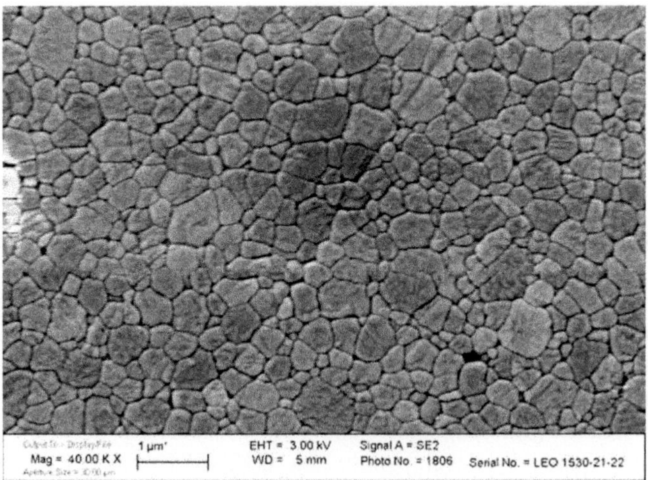

Figure 2.4 Microstructure of yttria tetragonal zirconia particles.
Reused from C. Piconi, A.A. Porporati, Bioinert ceramics: zirconia and alumina, in: Handbook of Bioceramics and Biocomposites, Springer, Cham, 2016, pp. 59–89. https://doi/org/10.1007/978-3-319-12460-5_4 after license via (copyright.com) number 4175321377496.

Ce-TZP. However, Y-TZP is preferred in orthopedics and restorative dentistry because of its better mechanical properties. On the other hand, increasing the temperature of all kinds of zirconia results in degradation of properties, thus the working temperatures of zirconia are below 800°C.

2.1.5 Zirconia-toughened alumina

The fully stabilized tetragonal zirconia nanoparticles may be added to an alumina matrix in uniform fashion to obtain a zirconia-toughened alumina (ZTA). The optimum fracture toughness and strength, which surpass that of stabilized zirconia, are usually obtained by inclusion of 17 vol% of zirconia to the alumina matrix. Thus ZTA composite is obtained to comply with the demanding requisite of arthroplasty. Table 2.2 presents the properties of ZTA compared with stabilized zirconia and alumina.

The ZTA composite can be further reinforced via the addition of chromia (Cr_2O_3). During sintering, an Al_2O_3:Cr_2O_3 solid solution is formed at the grain boundaries. This phase enhances the hardness of the sintered part and improves its wear properties. In addition, strontia (SrO) leads to a reaction with alumina during sintering and results in strontium hexaaluminate (SHA). The SHA grains have an elongated morphology and are deposited at the grain boundaries of the alumina matrix, as shown in Fig. 2.5. The figure shows that the SHA grains are uniformly distributed in the alumina matrix. These grains contribute to crack deflection and thus halt crack propagation and result in tougher solid material.

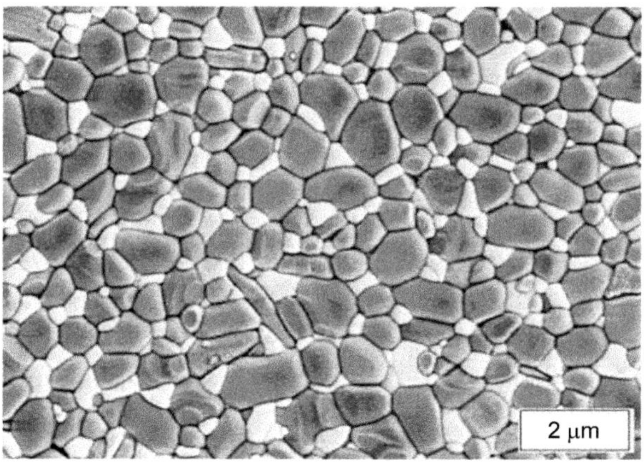

Figure 2.5 Scanning electron microscope image of the microstructure of the zirconia-toughened alumina composite ceramic BIOLOX Delta. The gray grains represent the alumina matrix, the white grains represent the zirconia phase, and the elongated grains consist of reinforcing strontium hexaaluminate platelets.
Reused from C. Piconi, A.A. Porporati, Bioinert ceramics: zirconia and alumina, in: Handbook of Bioceramics and Biocomposites, Springer, Cham, 2016, pp. 59–89. https://doi/org/10.1007/978-3-319-12460-5_4 after license via (copyright.com) number 4175321377496.

2.2 Calcium orthophosphates

Calcium phosphates are compounds of calcium (Ca^{2+}), phosphorus (P^{5+}), and oxygen (O^{2-}), hydrated and anhydrous. Calcium phosphates comprise a vast number of compounds, thus this section will be limited to the most celebrated category of calcium orthophosphates that contain Ca and PO_4. Calcium orthophosphates are found in the inorganic part of bones, teeth, and in various pathological calcifications. The following is an overview of the calcium orthophosphate compounds with their abbreviated names as used by the International Union of Pure and Applied Chemistry.

2.2.1 Monocalcium phosphates

Monocalcium phosphates are found as monohydrate ($Ca(H_2PO_4)_2 \cdot H_2O$) and called calcium dihydrogen orthophosphate monohydrate or monocalcium phosphate monohydrate (MCPM). MCPM releases a water molecule at ≈100°C and converts it into monocalcium phosphate anhydrous.

2.2.2 Octacalcium phosphate

Octacalcium phosphate is abbreviated as OCP, and the formula is $Ca_8(HPO_4)_2 \cdot 5H_2O$. The water content may be found with slight variation. OCP is found during the mineralization that occurs in bones and teeth as an intermediate to the formation of hydroxyapatite (HA).

2.2.3 Dicalcium phosphate dihydrate

Dicalcium phosphate dihydrate (DCPD) is also called calcium monohydrogen phosphate dihydrate, dibasic calcium phosphate dihydrate, and calcium hydrogen orthophosphate 2-hydrate with the formula $CaHPO_4 \cdot 2H_2O$. DCPD is also an intermediate in the precipitation of HA and bone mineralization.

2.2.4 Dicalcium phosphate anhydrous

Dicalcium phosphate anhydrous is abbreviated as DCPA. Other names are anhydrous dicalcium phosphate, dicalcium phosphate, and calcium hydrogen orthophosphate. It is less soluble than DCPD at all temperatures, and it is not detected in dental calculus or other pathological calcifications. DCPA may be found in fracture calluses and possibly in bone.

2.2.5 Anhydrous tricalcium phosphate

An alternative name for this compound is tricalcium orthophosphate (TCP), and the chemical formula is $Ca_3(PO_4)_2$. TCP exists in α and β forms. β-TCP is the low-temperature phase and transforms into α-TCP at 1125°C.

2.2.6 Tetracalcium phosphate

Tetracalcium phosphate, abbreviated as TetCP, is also called tetracalcium diphosphate monoxide. It is formed by the reaction of phosphorus, oxygen, and lime and has the chemical formula $Ca_4(PO_4)_2O$. Also, there is no evidence of formation in aqueous solutions at normal temperatures. Reaction of TetCP with either DCPD or DCPA and water sets to HA and suggested as bone cement.

2.2.7 Amorphous calcium phosphate

Amorphous calcium phosphate (ACP) often occurs as a transient phase during the formation of various calcium phosphates in aqueous systems. In view of this, ACP can have various chemical compositions with no definite short-range structure. The morphology of the ACP particles is mostly spherical, has a tendency to agglomerate, and forms branched clusters. In addition, the short-range order of the amorphous structure leads to the formation of so-called "Posner's clusters," as seen in Fig. 2.6. In addition, such clusters can also be found in crystalline calcium phosphate phases such as HA.

2.2.8 Hydroxyapatite

HA ($Ca_{10}(PO_4)6(OH)_2$) is hexagonal at ambient temperature and is converted to the high-temperature phase, monoclinic, above 250°C. HA is widely used in bioapplications such as orthopedic and dental implants, because HA is chemically similar to a large extent to bone and teeth.

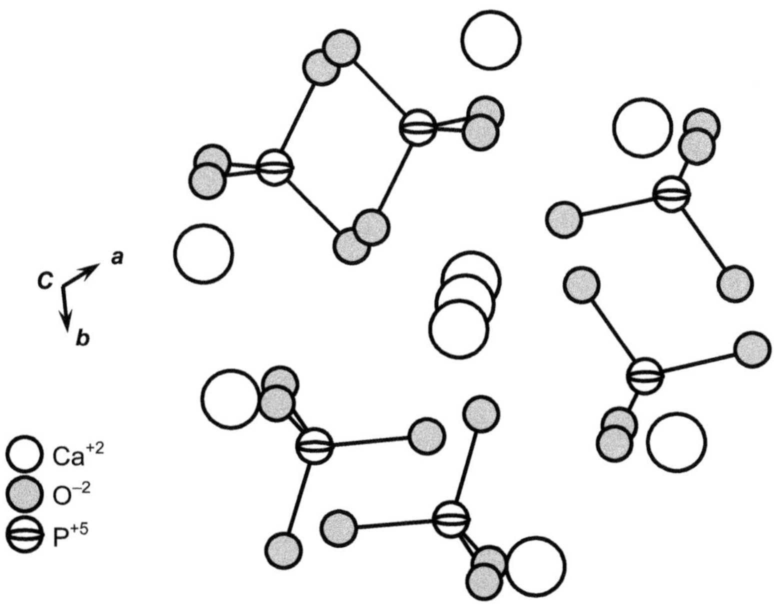

Figure 2.6 The "Posner's cluster" model for the short-range order of amorphous tricalcium phosphate.
Reused from C. Rey, C. Combes, C. Drouet, S. Somrani, 15-Tricalcium phosphate-based ceramics, in: T. Kokubo (Ed.), Bioceramics and Their Clinical Applications, Woodhead Publishing, 2008, pp. 326–366. https://doi.org/10.1533/9781845694227.2.326 after license via (copyright.com) Order number 501313698.

2.2.9 *Fluorhydroxyapatite*

Fluorhydroxyapatite (FA) is the most stable calcium orthophosphate phase until it reaches a melting point of ~1650°C. Also, it is the least soluble. The chemical formula is $Ca_{10}(PO_4)6F_2$. These properties may be attributed to the firm crystal structure of FA, where the F^- ion is positioned in the center of Ca triangles in compact configuration.

2.2.10 *Oxyapatite*

Oxyapatite (OA) is the least stable $CaPO_4$ and is not observed in biological systems or prepared in a pure state. OA ($Ca_{10}(PO_4)_6O$) may be detected in connection with the dehydration of HA and constitutes part of the OA–HA mixture. The only biomedical application of OA is its existence in the admixture phase in connection with plasma-sprayed coatings of $CaPO_4$.

Table 2.3 includes a summary of the crystallographic data for calcium orthophosphates.

Table 2.4 shows a comparison of composition and crystallography between the inorganic phases of adult human calcified tissues and HA. This table may illuminate the importance of the calcium orthophosphates category of materials and its relation to human hard tissues. Applications of calcium orthophosphates will be shown more explicitly in the next chapter. In this chapter, some microstructures are presented to show the bioactivity and functioning of calcium orthophosphates. The microstructure of bioceramics, whether classified as crystalline, amorphous, or composed of a combination of these (some composites and glass-ceramics), obviously plays a major role in determining the bioactivity and progress of the bioactivity process after implantation. The subject of the microstructure of bioceramics is diverse and fairly lengthy. A good introduction to the subject, e.g., for materials science educational purposes, may benefit from the following example of a microstructure. Fig. 2.7 shows a typical microstructure of calcium orthophosphate cement after setting. The microstructure is featured by calcium phosphate crystals interlocked with each other that give rise to mechanical stability. In addition, such a microstructure has a large surface area that helps in reactions of the formation of new tissue, which will be more obvious in the following chapters.

In general, bioactivity is the core strength of bioceramic materials. Another strength is that bioactive ceramic materials are already diverse and subject to an increase in numbers, new properties, and applications. An educative example is the synthesis of pseudowollastonite ($CaSiO_3$) (pW) by a solid-state reaction of a mixture of silica and calcium carbonate and the solid-state reaction synthesis of diopside ($CaMg(SiO_3)_2$) (D) of a mixture of silica. The diopside was synthesized by solid-state reaction from a mixture of high-purity silicon oxide, calcium carbonate, and MgO. The mixtures are certainly stoichiometric and composed of fine particle–sized powders. Finally, the eutectic composition of the wollastonite–diopside system (63.23 wt% of D and 36.77 wt% of pW) is reacted at 1250, 1300, and 1350°C to prepare a new bioceramic [9]. pW, which is a metastable high-temperature polymorph of wollastonite and diopside (pWD), was observed after reaction at 1250 and 1300°C, whereas, a

Table 2.3 Elementary crystallography for various calcium orthophosphates

CP_4	Space group	Unit cell parameters	Z	Density (g/cm^3)
MCPM	Triclinic $P\bar{1}$	a=5.6261(5), b=11.889(2), c=6.4731(8) Å, α=98.633(6)°, β=118.262(6)°, γ=83.344(6)°	2	2.23
MCPA	Triclinic $P\bar{1}$	a=7.5577(5), b=8.2531(6), c=5.5504(3) Å, α=109.87(1)°, β=93.68(1)°, γ=109.15(1)°	2	2.58
OCP	Triclinic $P\bar{1}$	a=19.692(4), b=9.523(2), c=6.835(2) Å, α=90.15(2)°, β=92.54(2)°, γ=108.65(1)°	1	2.61
DCPD	Monoclinic Ia	a=5.812(2), b=15.180(3), c=6.239(2) Å, β=116.25(2)°	4	2.32
DCPA	Triclinic $P\bar{1}$	a=6.910(1), b=6.627(2), c=6.998(2) Å, α=96.34(2)°, β=103.82(2)°, γ=88.33(2)°	4	2.89
α-TCP	Monoclinic $P2_1/a$	a=12.887(2), b=27.280(4), c=15.219(2) Å, β=126.20(1)°	24	2.86
β-TCP	Rhombohedral R3c	a=b=10.439(1), c=37.375(6) Å, γ=120°	21[a]	3.08
TetCP	Monoclinic $P2_1$	a=7.023(1), b=11.986(4), c=9.473(2) Å, β=90.90(1)°	4	3.05
ACP	–	Amorphous, described by "Posner's clusters"	–	–
HA	Monoclinic $P2_1/b$	a=9.4214(8), b=2a, c=6.8814(7) Å, γ=120°	4	3.16
	Hexagonal $P6_3/m$	a=b=9.4302(5), c=6.8911(2) Å, γ=120°	2	
FA	Hexagonal $P6_3/m$	a=b=9.367, c=6.884 Å, γ=120°	2	3.20
OHA	Pseudohexagonal $P\bar{6}$	a=b=9.432, c=6.881 Å, α=90.3°, β=90.0°, γ=119.9°	1	~3.2

ACP, amorphous calcium phosphate; *DCPA*, dicalcium phosphate anhydrous; *DCPD*, dicalcium phosphate dihydrate; *FA*, fluorhydroxyapatite; *HA*, hydroxyapatite; *MCPA*, monocalcium phosphate anhydrous; *OCP*, octacalcium phosphate; *TetCP*, tetracalcium phosphate.

[a]Calculated for hexagonal unit cell setting.

Reused from Chapter 1-general chemistry of the calcium orthophosphates, in: J.C. Elliott (Ed.), Studies in Inorganic Chemistry, Elsevier, 1994, pp. 1–62. https://doi.org/10.1016/B978-0-444-81582-8.50006-7 after license via (copyright.com) order number 501313707.

Table 2.4 **Typical composition and some crystallographic parameters of inorganic phases of adult human calcified tissues compared with hydroxyapatite**

Composition (wt%)	Enamel	Dentine	Bone	HA
Calcium	36.5	35.1	24.5	39.6
Phosphorus	17.7	16.9	11.5	18.5
Ca/P molar ratio	1.63	1.61	1.65	1.67
Sodium	0.5	0.6	0.7	–
Magnesium	0.44	1.23	0.55	–
Potassium	0.08	0.05	0.03	–
Carbonate (CO_3^{2-})	3.5	5.6	5.8	–
Fluoride	0.01	0.06	0.02	–
Chloride	0.30	0.01	0.10	–
Pyrophosphate ($P_2O_7^{4-}$)	0.022	0.10	0.07	–
Total inorganic	97	70	65	100
Total organic	1.5	20	25	–
Water	1.5	10	9.7	–
Ignition products 800°C	β-TCMP + HA	β-TCMP + HA	HA + CaO	
a-axis (Å)	9.441	9.421	9.419	9.422
c-axis (Å)	6.880	6.887	6.880	6.880
Crystallinity index	70–75	33–37	33–37	100

HA, hydroxyapatite; *β-TCMP*, magnesium-substituted β-TCP.
Reused from G. Daculsi, J.-M. Bouler, R.Z. LeGeros, Adaptive crystal formation in normal and pathological calcifications in synthetic calcium phosphate and related biomaterials, in: K.W. Jeon (Ed.), International Review of Cytology, Academic Press, 1997, pp. 129–191. https://doi.org/10.1016/S0074-7696(08)62360-8 after license via (copyright.com) number 4196380297977.

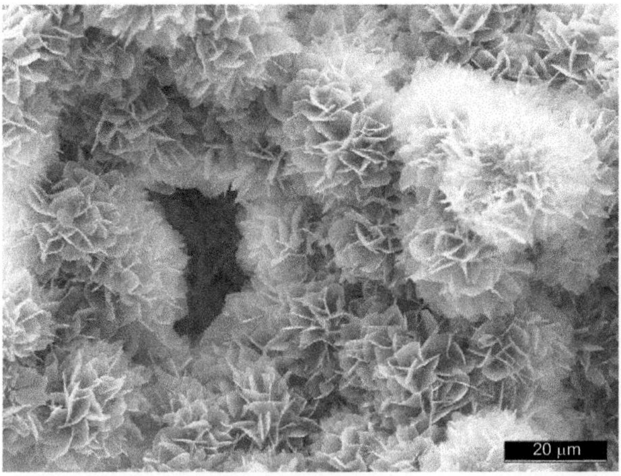

Figure 2.7 The microstructure of calcium orthophosphate cement after setting. Reused from M. Bohner, Resorbable biomaterials as bone graft substitutes, Materials Today 13 (2010) 24–30. https://doi.org/10.1016/S1369-7021(10)70014-6 after license via (copyright.com) number 4196381235311.

stable low-temperature polymorph wollastonite ($Ca_{0.83}Mg_{0.17}SiO_3$ (2M)) existed at 1350°C together with wollastonite and diopside as confirmed by X-ray diffraction (XRD) results, i.e., at 1350°C; the resulting system is a wollastonite-2M-diopside (W2MD) ceramic.

The bioactivity of pWD and W2MD systems was examined via soaking in simulated body fluid (SBF). SBF is an in vitro test that is frequently used to examine the potential of apatite formation at the surface of bioceramics, which indicates bioactivity in vivo [10]. The scanning electron microscope (SEM)–energy-dispersive X-ray spectroscopy (EDX) results confirmed the formation of apatite at the surface of both pWD and W2MD systems. Fig. 2.8 shows that the thickness of the apatite layer is increased by increasing the soaking time with a logarithmic behavior. The bioactivity of W2MD is slightly lower than that of the pWD system, but W2MD has higher mechanical stability and properties. The newly formed HA globular particles are shown in Fig. 2.9 in surface view, and the cross-section view is shown together with EDX analysis in Fig. 2.10.

In conclusion, the study of the microstructure of the prepared calcium orthophosphates before and after the bioactivity test is important to understand the behavior of the prepared material. The importance of the microstructural studies is crucial because of the recognition of the chemical composition. As a result, the selection of the preparation process evidently affects the properties of the final product.

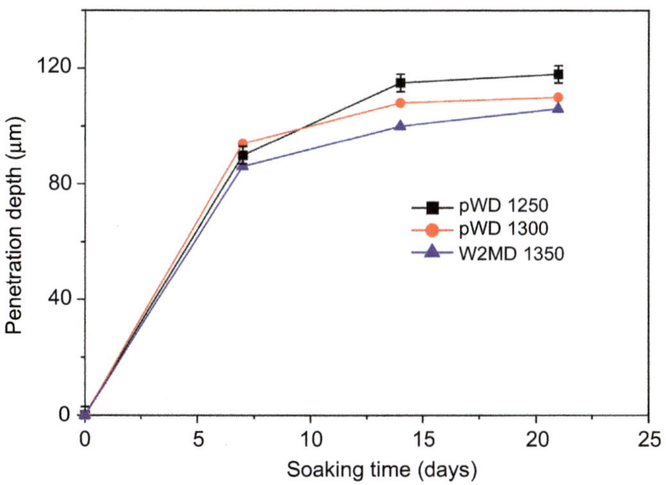

Figure 2.8 Thickness change of the formed porous layer as a function of soaking time in simulated body fluid. *pWD*, polymorph of wollastonite and diopside; *W2MD*, wollastonite-2M-diopside.
Reused from M.A. Sainz, P. Pena, S. Serena, A. Caballero, Influence of design on bioactivity of novel $CaSiO_3$–$CaMg(SiO_3)_2$ bioceramics: in vitro simulated body fluid test and thermodynamic simulation, Acta Biomaterialia 6 (2010) 2797–2807. https:doi.org/10.1016/j.actbio.2010.01.003 after license via (copyright.com) number 4280941493830.

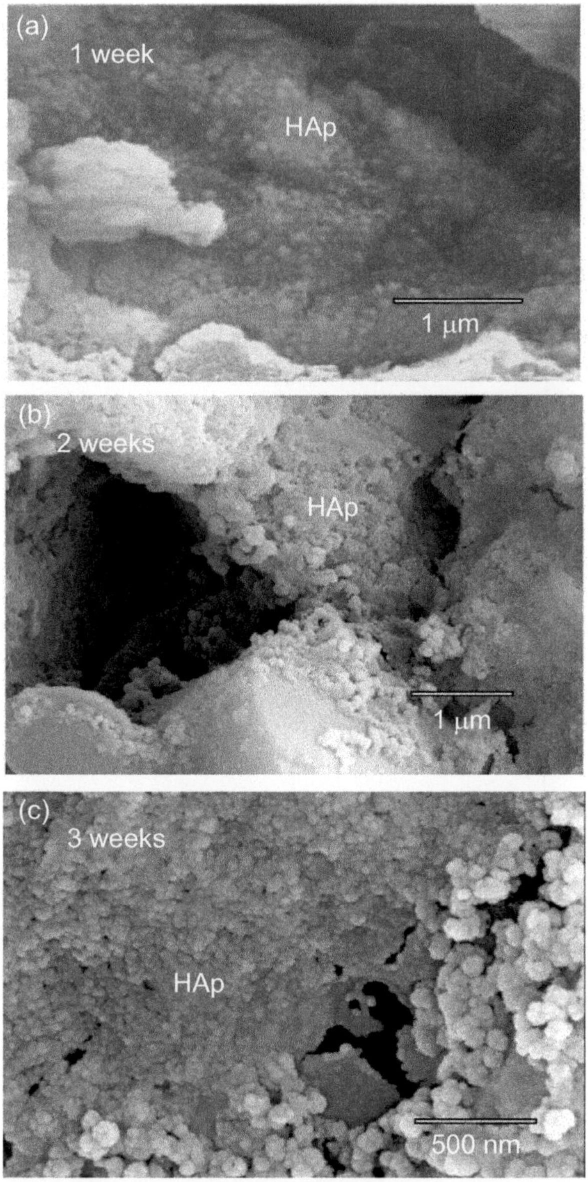

Figure 2.9 Scanning electron microscope surface views of wollastonite 2M-diopside (sintered at 1350°C/4 h) samples after soaking in simulated body fluid solution for (a) 7, (b) 14, and (c) 21 days. *HAp*, hydroxyapatite particles.

Reused from M.A. Sainz, P. Pena, S. Serena, A. Caballero, Influence of design on bioactivity of novel $CaSiO_3$–$CaMg(SiO_3)_2$ bioceramics: in vitro simulated body fluid test and thermodynamic simulation, Acta Biomaterialia 6 (2010) 2797–2807. https:doi.org/10.1016/j.actbio.2010.01.003 after license via (copyright.com) number 4280941493830.

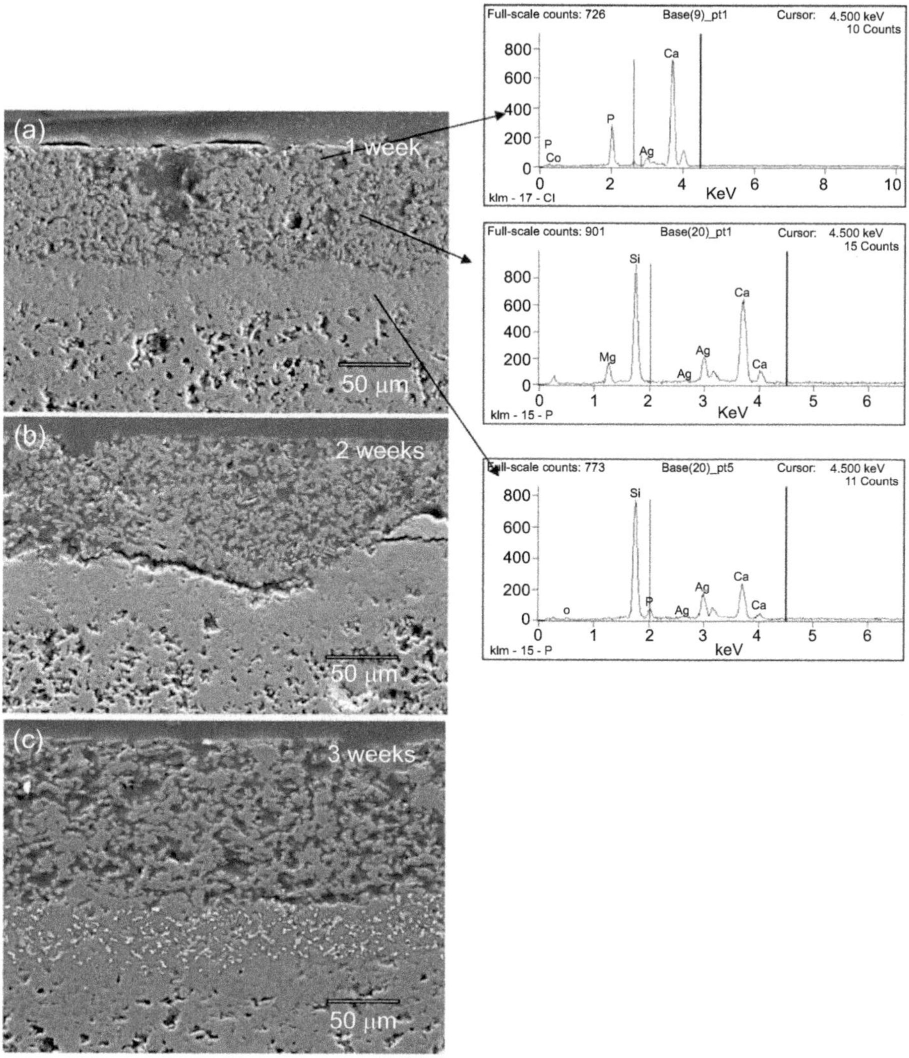

Figure 2.10 Scanning electron microscope micrographs of the cross-sections of simulated body fluid wollastonite-2M-diopside sample sintered at 1350°C/4 h interfaces after soaking for (a) 7, (b) 14, and (c) 21 days.
Reused from M.A. Sainz, P. Pena, S. Serena, A. Caballero, Influence of design on bioactivity of novel $CaSiO_3$–$CaMg(SiO_3)_2$ bioceramics: in vitro simulated body fluid test and thermodynamic simulation, Acta Biomaterialia 6 (2010) 2797–2807. https:doi.org/10.1016/j.actbio.2010.01.003 after license via (copyright.com) number 4280941493830.

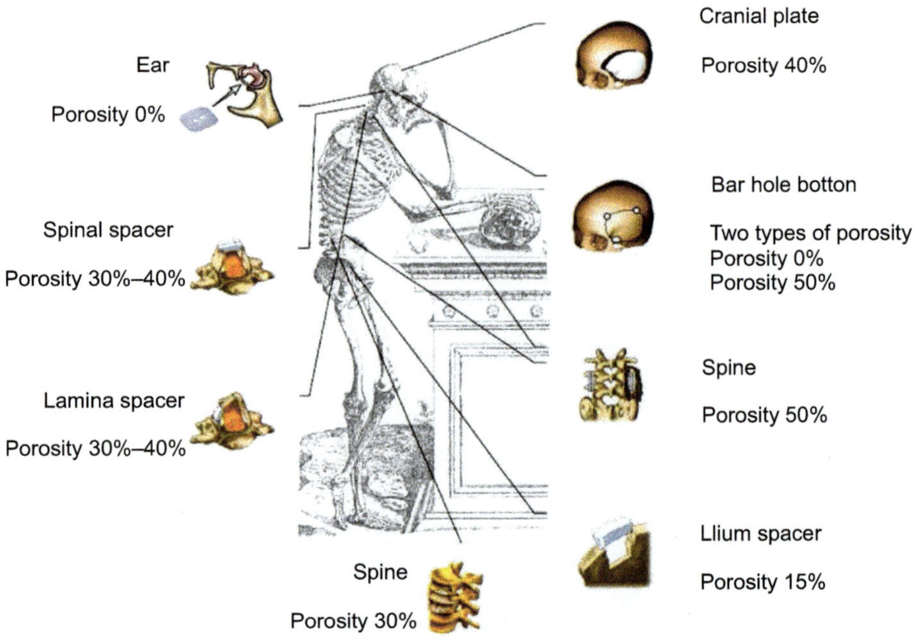

Figure 2.11 Schematic drawing that illustrates the potential application of hydroxyapatite according to the porosity %.

2.3 Glass and glass-ceramics

2.3.1 Glass

The structure of glass lacks long-range atomic order (crystallinity), i.e., it is described as amorphous. Accordingly, XRD does not show diffraction peaks that indicate crystallinity. On the other hand, techniques such as Fourier transform infrared spectroscopy (FTIR) and magic angle spinning nuclear magnetic resonance spectroscopy (MAS NMR) show that the glass has short-range order (nanometer range). The latter techniques allow the extraction of structural data from the glass. Glass is also described by its transition temperature range T_g at which a gradual decrease of viscosity of the glass takes place and results in the liquid state of the glass. On the other hand, the melting of the crystalline solid occurs in a very narrow temperature range at which the melting temperature can be defined. The melting of solids is related to the energies of bonding, which explains why the melting range is related to the degree of crystallinity of the solid. Fig. 2.12 compares the structure of long-range order (crystalline) silica with short-range order (vitreous) silica.

The amorphous state of silica is visualized via atomic resolution scanning tunneling microscopy, as shown in Fig. 2.13(a), which confirms the description of the

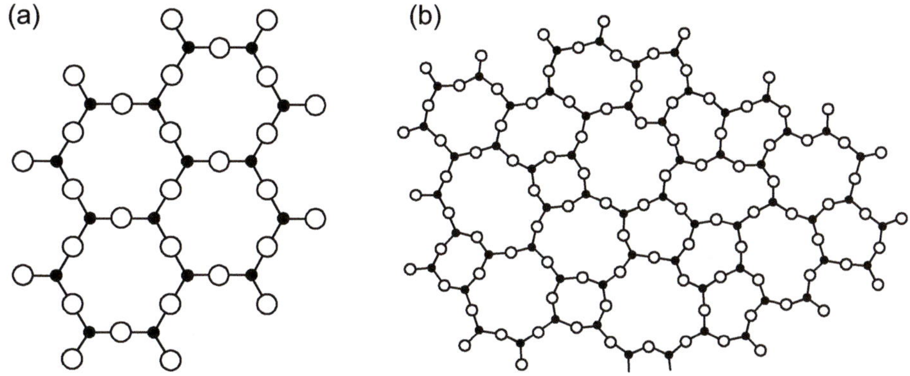

Figure 2.12 (a) The crystalline structure of silica; the fourth atom of the SiO_4 tetrahedron is out of plane. The *white circles* represent the oxygen atoms and the *black dots* represent the silicon atoms. (b) The amorphous state of silica.
Adapted with permission from W.H. Zachariasen, The atomic arrangement in glass, Journal of the American Chemical Society 54 (1932) 3841–3851. https:doi.org/10.1021/ja01349a006. Copyright (1932) American Chemical Society.

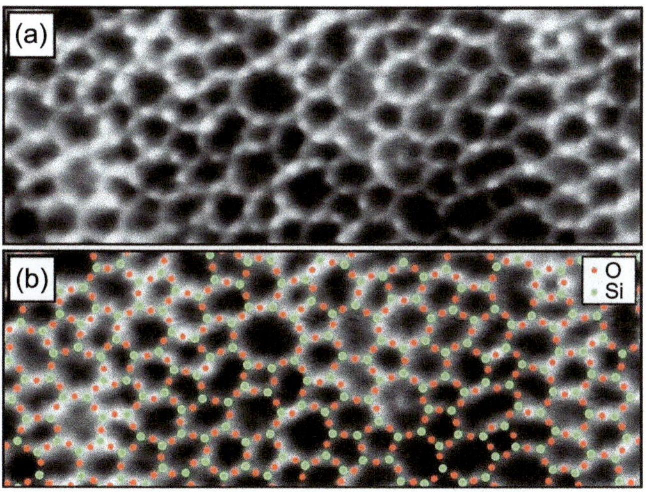

Figure 2.13 (a) Scanning tunneling microscope micrograph of SiO_2 in the amorphous state. (b) The same as (a) with the oxygen and silicon atomic position shown in the vitreous network.
Reused from L. Lichtenstein, C. Büchner, B. Yang, S. Shaikhutdinov, M. Heyde, M. Sierka, R. Włodarczyk, J. Sauer, H.-J. Freund, The atomic structure of a metal-supported vitreous thin silica film, Angewandte Chemie International Edition 51 (2012) 404–407. https://doi.org/10.1002/anie.201107097 after license via (copyright.com) number 4185541273471.

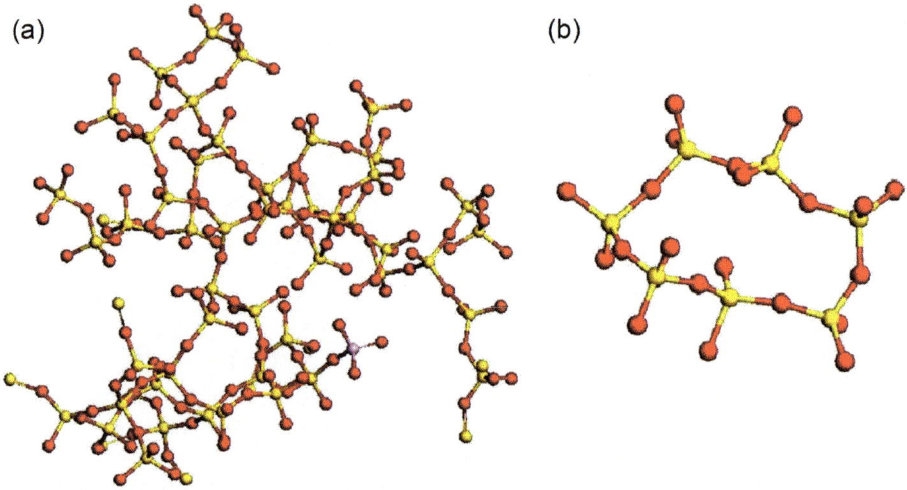

Figure 2.14 The structure of Bioglass. (a) Both the silicon and phosphorous oxides build the glass backbone (O red, Si yellow, P purple). (b) Short chain of the glassy network. Adapted with permission from Y. Xiang, J. Du, Effect of strontium substitution on the structure of 45S5 bioglasses, Chemistry of Materials 23 (2011) 2703–2717. https://doi.org/10.1021/cm102889q. Copyright (2010) American Chemical Society.

amorphous state of silica obtained via MAS NMR. The oxygen and silicon atomic position are labeled in Fig. 2.13(b).

The structure of silicate glass can be described by the network formers, network modifiers, and intermediate oxides. The network former is the building unit of silicate glasses and is the SiO_4 tetrahedron, which is connected via bridging oxygen atoms. Phosphorous pentoxide (P_2O_5) and boron trioxide (B_2O_3) are also network formers and can coexist with silica. The network modifiers include the oxides of alkali or alkaline earth metals. They modify the glass network structure by breaking the bonds of the bridging oxygen atoms and cause a decrease in glass viscosity. The intermediate oxides behave as network modifiers similar to a network former according to the composition of the glass. In the case of Bioglass, two types of network formers exist, which are the silicon and phosphorous oxides. Both of these network formers have tetrahedron profiles.

Fig. 2.14 shows the structure of Bioglass 45S5 obtained using molecular dynamic simulation. The important properties of Bioglass are listed in Table 2.5. Recalling the important mechanical properties of the cortical bones (tensile strength 50–150 MPa and Young's modulus 7–30 GPa), it is obvious that Bioglass has poor mechanical properties. Accordingly, Bioglass is either used to repair defects of bones, incorporated as scaffolds or fibers within composite or hybrid structures, or to enhance the formation of apatite at the surface of the implant.

In addition to glass composition, glass can also be described by the network connectivity (NC) model. NC is a number that represents the average number of bridging oxygen atoms per network-forming element; for silicon it is denoted as NC_{Si}. For pure silica

Table 2.5 Properties of Bioglass

Property	Value
Density	2.7 g/cm^3
Glass transition temperature	538°C
Crystallization onset temperature	677°C
Melting temperature	1224–1264°C
Thermal expansion coefficient	15.1×10^{-6}°C^{-1}
Refractive index	1.59
Tensile strength	42 MPa
Young's modulus	35 MPa
Shear modulus	30.7 GPa
Fracture toughness	0.6 MPa·m$^{1/2}$
Vickers hardness	5.75 GPa

Reused from M.D. O'Donnell, Melt-Derived bioactive glass, in: J.R. Jones, A.G. Clare (Eds.), Bio-glasses, John Wiley & Sons, Ltd., 2012, pp. 13–27. https://doi.org/10.1002/9781118346457.ch2 after license via (copyright.com) number 4196740353484.

glass, the NC is four. This number decreases with the increase in the network modifier. Usually, NC values for bioactive glasses range between 2 and 3, and 45S5 Bioglass is 2.11. Thus NC describes the average polymerization of the glass network. Hence it is a useful tool for estimating or forecasting the properties of Bioglass such as the glass transition temperature and bioactivity. Other models that describe the glass exist, but it seems that NC is best for the early introduction of Bioglass and estimating its properties based on the glass composition because it is directly connected to the glass structure.

Low NC of bioactive glasses means that it has an open network structure that facilitates the penetration of water molecules when in contact with body fluids. The penetration of water molecules and the existence of nonbridging oxygen atoms and modifier cations (e.g., Na^+) at the surface of the bioactive glass enhance its dissolution process; see Fig. 2.15. The result is ion release of calcium and phosphate, which accordingly stimulates the formation of apatite at the surface of the glass or the contact area. The formation of the apatite layer is, to a large extent, what is meant by bioactivity. Fig. 2.16 shows that water molecules start to diffuse into the bioactive glass network creating an interface area.

Other types of bioactive glass exist and are designed for specific purposes. 13-93 bioactive glass, for example, benefits from increased silica content with the addition of potassium and magnesium oxide. This type of glass is found to enhance the healing ability of the body. Another example of bioactive glass is a variation of 13-93 bioactive glass that replaces silica with other glass formers, namely, boron oxide (B_2O_3), and is coded 13-93B3. 13-93B3 bioactive borate glass suppresses the formation of the silica layer at the surface of the glass and facilitates direct bonding to hard tissue. Fig. 2.17 illustrates the formation of hydroxycarbonate apatite (HCA) at the surface of bioactive borate glass in an in vivo environment. The bioactive glass has been used for a long time in nonload-bearing implants such as small bone replacements, bone cements, and mesoporous nanoparticles for controlled drug delivery.

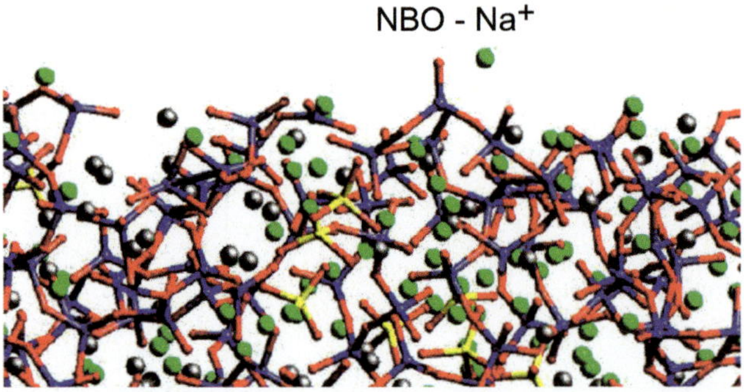

Figure 2.15 Molecular dynamic simulation of the open network of bioactive glass. Color codes: O red, Si blue, Na green, Ca dark gray, and P yellow. *NBO*, nonbridging oxygen atoms. The figure is cropped and adapted with permission from A. Tilocca, A.N. Cormack, Surface signatures of bioactivity: MD simulations of 45S and 65S silicate glasses, Langmuir 26 (2010) 545–551. https://doi.org/10.1021/la902548f. Copyright (2009) American Chemical Society.

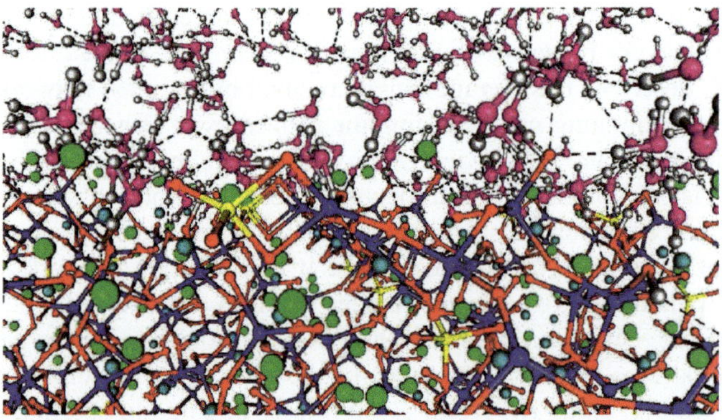

Figure 2.16 Interface of the Bioglass network with water. Color codes: purple O (water), H (water) white, O (glass) red, Si blue, Na green, and Ca turquoise.
The figure is cropped and adapted with permission from A. Tilocca, A.N. Cormack, Modeling the water–bioglass interface by Ab initio molecular dynamics simulations, ACS Applied Materials and Interfaces 1 (2009) 1324–1333. https://doi.org/10.1021/am900198t. Copyright (2009) American Chemical Society.

2.3.2 Glass-ceramics

The outcome of a controlled crystallization of the melt of a glass recipe is called glass-ceramics. Several advantages of glass-ceramics are mentioned in Chapter 1. The controlled crystallization process is achieved by controlling the nucleation of the crystalline phase or phases during the cooling period. Two types of the controlled crystallization process exist. The first is called internal processes or bulk processes in

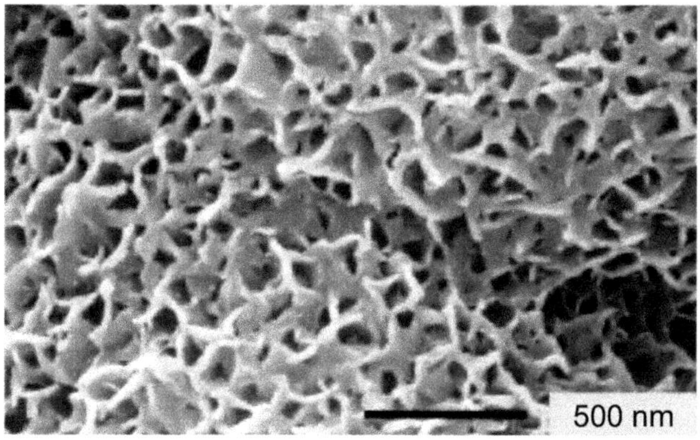

Figure 2.17 Scanning electron microscope micrograph shows the formation of a porous nano-crystalline needle-like microstructure of hydroxycarbonate apatite on the surface of bioactive borate glass after in vivo reaction.
Reused from S.B. Jung, Bioactive borate glasses, in: J.R. Jones, A.G. Clare (Eds.), Bio-glasses, John Wiley & Sons, Ltd., 2012, pp. 75–95. https://doi.org/10.1002/9781118346457.ch6 after license via (copyright.com) number 4196660427874.

which the base glass is seeded with crystalline oxide such as TiO_2 and is called nucleation sites or crystallization centers. The crystallization process starts and develops at the bulk with controlled cooling technology. The other technique of the bulk process allows phase separation of the melt glass via the design of the composition. When phase separation occurs, one of the phases will contain the nucleation oxides at higher concentration. Accordingly, the nucleation process starts at that phase. The second type of controlled crystallization process relies on the surface treatment of a bulk of solid glass with certain composition. The crystallization process starts at the surface and proceeds to the bulk. It is clear that the method of controlled crystallization determines the types and amounts of crystalline phases and their structure and establishes the final microstructure and final properties of glass-ceramics. The controlled nucleation–crystallization process is utilized to produce a wide variety of new materials for a broad range of applications, including bioceramics.

The motivation for employing glass-ceramics in biomaterials is to overcome drawbacks found with both Bioglass and bioceramics in some applications. Bioglass suffers from deficient tension strength or undercyclic loading, and bioceramics are generally limited to biocompatibility, but not bioactivity, which is required in many applications. Accordingly, apatite–wollastonite (A–W) glass-ceramics are utilized for their mechanical properties and bioactivity. In addition, the bioactivity of A–W glass-ceramics does not include the formation of a silica gel layer on the surface of the implant then the HCA layer on the gel layer. The gel layer noticeably reduces the implant's mechanical properties. With A–W glass-ceramics, the HCA layer directly formed on the implant surface that ensures better mechanical properties and wider applications.

The interesting crystalline phase in this type of glass-ceramic is β-wollastonite ($CaO{\cdot}SiO_2$), which has chains of SiO_4 tetrahedra included in its structure and exists

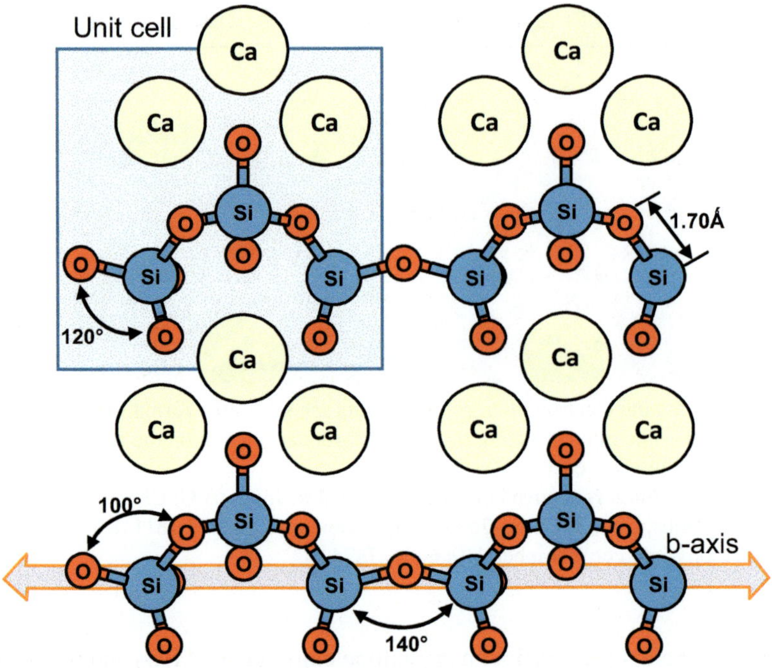

Figure 2.18 The crystal structure of wollastonite.
Adapted with permission from N. Giraudo, P. Krolla-Sidenstein, S. Bergdolt, M. Heinle, H. Gliemann, F. Messerschmidt, P. Brüner, P. Thissen, Early stage hydration of wollastonite: kinetic aspects of the metal-proton exchange reaction, Journal of Physical Chemistry C. 119 (2015) 10493–10499. https://doi.org/10.1021/acs.jpcc.5b02327. Copyright (2015) American Chemical Society.

up to 2000°C. Accordingly, β-wollastonite forms a strong fibrous phase because of its silicate chain structure. The crystal structure of β-wollastonite is triclinic $P\bar{1}$ with axes of $a=7.94$, $b=7.32$, and $c=7.07$ Å, angles of $\alpha=90.03$, $\beta=95.37$, and $\gamma=103.43$ degrees, and $Z=6$. Fig. 2.18 shows the crystal structure of wollastonite and the chain of the SiO_4 tetrahedra.

A typical and clear example of bioactive glass-ceramics is that based on the Na_2O–K_2O–CaO–SiO_2–F glass system [20]. Various mixtures were investigated and three of them are shown in Table 2.6. The control composition is that coded G1, which is modified by replacing K_2O with Na_2O to produce G4. Also, CeO_2 is introduced at the expense of CaO of the composition G1 to produce G1Ce.

After controlled heat treatment, different microstructures are observed, as shown in Fig. 2.19. Rod-shaped wollastonite crystals with G1, larger rods with G4, and prismatic crystals emerge with G1Ce, i.e., the microstructure can be controlled via the composition and heat treatment of the glass-ceramics, which makes glass-ceramics tailorable for various applications, including biomedical applications.

The bioactivity of the produced glass-ceramics should be tested. In vitro tests include immersion in SBF for different periods and observe whether the apatite phase

Table 2.6 The composition of selected model glasses in mol%

Code	K_2O	Na_2O	CaO	SiO_2	CaF_2	CeO_2
G1	5.17	–	29.31	55.18	10.34	–
G4	0.0	5.17	29.31	55.18	10.34	–
G1Ce	5.17	–	28.31	55.18	10.34	1.0

Reused from S.M. Salman, S.N. Salama, H.A. Abo-Mosallam, The crystallization behaviour and bioactivity of wollastonite glass-ceramic based on Na_2O–K_2O–CaO–SiO_2–F glass system, Journal of Asian Ceramic Societies 3 (2015) 255–261. https://doi.org/10.1016/j.jascer.2015.04.004 after written permission from the Journal of Asian Ceramic Societies.

begins to appear and the amount of this phase. Fig. 2.20 shows the growth of the apatite phase on the glass-ceramics mentioned in Table 2.6 and Fig. 2.20.

2.4 Bone cements and substitutes

The aim of bone cements is to perform fixation of prostheses and/or substitution of a missing part of a bone. Certainly, these cements are required to last a long time, have good biological properties, and can be applied without problems. In fact, there are design criteria for bone cements, listed in Table 2.7 [21], which should be satisfied to an acceptable extent. It is hard to select a cement type for a specific situation. Thus the surgeon should have sufficient knowledge of the various types of bone cements to help decide which cement type is best for each case. The materials scientist and engineer should be equipped with detailed knowledge of the properties of various cements and must listen attentively to surgeons and other physicians to deduce the aims of their future research. In this section, preliminary information of the types of bone cement and their properties is introduced.

Two properties of cement should be introduced first: the working time and the setting time. The working time is the time that the cement has sufficient plasticity, which helps during application of the cement. The setting time is the period required for plasticity to be diminished and the cement to reach the solid state and gain most of its mechanical properties. Obviously, increasing the working time and decreasing the setting time make the cement more practicable in applications.

The working and setting times may be estimated via the Vicat needle and Gillmore needle techniques. However, the American Dental Association [22] developed a modified technique for measuring the working and setting times, which seems based on stronger scientific findings. This technique relies on the exothermic heat produced during the setting of the cement. The time needed to attain the maximum temperature, measured via a certain thermocouple, denotes the setting time. This temperature is called the setting temperature. Halfway between the initial temperature and the setting temperature is called the working temperature. Accordingly, the time elapsed to reach the working temperature is called the working time. The time–temperature trajectory is not linear and thus the working time is more than the half the setting time. Certainly, the working and setting times of the cement are affected by the ambient temperatures and these times are shorter at higher temperatures.

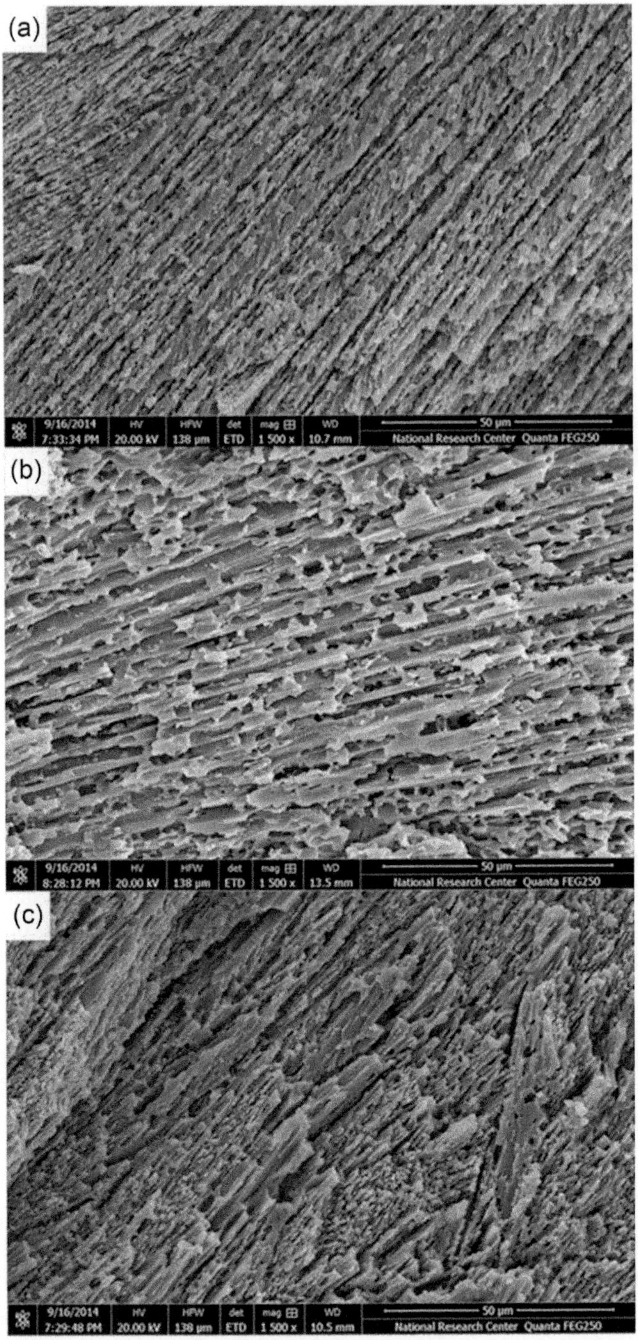

Figure 2.19 Scanning electron microscope micrograph of the fracture surface of the glass-ceramics shown in Table 2.6. (a) G1, (b) G4, and (c) G1Ce.
Reused from S.M. Salman, S.N. Salama, H.A. Abo-Mosallam, The crystallization behaviour and bioactivity of wollastonite glass-ceramic based on Na_2O–K_2O–CaO–SiO_2–F glass system, Journal of Asian Ceramic Societies 3 (2015) 255–261. https://doi.org/10.1016/j.jascer.2015.04.004 after written permission from the Journal of Asian Ceramic Societies.

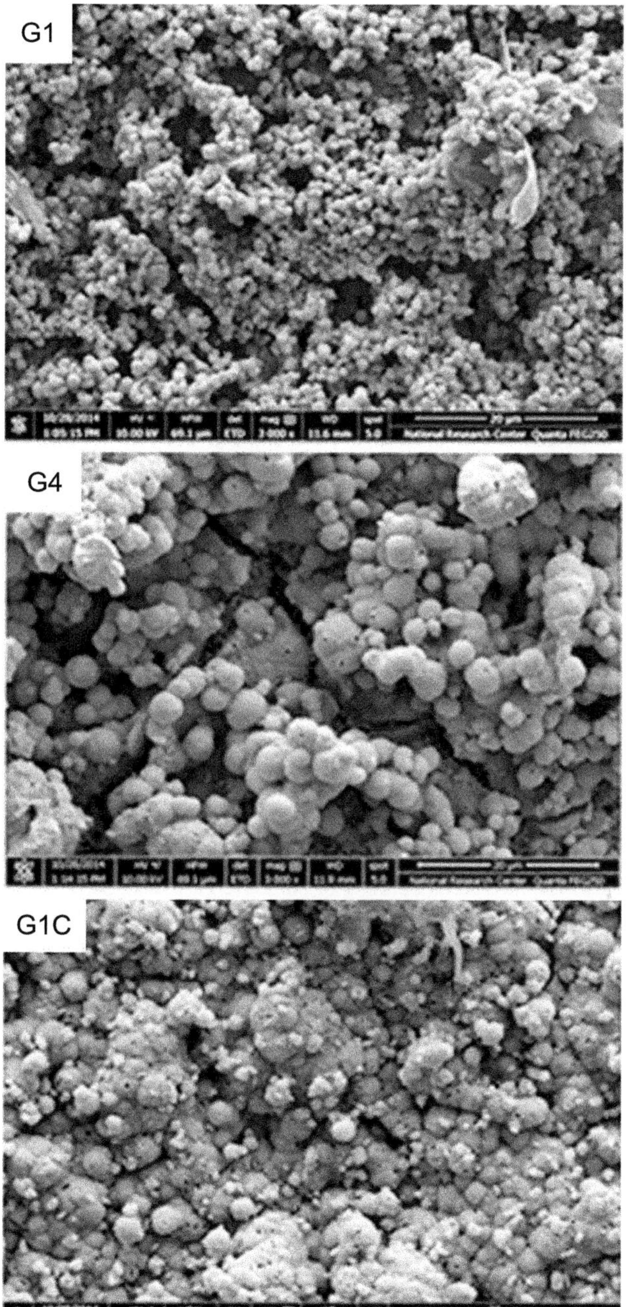

Figure 2.20 Scanning electron microscope micrographs of the glass-ceramics shown in the previous figure exposed to simulated body fluid solution for 21 days.
Reused from M. Salman, S.N. Salama, H.A. Abo-Mosallam, The crystallization behaviour and bioactivity of wollastonite glass-ceramic based on Na_2O–K_2O–CaO–SiO_2–F glass system, Journal of Asian Ceramic Societies 3 (2015) 255–261. https://doi.org/10.1016/j.jascer.2015.04.004 after written permission from the Journal of Asian Ceramic Societies.

Table 2.7 **Target properties in the design of new bone cement**

Criterion	Purpose
Mechanical properties to match that of bone	Enhance the elimination of the phenomenon known as stress shielding
Quick setting (5–15 mm)	To assist in clinical use and aftercare of the patient
In situ setting at body temperature	Elimination of necrosis of the adjacent tissue
Bonding to bone and medical grade alloys	Elimination of fibrous capsule and thus loosening of the implant
Bioactive bone in-growth	Enhancement of both stress transfer and chemical attachment of the implant
Radioopaque	Subsequent monitoring of the implant

Reused from S.M. Kenny, M. Buggy, Bone cements and fillers: a review, Journal of Materials Science: Materials in Medicine 14 (2003) 923–938. https://doi.org/10.1023/A:1026394530192 after license via (copyright.com) number 4198601415125.

2.4.1 The types of bone cements and substitutes

The major type of bone cements and substitutes can be introduced in short by the following classification:

1. Synthetic HA: The need for bone graft substitute material that supports the bone regeneration process is the motivation to use synthetic HA. Also, synthetic HA is used to overcome the problems accompanying the use of autogenous bone. Synthetic HA is one of the most studied materials with their different Ca/P ratios (1.55–2.2), forms, composites, etc.
2. Bioactive glass: The interfacial bonding of bioactive glass with hard tissue is one aspect of the bioactivity of bioactive glass. A range of bioactive glass formulations exists with the prime property of forming strong chemical bonds at the interface of the bioactive glass and the hard tissue. Accordingly, bioactive glass is classified as one of the bone substitutes. On the other hand, the term "bioactive fixation" is used to denote the strong chemical bonds formed with bone that can efficiently transfer stress to the bone. It should be noted that stimulated bone growth beyond the interface ("osteoinductivity") is not discussed here.
3. A–W glass-ceramics: Because of the known strong chemical bonds of A–W glass-ceramics to bone and its high fracture toughness, it is used as a bone substitute. This type of material is especially used for filling defects and irregularities in the bone skeleton. Porous granules are used for such purposes, which can be easily molded into the desired shape for better bioactivity because of the high surface area of the porous granules. These properties also qualify A–W glass-ceramics for use as an intramedullary plug in total hip replacement. In addition, A–W glass-ceramics are used as an additive to enhance the bioactivity of cements such as glass ionomer cements.
4. Calcium phosphate cements (CPCs): Bone consists of apatite as a major inorganic component, which belongs to calcium phosphate compounds. Accordingly, various calcium phosphates are studied for potential use as substitute materials, their bioactivity, and the final properties of newly generated bone. Calcium phosphates can also be formulated as cements. CPCs are a designed combination of calcium phosphate phases (see Section 2.2) as the solid part of the cement and water or an aqueous solution as the liquid part. On mixing the solid and liquid parts, a workable paste is produced with working and setting times that depend on the composition and initial particle sizes. Bioactivity and consequent bone substitution or tissue regeneration are shown significantly through vast research activities.

5. Poly(methyl methacrylate) (PMMA) cement: This cement is a two-part, room temperature-curing PMMA polymer. It has been used for prosthetic operations to ensure efficient load transfer from the implant to the bone. The working time (5–8 min) is comfortably long, but the setting time is comparable to the working time (8–10 min). The reported failure of this type of cement is caused by mechanical failure of the bond between implant and bone not because of infection, and is called aseptic loosening.
6. Zinc phosphate cements: This type of cement has a solid part and a liquid part. The solid part consists of zinc oxide and minor MgO addition. The liquid part is diluted phosphoric acid. It is difficult to control or manipulate the short working and setting times of this type of cement. In addition, there are no adhesive properties of the reaction product but it relies on the mechanical interlocking that is degraded with time when exposed to body liquids. The heat developed during setting caused by exothermic reaction may affect the surrounding tissue. Accordingly, zinc phosphate cements have limited applications in dentistry.
7. Zinc polycarboxylate cements: To overcome the problems associated with zinc phosphate cements, a modified version is introduced. In this cement, phosphoric acid is replaced with a type of polycarboxylic acid. The working and setting times of this cement (both 2–4 min) are far better than those of zinc phosphate cements. Other minor additions may be found for further improvement of the working and setting times. Zinc phosphate and zinc polycarboxylate cements are called acid-base cements.
8. Glass ionomer cements: Replacing zinc oxide with an ion-leachable glass (generally, a calcium aluminosilicate glass) and adding a polycarboxylic acid to it makes glass ionomer cement. The addition of polycarboxylic acid leads to the destruction of the glass network and leaching of Al and Ca ions. These ions bond with carboxylate groups forming a chelate (multiple-bonded ligands to these ions). The subsequent cross-linking process between these groups leads to the gradual setting of the cement. Originally, this type of cement is called "polyalkenoate" cement, but the cross-linking process stimulated by ions leached from the glass gives it the name glass ionomer. Various working and setting times are reported for glass ionomer cement that depends on the composition. A first estimate is that the working time is 2 min and the setting time is 8 min. Addition of tartaric acid increases the working time and reduces the setting time. Other additives with the same functioning can be found in the literature.
9. Resin-modified glass ionomer cement: This type of cement is suggested as an improvement to the previous glass ionomer cement in terms of stability, aesthetics, and final mechanical properties. The addition of a polyalkenoic acid, such as a poly(acrylic acid), gives rise to two different simultaneous chemical setting reactions of the cement. These reactions are the acid–base setting reaction and the free-radical polymerization reaction, which can be initiated with photocuring via a (blue) light-emitting diode halogen lamp. The effect of the wavelength of the curing light and curing time is subjected to numerous studies.
10. Composite cements: Polymer matrix glass or ceramic composite is prepared to overcome the problem of Young's modulus or stiffness mismatch between the implant and the bone. The mismatch leading to inefficient load transfer from the implant and the bone is called stress shielding. This phenomenon causes harmful changes in bone chemistry and microstructure. Accordingly, the polymer composite cements are designed to fulfill the requirement of bone-implant matching of the mechanical properties. Various polymers are utilized for this purpose such as PMMA and high-density polyethylene, and a variety of fillers such as HA and Bioglasses. Tuning of the mechanical properties can be achieved via controlling the type of fillers, their volume fractions, and morphologies. One or more types of filler may be incorporated in the design of the composite. Bioactivity of the composite is certainly assured in the stage of materials selection.

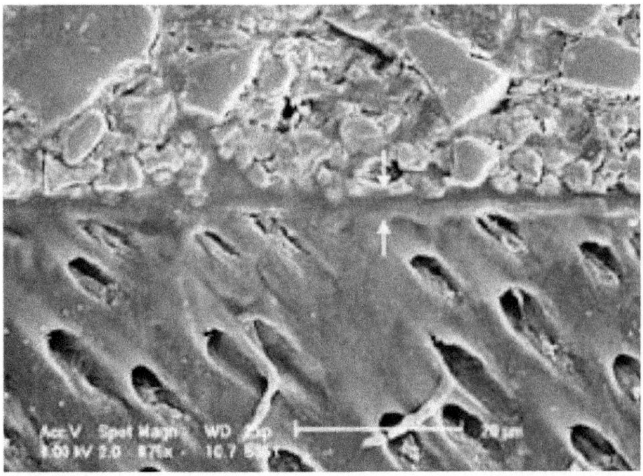

Figure 2.21 Conventional glass ionomer cement (*upper side*) with the "ion-exchange" layer indicated by *white arrows*.
Reused from M. Tyas, M. Burrow, Adhesive restorative materials: a review, Australian Dental Journal 49 (2004) 112–121. https://doi.org/10.1111/j.1834-7819.2004.tb00059.x after license via (copyright.com) number 4203580898028.

2.4.2 Example microstructures before and after in vitro tests

It is important for the materials scientist to examine the microstructure of the studied bone cements and substitutes before and after in vitro tests. This is done to evaluate the integrity of the microstructure and its functioning as a biomaterial. A number of example microstructures for bone substitutes have already been mentioned in this chapter. The following example microstructures are for bone cements that may be suitable for the objective of a textbook.

The first example microstructure is a simple photograph showing the bonding of cement (glass ionomer) to a tooth and is presented in Fig. 2.21. When the glass ionomer cement is applied, the phosphate and calcium ions are gradually absorbed from the HA of the living tissue by the acidic media of the cement. Thus an "ion-exchange" layer is formed, which also contains ions from the glass component of the cement such as aluminum, silicic acid, fluoride, and calcium. This layer serves as an isolation layer from organisms and is called an acid–base-resistant layer.

Table 2.8 shows the composition of different wollastonite-containing PMMA cements [24]. The microstructure of these five cement compositions, before and after immersion in SBF, is shown in Fig. 2.22.

The left side of the figure shows well-developed wollastonite grains that constitute the microstructure in the absence of PMMA addition (refer to Table 2.8). However, the gradual increase in PMMA in the cement leads to a composite microstructure of PMMA beads and wollastonite grains at the boundaries of the polymer beads. The morphology of the wollastonite grains is gradually concealed by the polymer as the polymer content is increased. The corresponding photos at the right side of the figure

Table 2.8 The composition of prepared wollastonite-containing PMMA cements

	Powder (wt%)			Liquid (wt%)	
ID	PMMA	BPO	W	MMA	DMPT
W-97	–	2.9	97.1	99.2	0.8
W-68	29.1	2.9	68	99.2	0.8
W-49	48.6	2.9	48.6	99.2	0.8
W-39	58.3	2.9	38.8	99.2	0.8
W-19	77.7	2.9	19.4	99.2	0.8

BPO, Benzoyl peroxide as a polymerization initiator; *DMPT*, *N*,*N*-dimethyl-*p*-toluidine, a polymerization accelerator; *MMA*, methyl methacrylate monomers.
Reused from D. Rentería-Zamarrón, D.A. Cortés-Hernández, L. Bretado-Aragón, W. Ortega-Lara, Mechanical properties and apatite-forming ability of PMMA bone cements, Materials and Design 30 (2009) 3318–3324. https://doi.org/10.1016/j.matdes.2008.11.024 after license via (copyright.com) number 4202650080226.

for the cements after immersion in SBF show a newly formed layer. This layer is identified as apatite, in the same study [24], via XRD. The formation of apatite, as already known, proves the bioactivity of the designed cements. The morphology of the newly formed apatite resembles a thick agglomerated layer, which becomes thinner as the PMMA content increases at the expense of the wollastonite.

Another research work [25] produced wollastonite via solid-state reaction of limestone and silica at 1450°C. An in vitro test of the sintered sample was carried out in SBF solution for different times. The resultant Ca/P ratios via SEM/EDX were all below 1.67, as shown in Table 2.9. This result indicates that the formed apatite layer on the surface of the wollastonite, Fig. 2.23, is calcium-deficient hydroxyapatite.

In the case of magnesia-doped wollastonite [26], the final value of the Ca/P ratio, after soaking in SBF solution for different periods, is changed according to the amount of magnesia in the magnesia-doped wollastonite. Fig. 2.24 shows that the Ca/P ratio is closer to that of the stoichiometric apatite (1.67) as the amount of dopant increased. Magnification of the SEM micrograph does not appear in the original reference probably because of the cropping of the micrographs to save space. However, the micrographs clearly show the gradual formation of the apatite layer. Globular precipitates are shown in some dopant concentrations and soaking periods in SBF, but the morphology of the needle-like apatite agglomerates is obvious.

An important biomaterial is the injectable bioactive cement filler that is composed of β-dicalcium silicate (β-Ca_2SiO_4) [27]. This cement is self-setting and can be used as bone repair material and a host for drug release. The cement is injected as paste after mixing with water. Fig. 2.25 shows the apatite precipitated at the surface of the cement after 7 days of immersion in SBF. Once more, needle-like agglomerates (≈150 nm × 300 nm) are shown covering the cement spherical particles (2–5 μm). Both the morphology of the set cement and the apatite formation are the same for the different cement liquid-to-powder ratios.

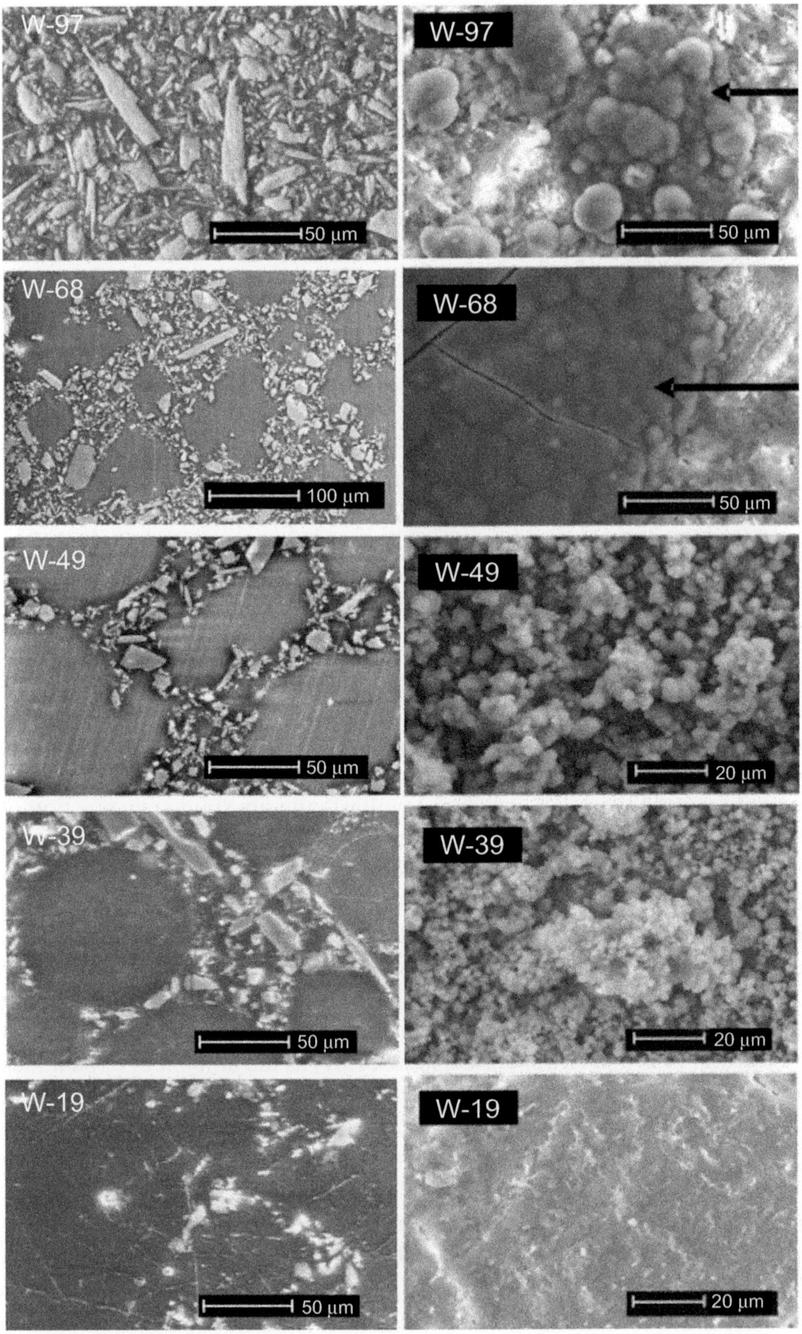

Figure 2.22 Scanning electron microscope micrographs showing the microstructure of the cements mentioned in Table 2.8. *Left*: before immersion in simulated body fluid (SBF), *right*: after immersion in SBF.
Reused from D. Rentería-Zamarrón, D.A. Cortés-Hernández, L. Bretado-Aragón, W. Ortega-Lara, Mechanical properties and apatite-forming ability of PMMA bone cements, Materials and Design 30 (2009) 3318–3324. https://doi.org/10.1016/j.matdes.2008.11.024, Fig. 3 and Fig. 6, after license via (copyright.com) number 4202650080226.

Table 2.9 **Ca/P ratios of the apatite layer on the produced wollastonite for different soaking times in SBF**

Soaking period (day)	Ca/P ratio
1	1.48
3	1.27
5	1.17
7	1.15

Reused from R. Abd Rashid, R. Shamsudin, M.A. Abdul Hamid, A. Jalar, In-vitro bioactivity of wollastonite materials derived from limestone and silica sand, Ceramics International 40 (2014) 6847–6853. https://doi.org/10.1016/j.ceramint.2013.12.004 after license via (copyright.com) number 4203730963445.

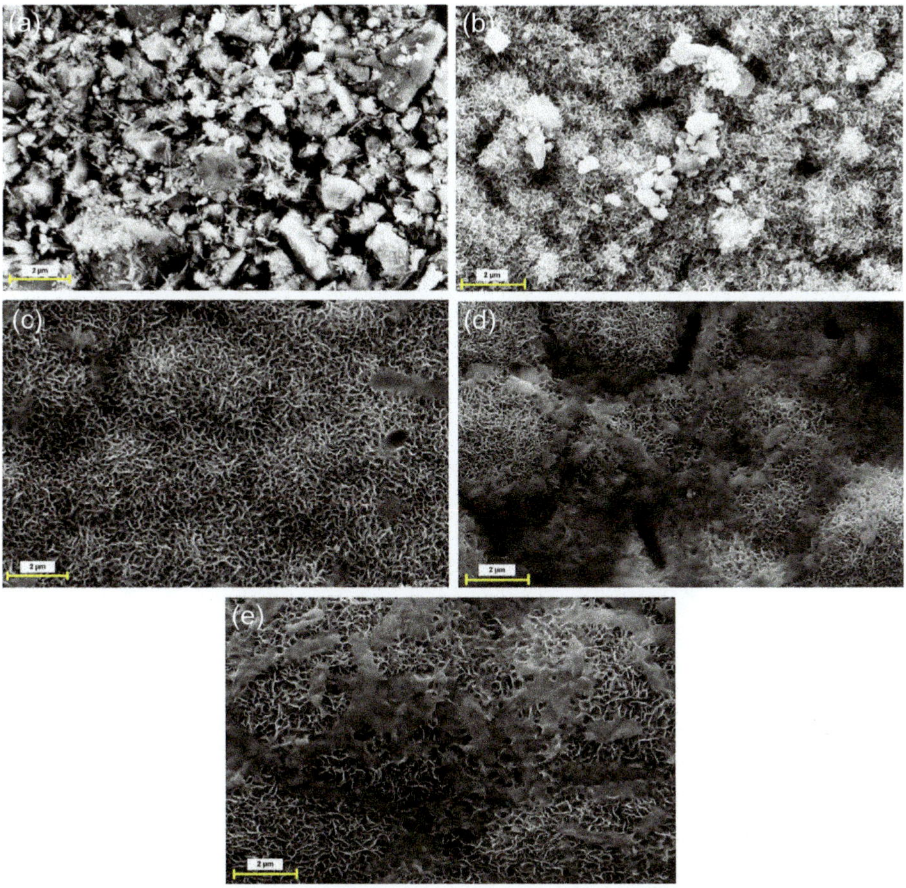

Figure 2.23 Scanning electron microscope micrographs of wollastonite before immersion in simulated body fluid solution (a) and after immersion for 1, 3, 5, and 7 days (b), (c), (d), (e), respectively. The apatite is gradually formed as agglomerates of needle-like granules. Reused from R. Abd Rashid, R. Shamsudin, M.A. Abdul Hamid, A. Jalar, In-vitro bioactivity of wollastonite materials derived from limestone and silica sand, Ceramics International 40 (2014) 6847–6853. https://doi.org/10.1016/j.ceramint.2013.12.004 after license via (copyright.com) number 4203730963445.

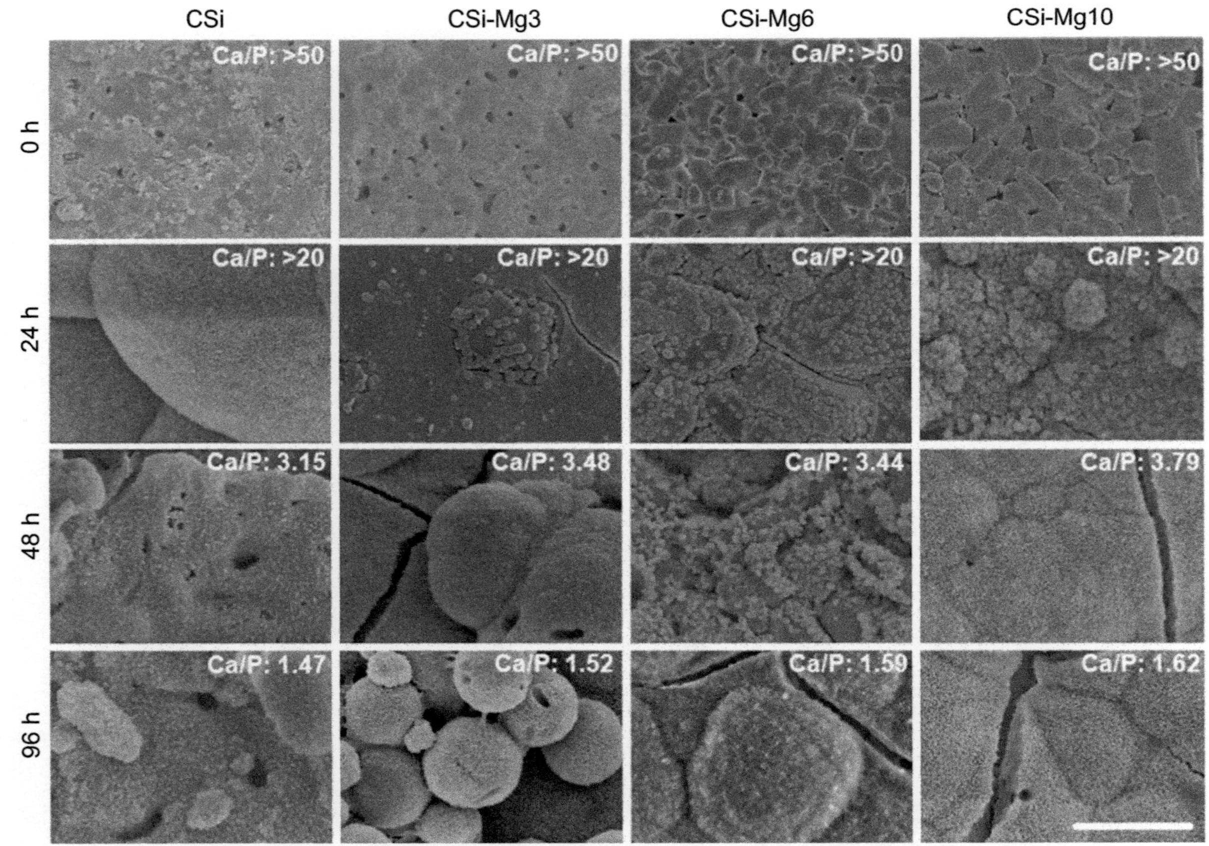

Figure 2.24 Scanning electron microscope micrographs of wollastonite after immersion in simulated body fluid solution for different soaking periods. *CSi*, undoped wollastonite; *CSi-Mgx*, x mol% doped wollastonite.

Reused from J. Xie, X. Yang, H. Shao, J. Ye, Y. He, J. Fu, C. Gao, Z. Gou, Simultaneous mechanical property and biodegradation improvement of wollastonite bioceramic through magnesium dilute doping, Journal of the Mechanical Behavior of Biomedical Materials 54 (2016) 60–71. https://doi.org/10.1016/j.jmbbm.2015.09.012 after license via (copyright.com) number 4204070395196.

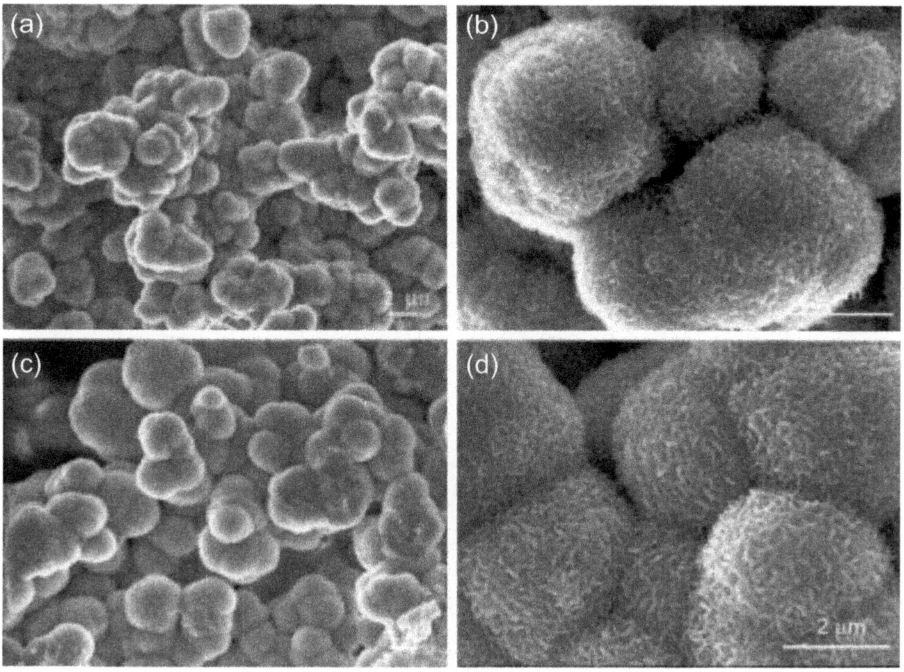

Figure 2.25 Scanning electron microscope micrographs of the β-dicalcium silicate cement after 7 days' soaking in simulated body fluid. The liquid-to-powder ratios are (a) 1.0 and (c) 1.4. (b) and (d) are high-magnification images of (a) and (c).
Reused from Z. Gou, J. Chang, W. Zhai, J. Wang, Study on the self-setting property and the in vitro bioactivity of β-Ca_2SiO_4, Journal of Biomedical Materials Research 73B (2005) 244–251. https://doi.org/10.1002/jbm.b.30203 after license via (copyright.com) number 4204310327181.

A final example in this section is the microstructures of self-setting bioactive CPC–magnesium phosphate cement (MPC) [28]: (1) MPC, (2) CPC, and (3) a combination of MPC and CPC with a 1/1 ratio $CMPC_{1/1}$. Fig. 2.26 shows the microstructure of the set cements. A xerogel-like morphology is shown for MPC, and a porous grained microstructure is shown for CPC. The combination $CMPC_{1/1}$ shows a dense microstructure and the micropores of CPC are filled with the xerogel of MPC. This is an ideal technique to obtain a dense microstructure. These microstructures influence the results after immersion in SBF. Fig. 2.27 shows different morphologies of the apatite agglomerates for MPC, CPC, and $CMPC_{1/1}$ cements. The degradation that the cement undergoes after immersion in SBF is most rapid in the case of MPC because of the originally porous microstructure, and it leads to obvious cracks. On the other hand, degradation is slowest in the case of CPC because of minimum interconnected porosity of the grained microstructure. Finally, the degradation of $CMPC_{1/1}$ is between that of MPC and CPC.

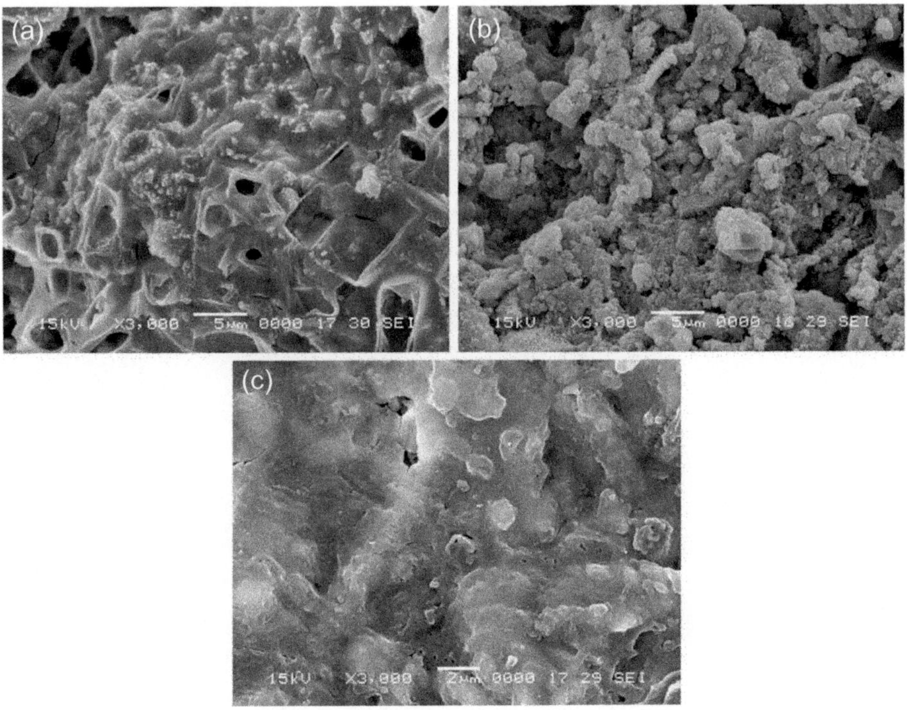

Figure 2.26 Scanning electron microscope micrographs of the fracture surfaces of the cement samples hardened for 24 h: (a) magnesium phosphate cement, (b) calcium phosphate cement, and (c) $CMPC_{1/1}$.
Reused from F. Wu, J. Wei, H. Guo, F. Chen, H. Hong, C. Liu, Self-setting bioactive calcium–magnesium phosphate cement with high strength and degradability for bone regeneration, Acta Biomaterialia 4 (2008) 1873–1884. https://doi.org/10.1016/j.actbio.2008.06.020 after license via (copyright.com) number 4204310865403.

Review questions

2.1 Oxide ceramics

1. Describe the structure of α-alumina and draw an illustrative figure.
2. What are the properties arising from the strong chemical bonds of alumina?
3. Briefly describe why α-alumina is suitable for use as a biomaterial.
4. What are the microstructural factors that affect the properties of solid ceramics?
5. How can the best compressive and flexural strength of alumina be achieved?
6. Describe the typical microstructure properties for alumina intended for bioapplications.
7. Why does α-alumina represent a typical implant material for wear applications?
8. What is the role of grain-size distribution of α-alumina in joint replacement bearings?
9. What are the environmental impacts for the production of alumina powder and synthesis of alumina parts?
10. Why do manufacturers attempt to produce zero-porosity sintered alumina parts?
11. Describe the zirconia polymorphs and state the associated densities.
12. What is the effect of the phase transformations on the sintering of zirconia?

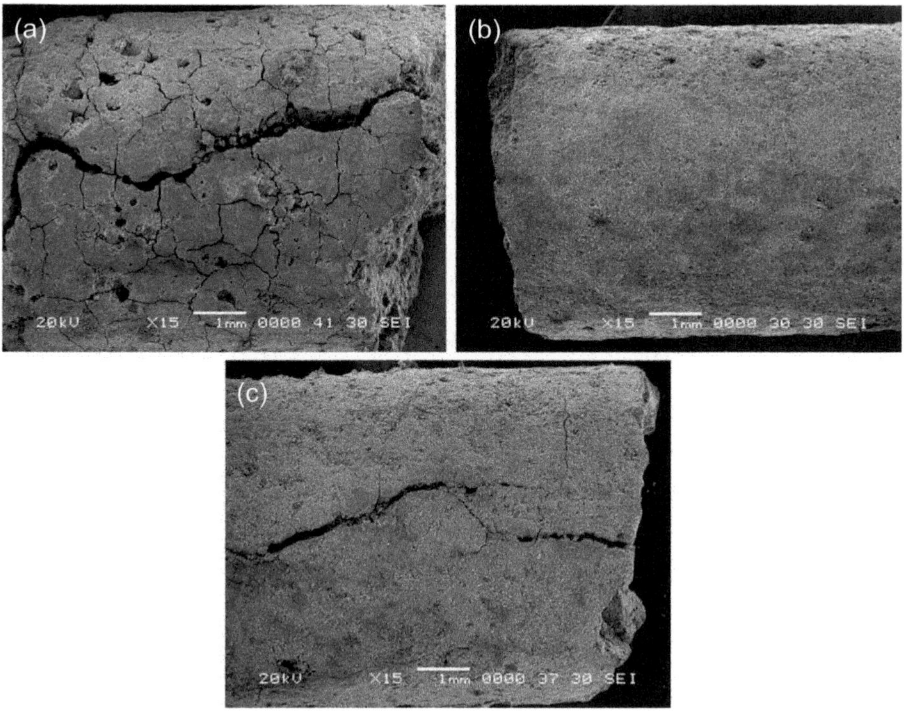

Figure 2.27 Scanning electron microscope micrographs of surface morphologies of samples immersed in simulated body fluid for 30 days: (a) magnesium phosphate cement, (b) calcium phosphate cement, and (c) $CMPC_{1/1}$.
Reused from F. Wu, J. Wei, H. Guo, F. Chen, H. Hong, C. Liu, Self-setting bioactive calcium–magnesium phosphate cement with high strength and degradability for bone regeneration, Acta Biomaterialia 4 (2008) 1873–1884. https://doi.org/10.1016/j.actbio.2008.06.020 after license via (copyright.com) number 4204310865403.

13. Describe renowned additives to zirconia and their effect in the stabilization of its high-temperature phase.
14. Describe the material design parameters that affect phase distribution in PSZ.
15. Describe transformation toughening in zirconia.
16. How can full stabilization of zirconia be achieved?
17. What are the prime mechanical properties of zirconia and why does it exist in metal–ceramic joints?
18. How can the best mechanical properties of zirconia be attained?
19. What are the drawbacks associated with the low thermal conductivity of zirconia? Describe.
20. Review the literature and assign major techniques to improve the hardness and wear resistance of zirconia.
21. Describe a typical microstructure of the sintered stabilized zirconia shown in Fig. 2.4.
22. Describe the LTD of zirconia and the techniques used to reduce its rate.
23. State the advantage of composing ZTA and its use as a bioceramic.
24. Describe the advantages of including Cr_2O_3 and SrO in ZTA.
25. Construct a table that includes the names of the important calcium orthophosphates, their abbreviated names, and chemical formulas.

26. Define Posner's cluster.
27. Analyze Table 2.4 to indicate the important chemical similarities between the inorganic phases of adult human calcified tissues and HA.
28. Based on Fig. 2.7, describe the typical microstructure of calcium orthophosphate cement after setting.
29. Write a summary of what you learned from Figs. 2.9 and 2.10. You may refer to its original article.
30. Suggest applications of the biomaterials presented in Figs. 2.9 and 2.10 separately.
31. Allocate potential applications of the biomaterials presented in Figs. 2.9 and 2.10 to Fig. 2.11.
32. Why is EDX analysis sometimes mandatory with SEM observations of calcium phosphate biomaterials?
33. Distinguish between the long-range atomic order and short-range atomic order of solids.
34. Why does XRD not show diffraction peaks for short-range atomic order, whereas FTIR does?
35. How does the melting behavior of glass differ from that of crystalline solid?
36. Explain the role of network formers, network modifiers, and the intermediate oxides in the structure of silicate glass. What are the network formers of Bioglass.
37. What are the limitations of the use of Bioglass according to its mechanical properties.
38. Explain the NC model to describe glass. How is the NC number connected to the properties of glass?
39. In what circumstances is the dissolution process of bioactive glass facilitated?
40. What are the observable events that are indicative of the bioactivity of glass?
41. Explain the 13-93 and 13-93B3 variations of Bioglass and their applications.
42. Briefly explain the controlled crystallization process in the production of glass-ceramics.
43. Explain the bulk crystallization process of glass-ceramics.
44. Explain the surface crystallization process of glass-ceramics.
45. What is the consequence of the choice of the type of controlled crystallization process of produced glass-ceramics?
46. What was the motivation for employing glass-ceramics in biomaterials?
47. What are the advantages of the utilization of A–W glass-ceramics as bioceramics?
48. Introduce the β-wollastonite phase into glass-ceramics and state its advantage as a bioceramic.
49. Use Table 2.6 to explain an example of the tailoring of properties of glass-ceramics by controlling their composition.
50. Explain the difference in the growth of the apatite phase on the surface of the glass-ceramic mentioned in Table 2.6 and Fig. 2.20.
51. What are the design criteria for bone cements? Explain.
52. What are the twofold responsibilities of the materials scientist in the selection and design of bone cements?
53. Introduce the working time and setting time of cements and the methods to measure them.
54. Construct a table that includes the type of biocement, composition, and major uses.
55. What are the major spot points examined in the course of evaluation of an SEM micrograph of biocement?
56. What are the benefits of utilizing wollastonite-containing PMMA cements?
57. The Ca/P ratios of the apatite layer on wollastonite ceramics immersed in SBF solution are reduced over time; explain why.
58. What is the expected morphology of an apatite formed on the surface of a bioceramic after soaking in SBF solution?
59. Explain injectable bioactive cement.
60. Give an example of the correlation between the degradation of biocement in SBF solution and its morphology.

References

[1] K.C. Popat, T.A. Desai, B - alumina, in: B.D. Ratner, A.S. Hoffman, F.J. Schoen, J.E. Lemons (Eds.), Biomaterials Science, third ed., Academic Press, 2013, pp. 162–166, https://doi.org/10.1016/B978-0-08-087780-8.00018-8.

[2] C. Piconi, A.A. Porporati, Bioinert ceramics: zirconia and alumina, in: Handbook of Bioceramics and Biocomposites, Springer, Cham, 2016, pp. 59–89, https://doi.org/10.1007/978-3-319-12460-5_4.

[3] J. Chevalier, L. Gremillard, 1.106-Zirconia as a biomaterial, in: P. Ducheyne (Ed.), Comprehensive Biomaterials, Elsevier, Oxford, 2011, pp. 95–108, https://doi.org/10.1016/B978-0-08-055294-1.00017-9.

[4] C. Piconi, Oxide ceramics for biomedical applications, in: K.H.J. Buschow, R.W. Cahn, M.C. Flemings, B. Ilschner, E.J. Kramer, S. Mahajan, P. Veyssière (Eds.), Encyclopedia of Materials: Science and Technology, second ed., Elsevier, Oxford, 2001, pp. 6595–6601, https://doi.org/10.1016/B0-08-043152-6/01165-7.

[5] C. Rey, C. Combes, C. Drouet, S. Somrani, 15-Tricalcium phosphate-based ceramics, in: T. Kokubo (Ed.), Bioceramics and Their Clinical Applications, Woodhead Publishing, 2008, pp. 326–366, https://doi.org/10.1533/9781845694227.2.326.

[6] Chapter 1-general chemistry of the calcium orthophosphates, in: J.C. Elliott (Ed.), Studies in Inorganic Chemistry, Elsevier, 1994, pp. 1–62, https://doi.org/10.1016/B978-0-444-81582-8.50006-7.

[7] G. Daculsi, J.-M. Bouler, R.Z. LeGeros, Adaptive crystal formation in normal and pathological calcifications in synthetic calcium phosphate and related biomaterials, in: K.W. Jeon (Ed.), International Review of Cytology, Academic Press, 1997, pp. 129–191, https://doi.org/10.1016/S0074-7696(08)62360-8.

[8] M. Bohner, Resorbable biomaterials as bone graft substitutes, Materials Today 13 (2010) 24–30, https://doi.org/10.1016/S1369-7021(10)70014-6.

[9] M.A. Sainz, P. Pena, S. Serena, A. Caballero, Influence of design on bioactivity of novel $CaSiO_3$–$CaMg(SiO_3)_2$ bioceramics: in vitro simulated body fluid test and thermodynamic simulation, Acta Biomaterialia 6 (2010) 2797–2807, https://doi.org/10.1016/j.actbio.2010.01.003.

[10] T. Kokubo, H. Takadama, How useful is SBF in predicting in vivo bone bioactivity? Biomaterials 27 (2006) 2907–2915, https://doi.org/10.1016/j.biomaterials.2006.01.017.

[11] M. Sakamoto, T. Matsumoto, Development and Evaluation of Superporous Ceramics Bone Tissue Scaffold Materials with Triple Pore Structure A) Hydroxyapatite, B) Beta-Tricalcium Phosphate, 2012https://doi.org/10.5772/33901.

[12] W.H. Zachariasen, The atomic Arrangement in glass, Journal of the American Chemical Society 54 (1932) 3841–3851, https://doi.org/10.1021/ja01349a006.

[13] L. Lichtenstein, C. Büchner, B. Yang, S. Shaikhutdinov, M. Heyde, M. Sierka, R. Włodarczyk, J. Sauer, H.-J. Freund, The atomic structure of a metal-supported vitreous thin silica film, Angewandte Chemie International Edition 51 (2012) 404–407, https://doi.org/10.1002/anie.201107097.

[14] Y. Xiang, J. Du, Effect of strontium substitution on the structure of 45S5 bioglasses, Chemistry of Materials 23 (2011) 2703–2717, https://doi.org/10.1021/cm102889q.

[15] M.D. O'Donnell, Melt-Derived bioactive glass, in: J.R. Jones, A.G. Clare (Eds.), Bio-glasses, John Wiley & Sons, Ltd., 2012, pp. 13–27, https://doi.org/10.1002/9781118346457.ch2.

[16] A. Tilocca, A.N. Cormack, Surface signatures of bioactivity: MD simulations of 45S and 65S silicate glasses, Langmuir 26 (2010) 545–551, https://doi.org/10.1021/la902548f.

[17] A. Tilocca, A.N. Cormack, Modeling the water–bioglass interface by Ab initio molecular dynamics simulations, ACS Applied Materials and Interfaces 1 (2009) 1324–1333, https://doi.org/10.1021/am900198t.

[18] S.B. Jung, Bioactive borate glasses, in: J.R. Jones, A.G. Clare (Eds.), Bio-glasses, John Wiley & Sons, Ltd., 2012, pp. 75–95, https://doi.org/10.1002/9781118346457.ch6.

[19] N. Giraudo, P. Krolla-Sidenstein, S. Bergdolt, M. Heinle, H. Gliemann, F. Messerschmidt, P. Brüner, P. Thissen, Early stage hydration of wollastonite: kinetic aspects of the metal-proton exchange reaction, Journal of Physical Chemistry C 119 (2015) 10493–10499, https://doi.org/10.1021/acs.jpcc.5b02327.

[20] S.M. Salman, S.N. Salama, H.A. Abo-Mosallam, The crystallization behaviour and bioactivity of wollastonite glass-ceramic based on Na_2O–K_2O–CaO–SiO_2–F glass system, Journal of Asian Ceramic Societies 3 (2015) 255–261, https://doi.org/10.1016/j.jascer.2015.04.004.

[21] S.M. Kenny, M. Buggy, Bone cements and fillers: a review, Journal of Materials Science: Materials in Medicine 14 (2003) 923–938, https://doi.org/10.1023/A:1026394530192.

[22] ADA, Professional product review laboratory testing methods: core materials, The Journal of the American Dental Association 3 (2008) 1–18.

[23] M. Tyas, M. Burrow, Adhesive restorative materials: a review, Australian Dental Journal 49 (2004) 112–121, https://doi.org/10.1111/j.1834-7819.2004.tb00059.x.

[24] D. Rentería-Zamarrón, D.A. Cortés-Hernández, L. Bretado-Aragón, W. Ortega-Lara, Mechanical properties and apatite-forming ability of PMMA bone cements, Materials and Design 30 (2009) 3318–3324, https://doi.org/10.1016/j.matdes.2008.11.024.

[25] R. Abd Rashid, R. Shamsudin, M.A. Abdul Hamid, A. Jalar, In-vitro bioactivity of wollastonite materials derived from limestone and silica sand, Ceramics International 40 (2014) 6847–6853, https://doi.org/10.1016/j.ceramint.2013.12.004.

[26] J. Xie, X. Yang, H. Shao, J. Ye, Y. He, J. Fu, C. Gao, Z. Gou, Simultaneous mechanical property and biodegradation improvement of wollastonite bioceramic through magnesium dilute doping, Journal of the Mechanical Behavior of Biomedical Materials 54 (2016) 60–71, https://doi.org/10.1016/j.jmbbm.2015.09.012.

[27] Z. Gou, J. Chang, W. Zhai, J. Wang, Study on the self-setting property and the in vitro bioactivity of β-Ca_2SiO_4, Journal of Biomedical Materials Research 73B (2005) 244–251, https://doi.org/10.1002/jbm.b.30203.

[28] F. Wu, J. Wei, H. Guo, F. Chen, H. Hong, C. Liu, Self-setting bioactive calcium–magnesium phosphate cement with high strength and degradability for bone regeneration, Acta Biomaterialia 4 (2008) 1873–1884, https://doi.org/10.1016/j.actbio.2008.06.020.

Osteoinduction, osteoconduction, and osseointegration

3

There are many terms that are frequently used in connection with orthopedics and dentistry, which are not familiar in materials science and engineering, but are vital to the field of biomaterials. This chapter is named after the magnificent paper by Albrektsson and Johansson [1], which is strongly recommended for the newcomer to the field of biomaterials. The aim of this chapter is to start with the essential terminology of osteoinduction, osteoconduction, and osseointegration and proceed with related terms to facilitate a grasp of the concepts usually met in orthopedics and dentistry.

Workers in the field of materials science and engineering are already familiar with concepts such as growth and growth factors connected with chemical reactions, leaching of ions, bonding, mechanical interlock, phase formation, and phase transformations. The use of Greek words is limited. So, it is not insignificant to start with the definition of the Greek word "osteo" because it is a combining form that indicates bone or bones. In addition, the osteogenesis process indicates the formation of new bone tissue replacing defective or missing parts of bone, also called ossification. This process is accomplished via local stem cells or introduced via donor cells derived from either the host or graft donor.

Bone includes four types of cells: osteogenic cells, osteoblasts, osteocytes, and osteoclasts. Osteogenic cells are found in bone marrow and enveloping bone. Osteogenic cells are stem cells, i.e., they are continually generating new cells of their type and other types of bone cells. Osteogenic cells are stimulated by the dissolution products of bioactive glass (BG), i.e., BG promotes the osteogenesis process. This last sentence can act an alternative definition of the bioactivity of BG. The discovery of the bioactivity of bioglass is one of those historical moments where materials scientists and medical doctors shake hands.

The three remaining types of bone cells are osteoblasts, osteocytes, and osteoclasts. These cells serve bone repair by a consecutive destruct and reconstruct mechanism called bone remodeling. In other words, these cells control the decay and formation of bone. Bone structure can be visualized as connected cells, called osteocytes, that form the bone matrix filled with collagen and calcium phosphates. The function of osteoclasts is to decompose the bone matrix and resorb damaged or old matter at a site indicated by the osteocytes. The formation of a new bone matrix, including osteocytes, is performed by the osteoblasts. The balance between the number of osteoblasts and osteoclasts is controlled by secretion from the thyroid gland.

The terms osteoinduction, osteoconduction, and osseointegration are frequently used in research activity and scientific publications. These terms are often connected with bone grafting or implantation. In either case, bone tissue healing or implant fixation needs the formation of new tissue to accomplish the process and is called *osteoinduction*. This process is performed via the osteoblasts and can be accelerated via chemical means. The acceleration strategies are based on the requirement of supplying

Bioceramics: For Materials Science and Engineering. https://doi.org/10.1016/B978-0-08-102233-7.00003-3

the necessary balanced amounts of calcium and phosphorus required for the formation of bone tissue.

Essentially, osteoinduction is the in situ bone repair or attachment of an implant. If the growth of tissue continues outside the location implant surface, the process is called *osteoconduction*. With osteoconduction, bone ingrowth takes place in a way that depends on the structure and chemical composition of an implant or graft. Osteoconduction is also the process observed by implanting a scaffold that proceeds in three dimensions and develops a new bone or a missing part of a bone, or the new bone tissue develops on the surface of the scaffold if the implant is not resorbable.

As we have already learned the advantage of bioactive materials over biocompatibility is that there is no fibrous tissue developed at the interface with the implant. The accompanying advantage of this situation is that a direct structural and functional interface is developed with the orthopedic or dental implant. This type of interfacing is called *osseointegration*. In other words, osseointegration is a direct attachment of the implant surface to the bone that allows efficient load transfer from the load-carrying implant to the bone.

A prime demand from bioceramics in orthopedics and dentistry is the ability to promote osteoconduction. Certainly, the ceramic should be bioactive. Thus the first research step is to investigate bioactivity, which can be performed in vitro via several strategies such as soaking in simulated body fluid (SBF) solution and observing its ability to form an apatite layer on the surface. Fig. 3.1 shows the apatite formation on different silicate ceramics exposed to the SBF solution and the different surface morphology for different compositions of silicate ceramics.

In vivo investigation shows osteoblast attachment to the surface of silicate bioceramics, Fig. 3.2. The attachment of osteoblasts on the implant surface can be another definition of osseointegration. In the case of implanting a scaffold, usually made from porous bioceramics, osseointegration shows itself via the observation of osteoblasts attached to the pore walls, Fig. 3.3. In this case the utilized silicate bioceramics, are believed to be of moderate or slow degradation rather than showing rapid degradation such as wollastonite, bredigite, and tricalcium silicate [2].

Not all the published research can be easily employed in a textbook and/or used as examples by an instructor. Apart from scientific value, some published research can be utilized by the instructor because he or she can skip the details and utilize figures, tables, and illustrations to illuminate the subject matter in a lecture. The student should be able to find other literature that serves the same goal, and the instructor is encouraged to ask students to do so as part to their required activities.

Bioactive glass-ceramics (BGCs) are also utilized for the synthesis of scaffolds; however, there is no guarantee that osteoconduction is beneficial for successful scaffolds based on the suggested materials. BGC nanoparticles incorporated in poly(L-lactic acid) (PLLA) with different wt% are used to produce nanocomposite scaffolds. BGCs are prepared with a composition of SiO_2:CaO:$P_2O_5 \approx 55$:40:5 mol%, as shown in Fig. 3.4. The processing method for the preparation of porous scaffolds is described in [3]. A microstructure of continuous interconnected pores is shown with BGC content up to 20 wt%. The pore diameters are in the range of 200–400 μm, which is similar to the microstructure of the matrix of PLLA foam alone (BGC of 0 wt%). The microstructure is changed when the BGC content is increased to 30 wt% and the pore

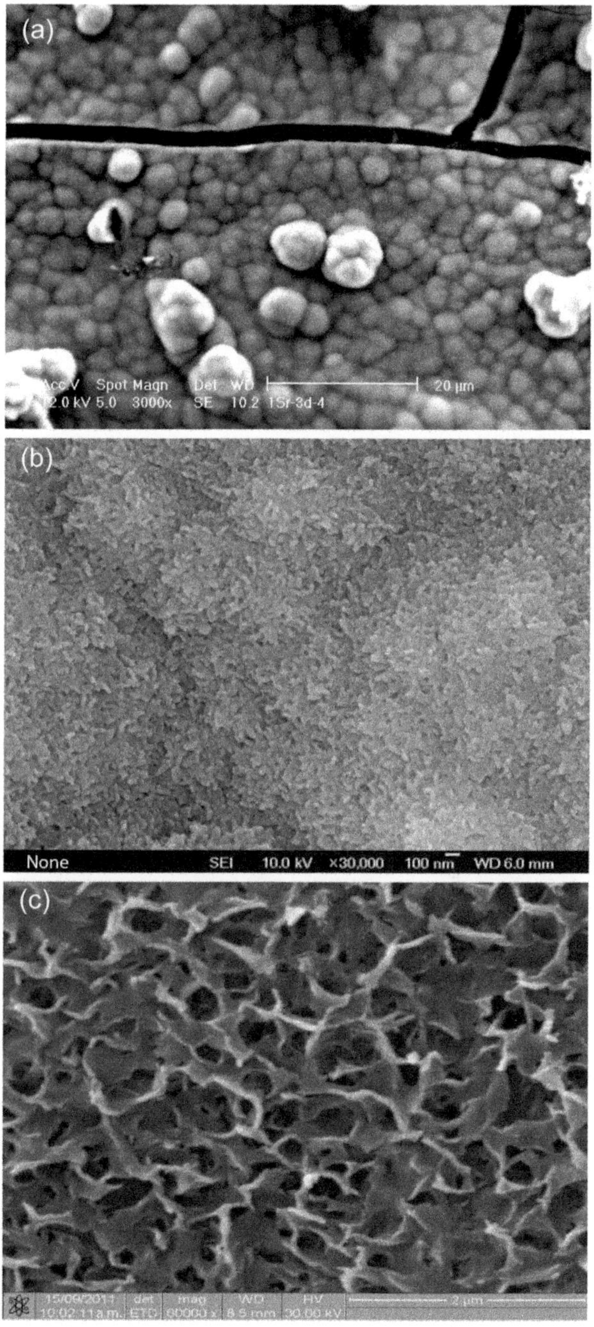

Figure 3.1 Scanning electron microscope micrographs for different silicate ceramics showing the different morphologies after the formation of the apatite layer. (a) Wollastonite ($CaSiO_3$); (b) akermanite ($Ca_2MgSi_2O_7$); and (c) nagelschmidtite ($Ca_7P_2Si_2O_{16}$).
Reused from C. Wu, J. Chang, A review of bioactive silicate ceramics, Biomedical Materials 8 (2013) 032001. https://doi.org/10.1088/1748-6041/8/3/032001 after license via (copyright.com) number 501318768.

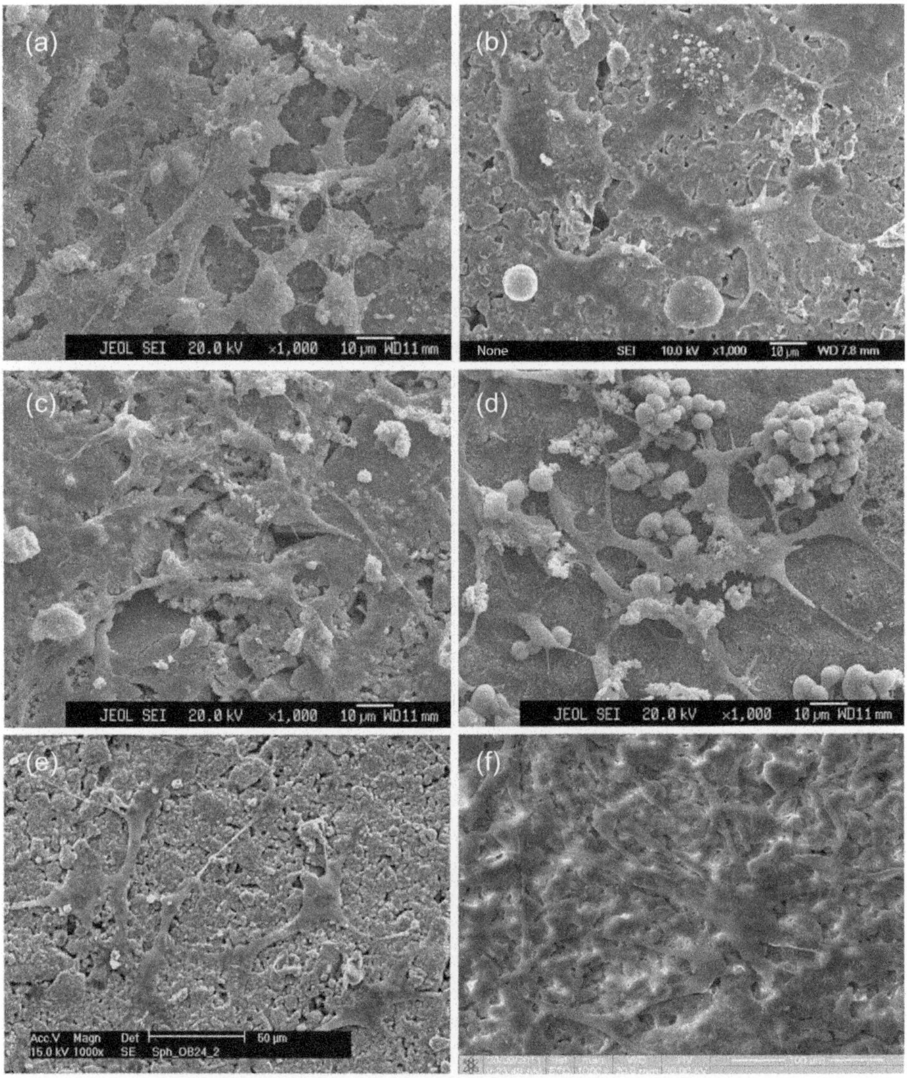

Figure 3.2 Scanning electron microscope micrographs for different silicate ceramics showing osteoblast attachment. (a) Akermanite ($Ca_2MgSi_2O_7$); (b) hardystonite ($Ca_2ZnSi_2O_7$); (c) diopside ($CaMgSi_2O_6$); (d) bredigite ($Ca_7MgSi_4O_{16}$); (e) sphene ($CaTiSiO_5$); and (f) nagelschmidtite ($Ca_7P_2Si_2O_{16}$).
Reused from C. Wu, J. Chang, A review of bioactive silicate ceramics, Biomedical Materials 8 (2013) 032001. https://doi.org/10.1088/1748-6041/8/3/032001 after license via (copyright.com) number 501318768.

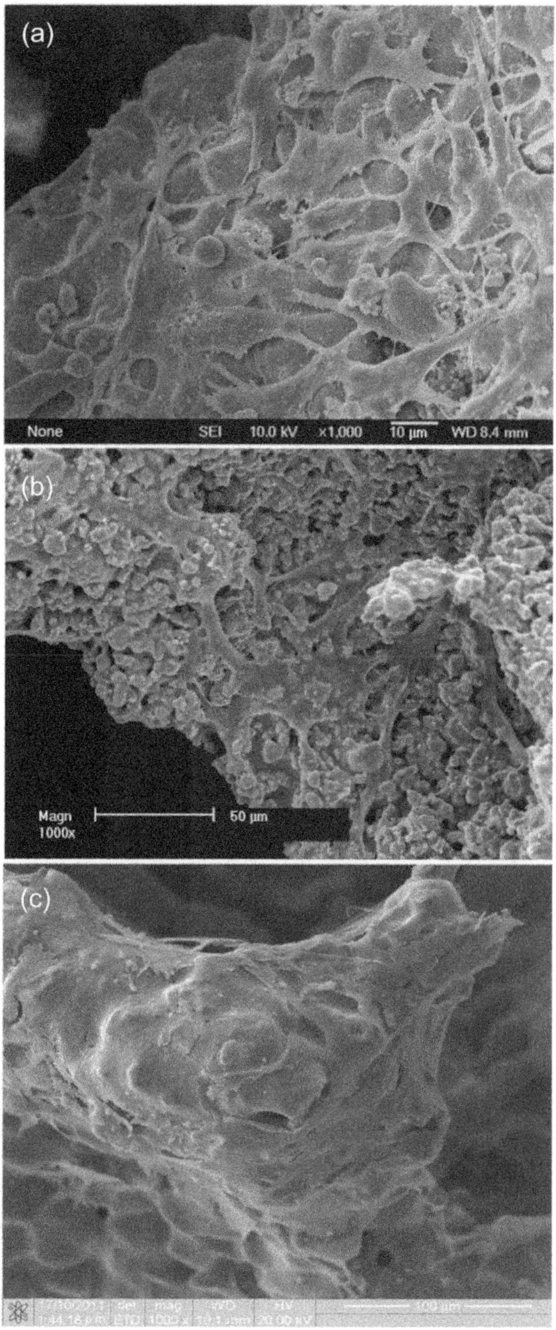

Figure 3.3 Scanning electron microscope micrographs for different silicate ceramics showing osteoblast ingrowth. (a) Akermanite ($Ca_2MgSi_2O_7$); (b) diopside ($CaMgSi_2O_6$); and (c) nagelschmidtite ($Ca_7P_2Si_2O_{16}$).
Reused from C. Wu, J. Chang, A review of bioactive silicate ceramics, Biomedical Materials 8 (2013) 032001. https://doi.org/10.1088/1748-6041/8/3/032001 after license via (copyright.com) number 501318768.

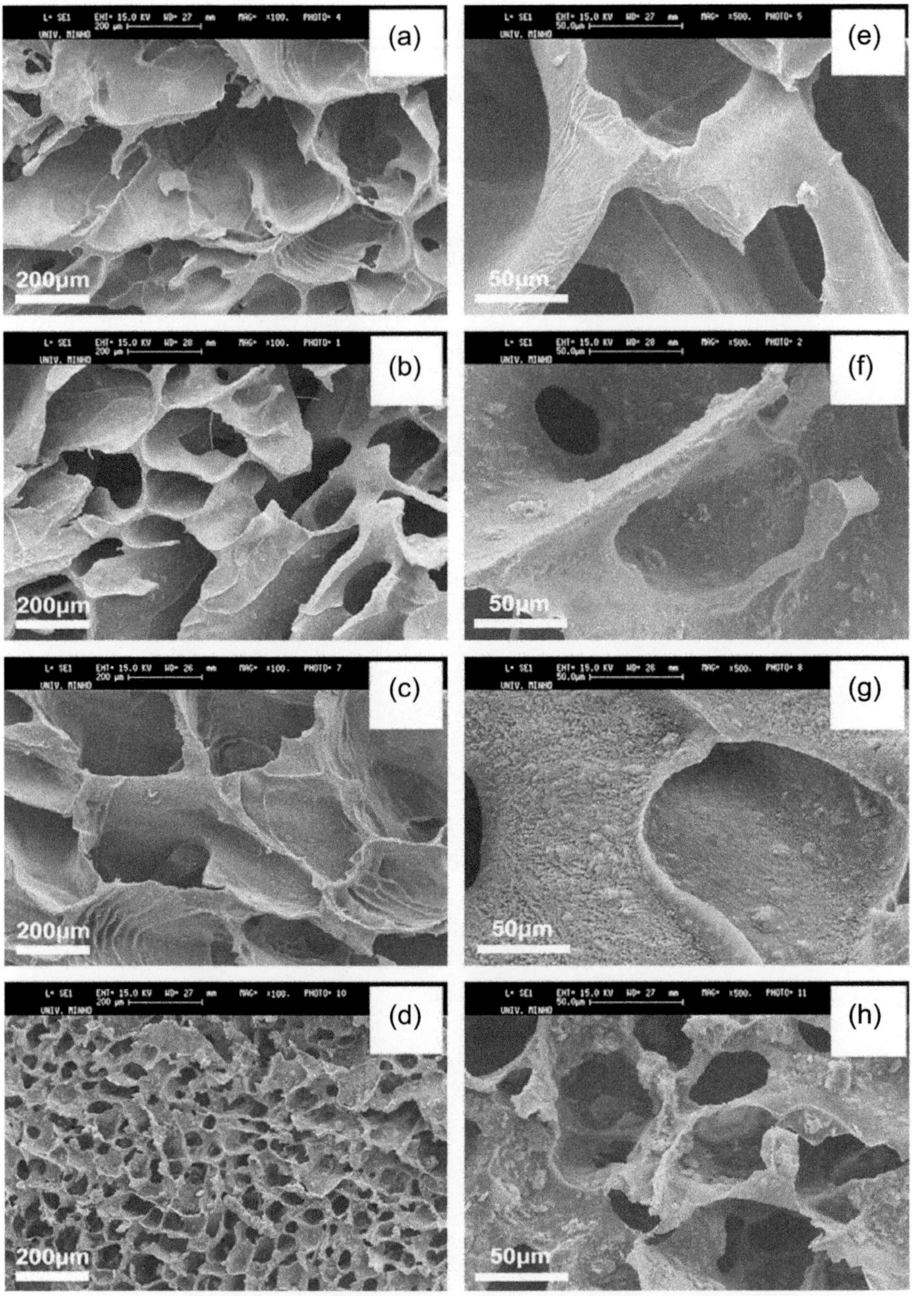

Figure 3.4 Scanning electron microscope morphology for the porous poly(L-lactic acid)/bioactive glass ceramic (BGC) scaffolds with different BGC contents: at low magnification (a) 0 wt%, (b) 10 wt%, (c) 20 wt%, and (d) 30 wt%; at high magnification (e) 0 wt%, (f) 10 wt%, (g) 20 wt%, and (h) 30 wt%.

Reused from Z. Hong, R.L. Reis, J.F. Mano, Preparation and in vitro characterization of scaffolds of poly(l-lactic acid) containing bioactive glass ceramic nanoparticles, Acta Biomaterialia 4 (2008) 1297–1306. https://doi.org/10.1016/j.actbio.2008.03.007 after license via (copyright.com) number 4212320112360.

size range is changed to 10–150 μm. This change of microstructure is expected to take place at some BGC filler loadings because of the reduction in matrix vol%.

To examine osteoconductivity, the prepared scaffolds are subjected to SBF solution for different periods. Fig. 3.5 demonstrates that the plain PLLA foam shows no bioactivity, whereas the composites show the formation of apatite clusters, which are enhanced with the increase in BGC content and also with the time of soaking in SBF solution. On the other hand, composites with 30 wt% BGC content show no complete coverage of the apatite on the surface of the scaffold. This can be attributed to the overloading of BGC and may affect the chemical balances with the SBF solution that lead to an inefficient formation of apatite.

Composites of BGs are also utilized for synthesizing porous scaffolds. BG nanoparticles of composition Si:P:Ca = 29:13:58 wt% were prepared by the sol–gel method and incorporated into BG/PLLA composites. A surface-grafted BG (g-BG) powder is also prepared by the method described in the original article [4]. The surface modification of BG to produce g-BG is performed to avoid phase separation often found at the surface of the glass that negatively affects the attachment between the matrix and the filler. The BG/PLLA and g-BG/PLLA composites were then prepared, and their tensile fracture surface was examined via scanning electron microscope (SEM), as shown in Fig. 3.6. The ductile deformation feature is more obvious in the case of the g-BG/PLLA compared with the BG/PLLA composite for two different wt% of the filler content. In addition, a particle aggregation at the fracture surface of the 20 wt% BG/PLLA composite, indicated by an arrow, may assign the harmful stress concentration to the mechanical properties.

Finally, scaffolds of pure PLLA and g-BG/PLLA were synthesized. The pure PLLA shows no evidence of bioactivity after soaking in SBF solution, Fig. 3.7. Alternatively, the g-BG/PLLA scaffold shows an initiation of the bioactivity after 3 days of soaking. The apatite-like deposits are clear and cover the whole of the surface of the scaffold after soaking for 7 days.

The choice of another composite may alter the preparation method. Commercial open-cell polyurethane sponges were utilized to prepare glass-coated foams via dipping the sponges in glass slurry followed by infiltration [5]. The polyurethane sponges are of three types, 45, 30, and 20 pores per inch (ppi), and the glass is a silicate bioactive glass of composition $45SiO_2$–$3P_2O_5$–$26CaO$–$15Na_2O$–$7MgO$–$4K_2O$ mol%. Fig. 3.8 shows the microstructure of the polymer templates. The figure shows a utilization of different pore densities for the scaffolds to simulate healthy and osteoporotic bone. The compact microstructure is for healthy bone, and it begins to loosen for unhealthy or elderly people. The loss of bone mass and accordingly bone strength with age is called osteoporosis. Thus utilizing scaffolds of different densities produces a better picture for different bone status. In addition, the scaffold should be synthesized similar to the living bone as much as possible. This is to ensure the best mechanical compatibility between the bone and the implant.

Fig. 3.9 shows the pore structure in the polymer and the impregnated sponge (template). Narrow size distribution of the pores may be observed with no large voids that can disturb the microstructure of the new bone. The scaffold is produced after a thermal treatment step to burn the polymeric template, followed by sintering to gain partial densification of the glass to enhance mechanical strength. The enhancement of

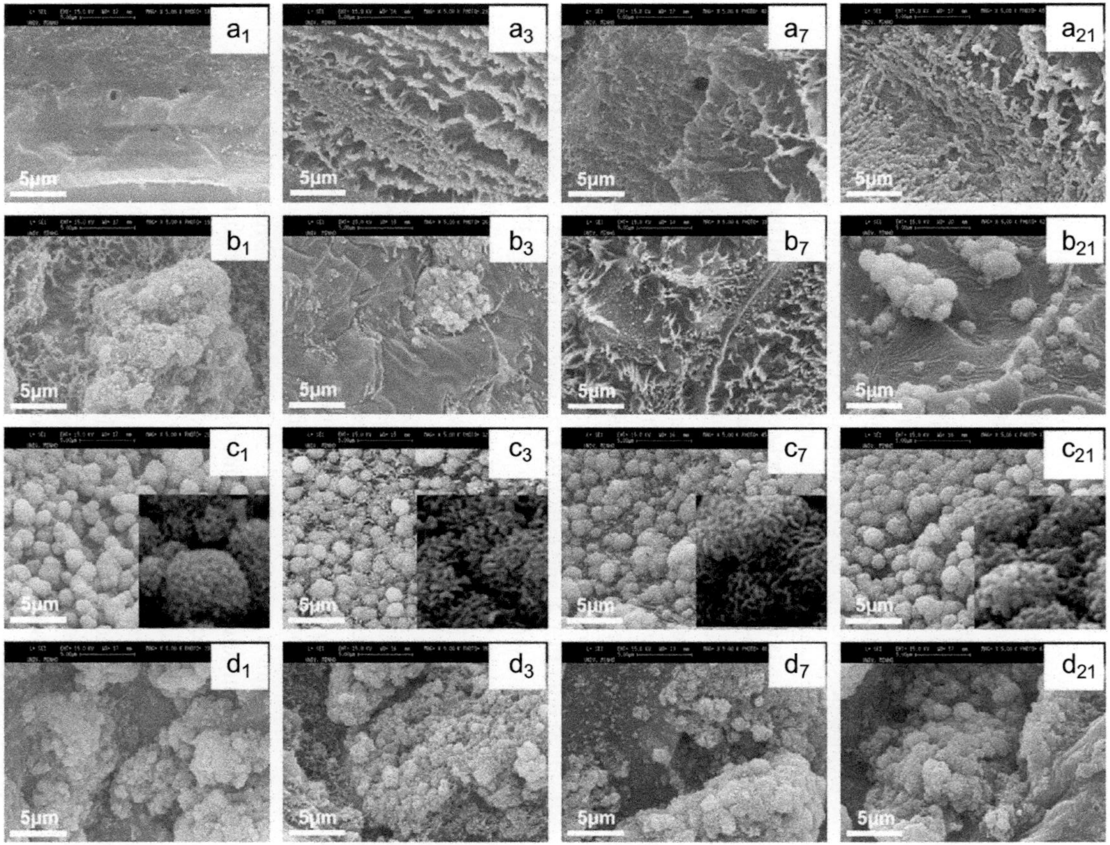

Figure 3.5 Morphology of the porous poly(L-lactic acid) (PLLA)/bioactive glass ceramic (BGC) composites with different contents of BGC particles after immersion in simulated body fluid (SBF) for different periods, observed by scanning electron microscope: (a) 0 wt%, (b) 10 wt%, (c) 20 wt%, and (d) 30 wt%. The subscripts indicate the incubation time in SBF (days). The images inserted in the C series are the high-magnification pictures of apatite clusters formed on the surface of PLLA/(20 wt%)BGC composites after different soaking times.

Reused from Z. Hong, R.L. Reis, J.F. Mano, Preparation and in vitro characterization of scaffolds of poly(l-lactic acid) containing bioactive glass ceramic nanoparticles, Acta Biomaterialia 4 (2008) 1297–1306. https://doi.org/10.1016/j.actbio.2008.03.007 after license via (copyright.com) number 4212320112360.

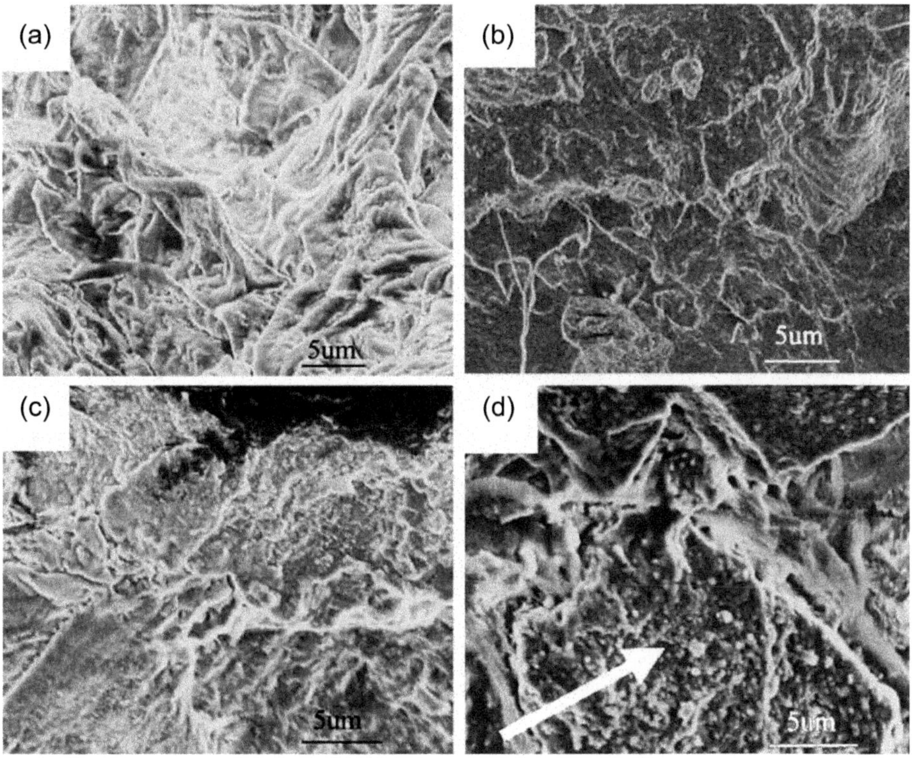

Figure 3.6 Scanning electron microscope micrographs showing the fracture surface of (a) 4 wt% g-BG, (b) 4 wt% BG, (c) 20 wt% g-BG, and (d) 20 wt% BG. *BG*, bioactive glass; *g-BG*, grafted BG powder.
Reused from A. Liu, Z. Hong, X. Zhuang, X. Chen, Y. Cui, Y. Liu, X. Jing, Surface modification of bioactive glass nanoparticles and the mechanical and biological properties of poly(l-lactide) composites, Acta Biomaterialia 4 (2008) 1005–1015. https://doi.org/10.1016/j.actbio.2008.02.013 after license via (copyright.com) number 4212340120919.

the mechanical strength is necessary to make it possible to handle the scaffold. In the course of sintering, a partial crystallization takes place, which should not affect the bioactivity of the glass. A look at the scaffold produced by the foregoing method, Fig. 3.10, shows that the strut thickness ranges between 430 and 450 μm, which indicates a rigid structure. At this point, it might be useful to compare the compression properties of the final scaffold with respect to their designed pore density. Fig. 3.11 shows that the scaffold with higher ppi has higher compressive strength and comparable strain to failure. For a materials scientist, it is a straightforward conclusion because the scaffold of higher ppi has a denser microstructure.

On the other hand, the strut thickness ranges can be altered via optimization of the slurry characteristics and the process of excess removal. A pore strut thickness of about 5–20 μm is obtained, as seen in Fig. 3.12. In this figure, the pore structure is close to the trabecular structure that resembles natural bone. This type of microstructure is

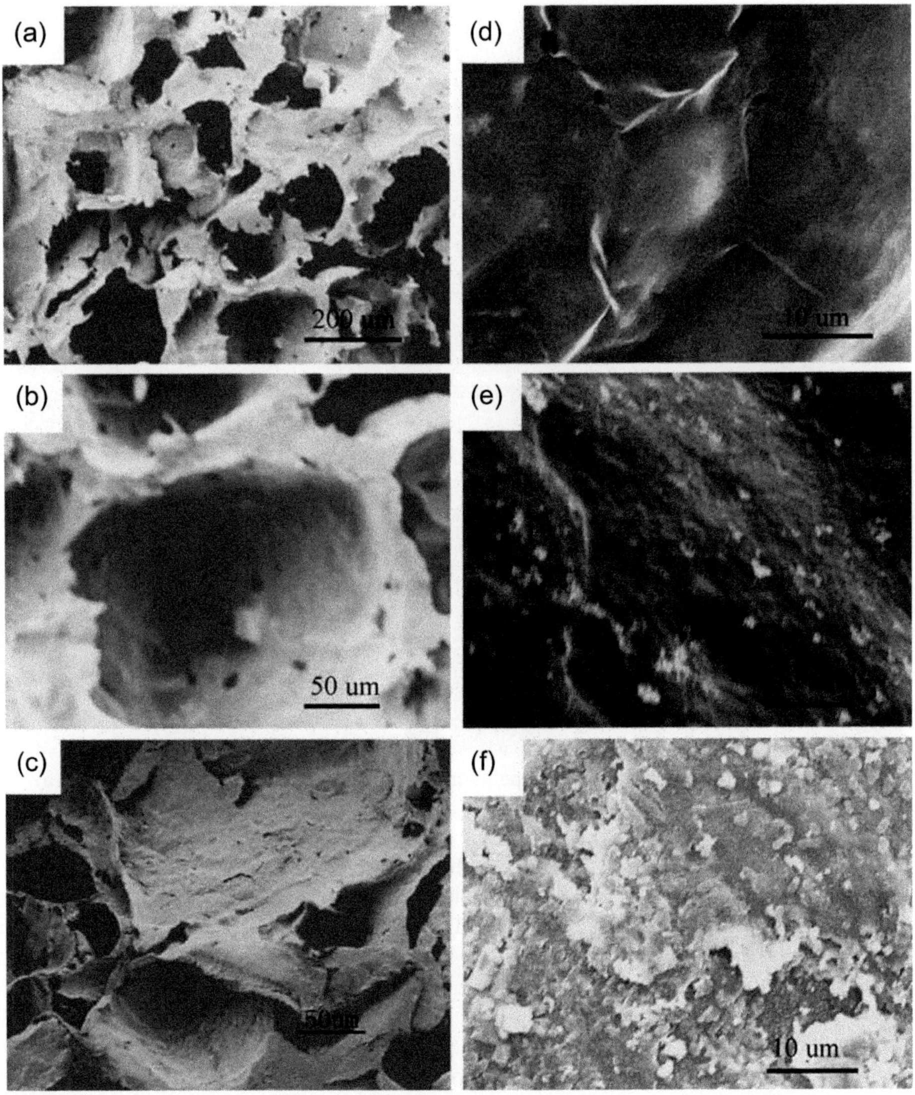

Figure 3.7 Scanning electron microscope micrographs showing scaffold morphology. (a and b) Poly(L-lactic acid) (PLLA) for 0 days, (c) PLLA for 7 days, (d) g-BG/PLLA composite for 0 days, (e) 3 days, and (f) 7 days. *g-BG*, grafted BG powder.
Reused from A. Liu, Z. Hong, X. Zhuang, X. Chen, Y. Cui, Y. Liu, X. Jing, Surface modification of bioactive glass nanoparticles and the mechanical and biological properties of poly(l-lactide) composites, Acta Biomaterialia 4 (2008) 1005–1015. https://doi.org/10.1016/j.actbio.2008.02.013 after license via (copyright.com) number 4212340120919.

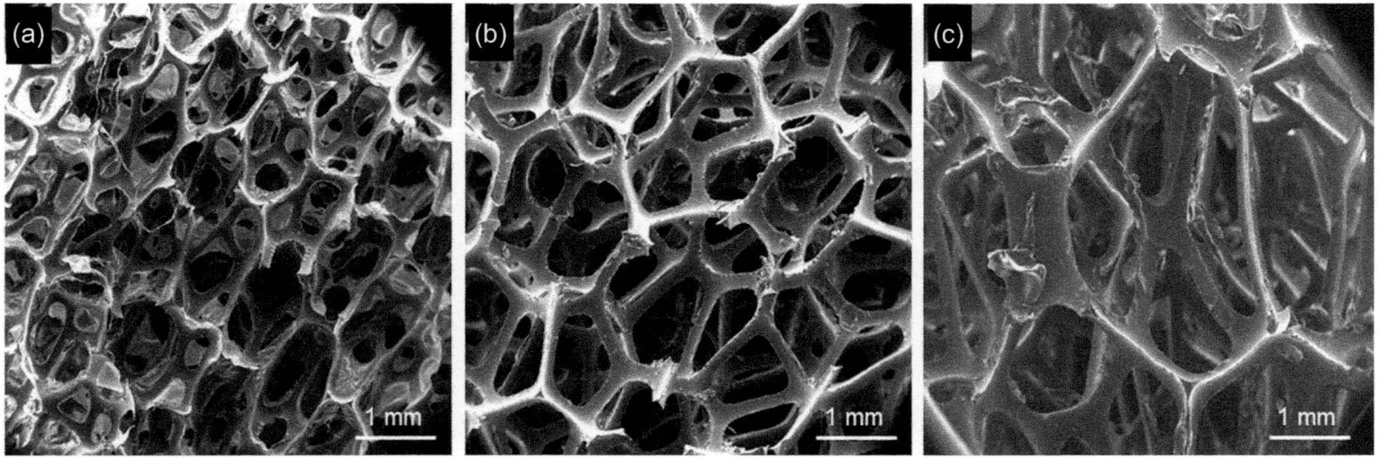

Figure 3.8 Scanning electron microscope micrographs (×50) showing starting polyurethane templates. (a) 45 pores per inch (ppi), (b) 30 ppi, and (c) 20 ppi.

Reused from F. Baino, S. Caddeo, G. Novajra, C. Vitale-Brovarone, Using porous bioceramic scaffolds to model healthy and osteoporotic bone, Journal of the European Ceramic Society 36 (2016) 2175–2182. https://doi.org/10.1016/j.jeurceramsoc.2016.01.011 after license via (copyright.com) number 4213570993566.

(a)

(b)

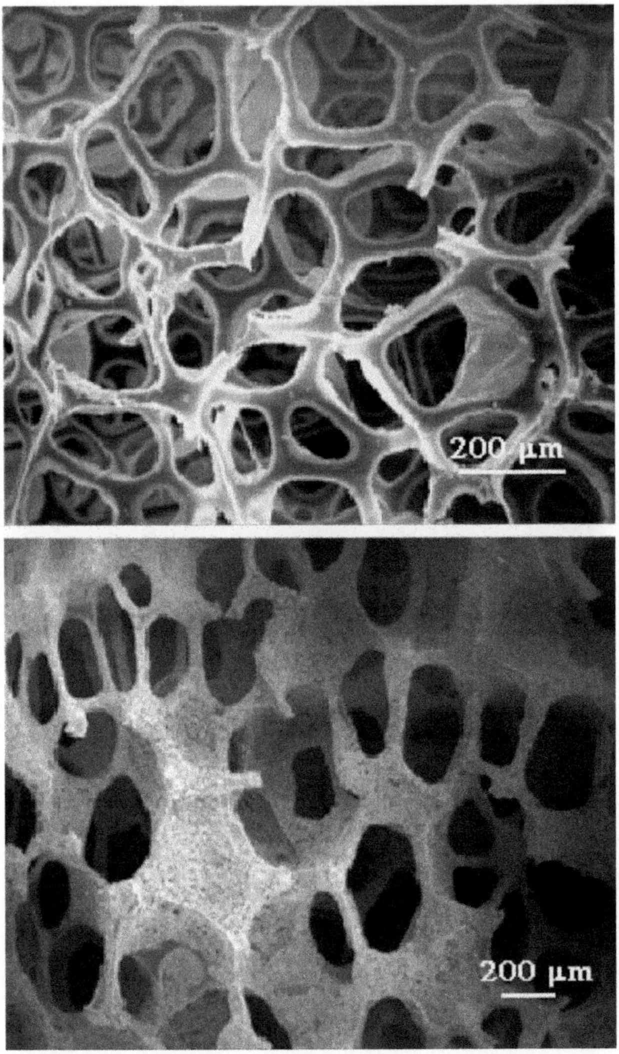

Figure 3.9 Scanning electron microscope micrograph showing (a) polymeric sponge and (b) impregnated sponge.
Reused from C. Vitale-Brovarone, E. Verné, L. Robiglio, P. Appendino, F. Bassi, G. Martinasso, G. Muzio, R. Canuto, Development of glass–ceramic scaffolds for bone tissue engineering: characterisation, proliferation of human osteoblasts and nodule formation, Acta Biomaterialia 3 (2007) 199–208. https://doi.org/10.1016/j.actbio.2006.07.012 after license via (copyright.com) number 4213751393189.

tested for osteoconductivity, as detailed in Ref. [6]. The osteoblasts were seeded on the pretreated scaffolds with SBF solution. The osteoblasts are proliferated, colonized, and adhered at the pore surfaces of the scaffold, as seen in Fig. 3.13. The figure also shows that increasing the incubation time from 10 to 20 days increases the cell growth and forms mineralized nodules.

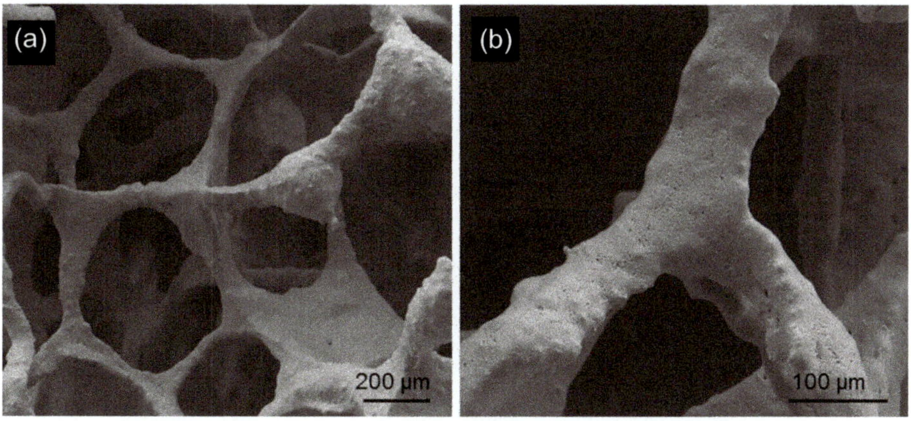

Figure 3.10 Scanning electron microscope micrograph, in two magnifications, of a scaffold produced from a 45-ppi template and sintered at 1000°C for 3 h. (a) scale bar 200 µm, (b) scale bar 100 µm.

Reused from F. Baino, S. Caddeo, G. Novajra, C. Vitale-Brovarone, Using porous bioceramic scaffolds to model healthy and osteoporotic bone, Journal of the European Ceramic Society 36 (2016) 2175–2182. https://doi.org/10.1016/j.jeurceramsoc.2016.01.011 after license via (copyright.com) number 4213570993566.

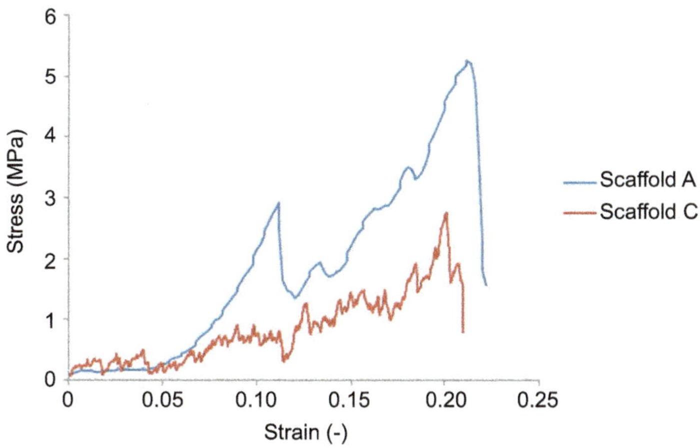

Figure 3.11 Comparison between compressive stress–strain curves of scaffolds A (45 ppi) and C (30 ppi).

Reused from F. Baino, S. Caddeo, G. Novajra, C. Vitale-Brovarone, Using porous bioceramic scaffolds to model healthy and osteoporotic bone, Journal of the European Ceramic Society 36 (2016) 2175–2182. https://doi.org/10.1016/j.jeurceramsoc.2016.01.011 after license via (copyright.com) number 4213570993566.

(a)

(b)

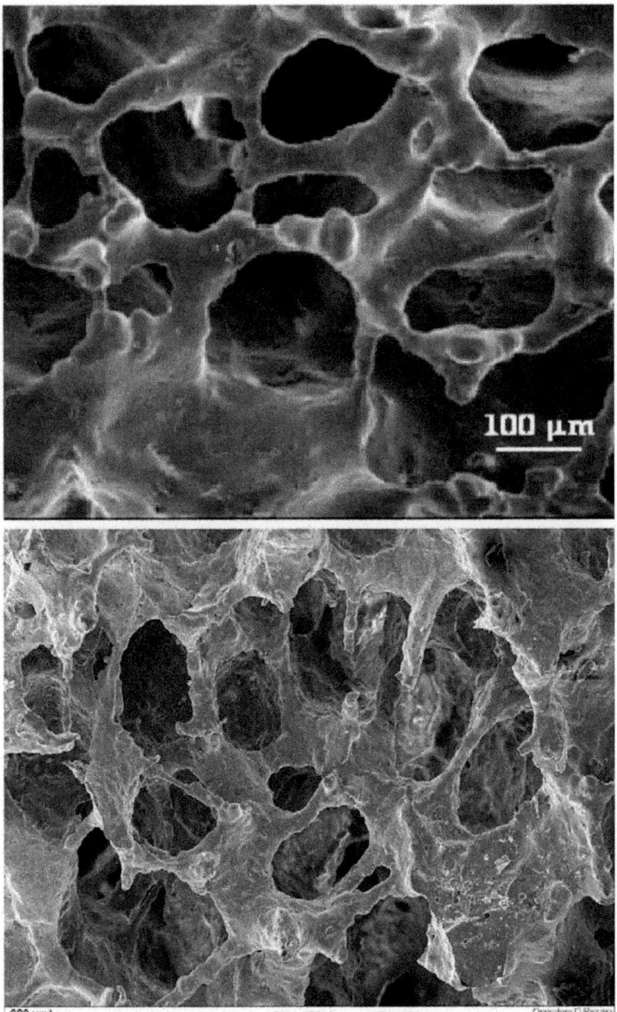

Figure 3.12 The pore structure of the scaffold resembles the trabecular texture of the bone. (a) scale bar 100 μm, (b) scale bar 200 μm.
Reused from C. Vitale-Brovarone, E. Verné, L. Robiglio, P. Appendino, F. Bassi, G. Martinasso, G. Muzio, R. Canuto, Development of glass–ceramic scaffolds for bone tissue engineering: characterisation, proliferation of human osteoblasts and nodule formation, Acta Biomaterialia 3 (2007) 199–208. https://doi.org/10.1016/j.actbio.2006.07.012 after license via (copyright.com) number 4213751393189.

Glass ionomer cement (GIC) has proven successful in practice; on the other hand, this type of cement needs to be modified to promote bioactivity. Wollastonite and mineral trioxide aggregate (MTA) (a mixture of dicalcium silicate [C_2S] and tricalcium silicate [C_3S]) have been added to GIC to examine their effect on the cement [7]. Figs. 3.14–3.16 show that the bioactivity of the modified cement depends on the

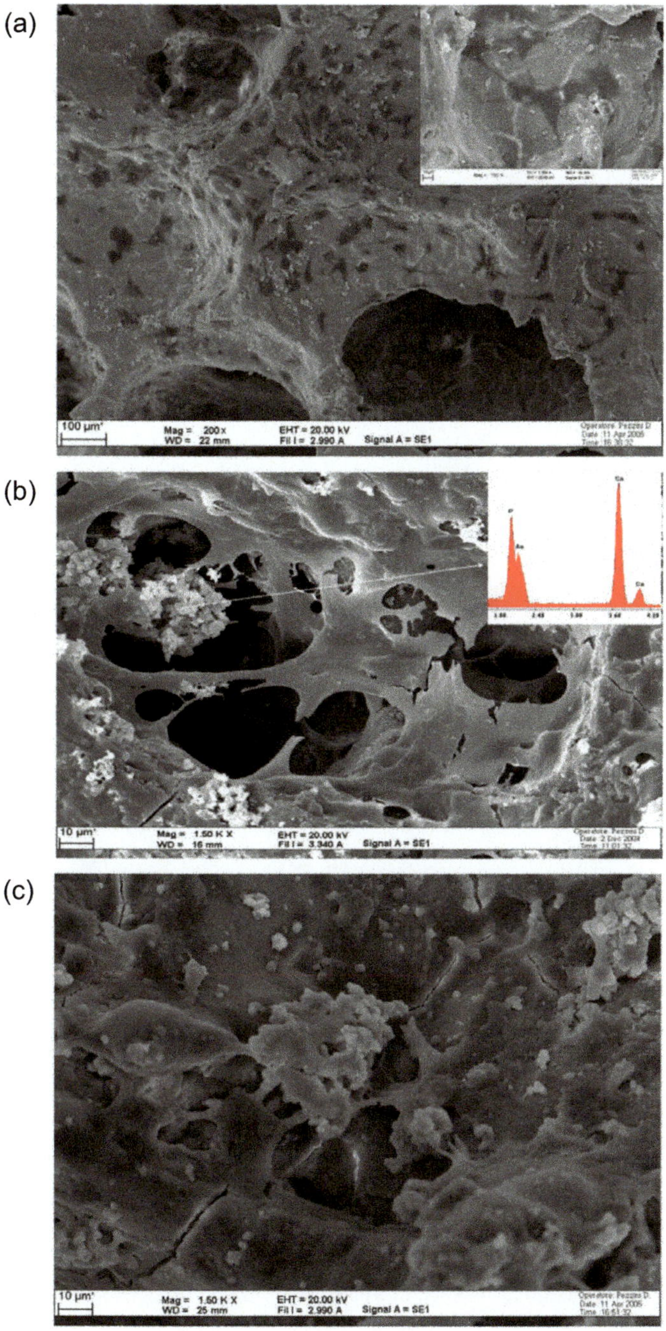

Figure 3.13 Scanning electron microscope micrographs of the osteoblasts cultured on the scaffolds of the previous figure. (a) Incubation of 10 days, (b) higher magnification of the same case, and (c) incubation of 20 days.
Reused from C. Vitale-Brovarone, E. Verné, L. Robiglio, P. Appendino, F. Bassi, G. Martinasso, G. Muzio, R. Canuto, Development of glass–ceramic scaffolds for bone tissue engineering: characterisation, proliferation of human osteoblasts and nodule formation, Acta Biomaterialia 3 (2007) 199–208. https://doi.org/10.1016/j.actbio.2006.07.012 after license via (copyright.com) number 4213751393189.

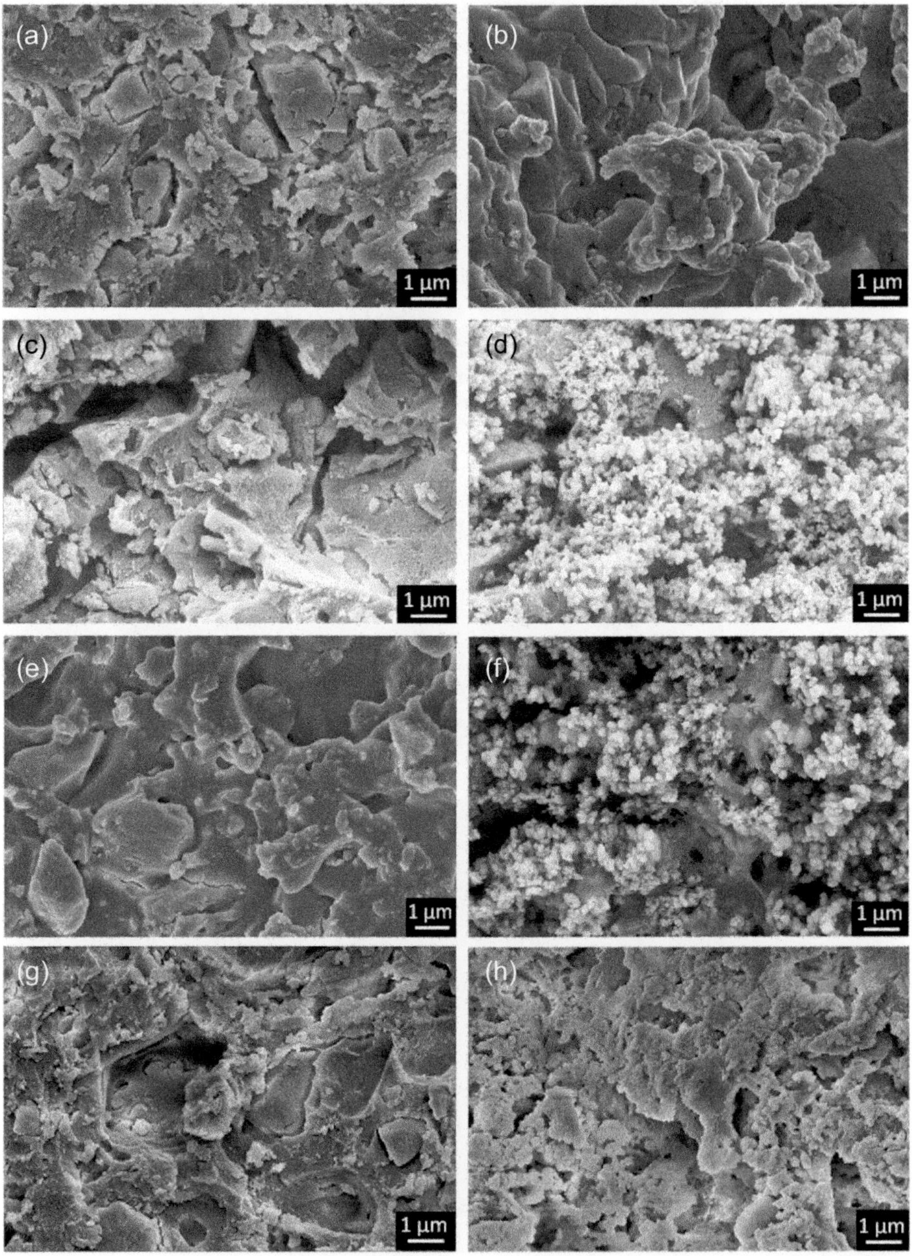

Figure 3.14 Scanning electron microscope micrographs of the glass ionomer cements (GICs) with different wollastonite content after soaking in simulated body fluid solution. (a) GIC after 1 h, (b) GIC after 7 days, (c) 10% wollastonite after 1 h, (d) 10% wollastonite after 7 days, (e) 20% wollastonite after 1 h, (f) 20% wollastonite after 7 days, (g) 30% wollastonite after 1 h, and (h) 30% wollastonite after 7 days.

Reused from S. Chen, Y. Cai, H. Engqvist, W. Xia, Enhanced bioactivity of glass ionomer cement by incorporating calcium silicates, Biomatter 6 (2016) e1123842. https://doi.org/10.1080/21592535.2015.1123842 according to STM opt out.

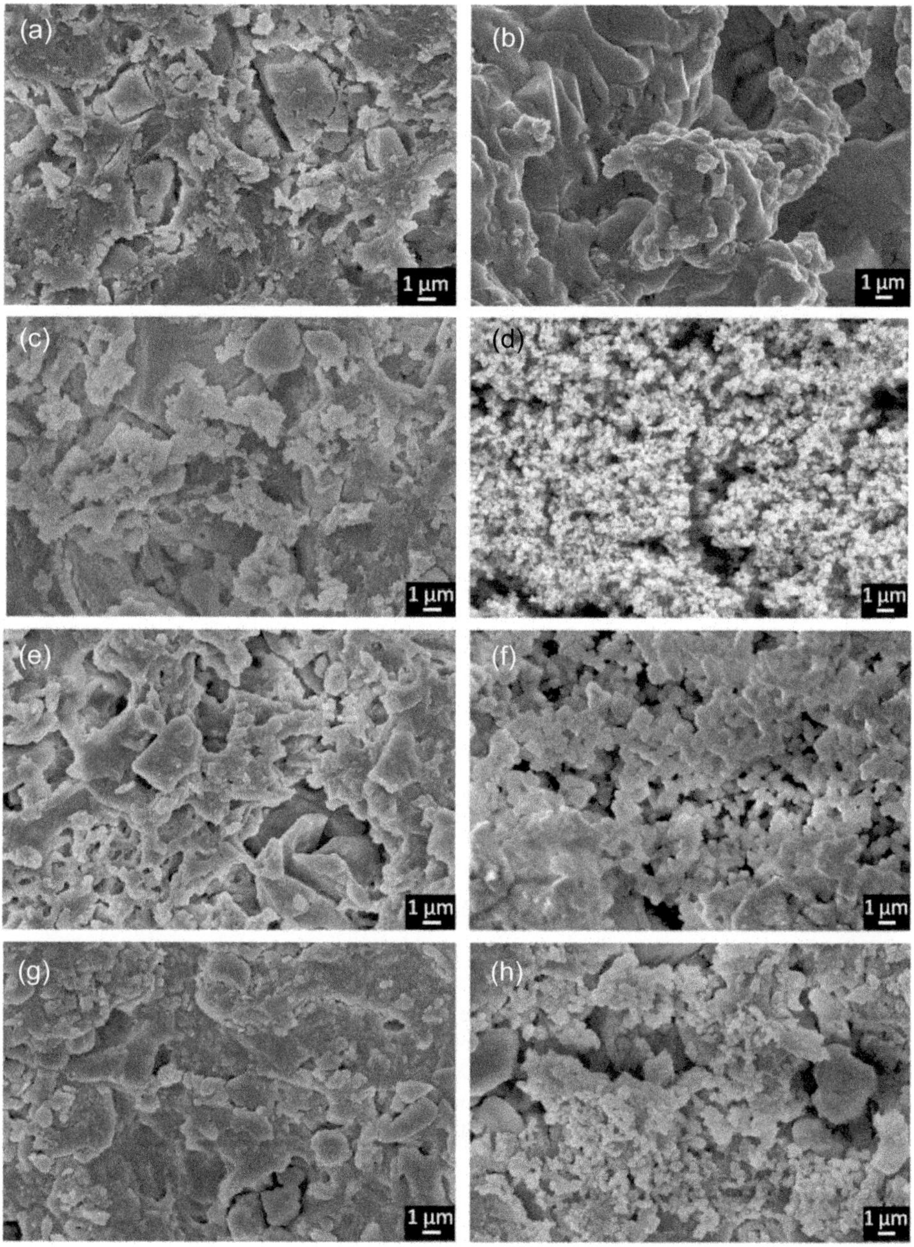

Figure 3.15 Scanning electron microscope images of the cements with mineral trioxide aggregate (MTA) after soaking in simulated body fluid solution. (a) Glass ionomer cement (GIC) after 1 h, (b) GIC after 7 days, (c) 10% MTA after 1 h, (d) 10% MTA after 7 days, (e) 20% MTA after 1 h, (f) 20% MTA after 7 days, (g) 30% MTA after 1 h, and (h) 30% MTA after 7 days.
Reused from S. Chen, Y. Cai, H. Engqvist, W. Xia, Enhanced bioactivity of glass ionomer cement by incorporating calcium silicates, Biomatter 6 (2016) e1123842. https://doi.org/10.1080/21592535.2015.1123842 according to STM opt out.

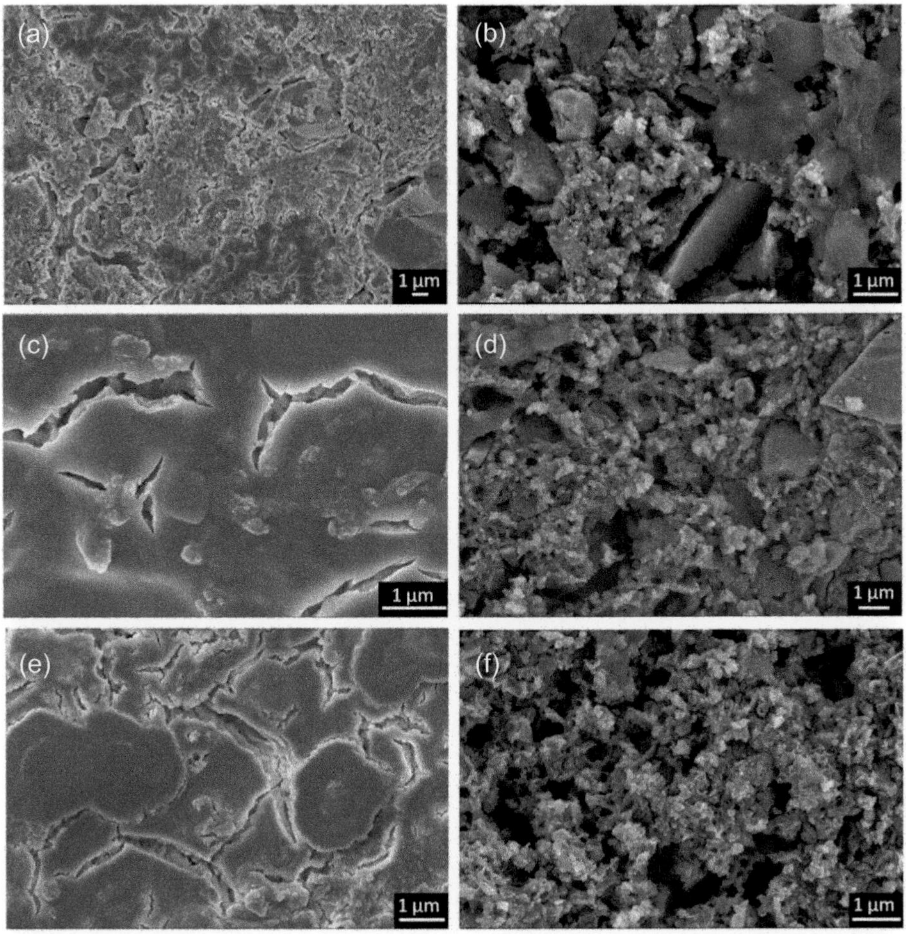

Figure 3.16 Scanning electron microscope images of the cements after soaking in simulated body fluid solution. (a) Glass ionomer cement (GIC) after 1 h, (b) GIC after 14 days, (c) 20% wollastonite after 1 h, (d) 20% wollastonite after 14 days, (e) 20% MTA after 1 h, and (f) 20% MTA after 14 days. *MTA*, mineral trioxide aggregate.
Reused from S. Chen, Y. Cai, H. Engqvist, W. Xia, Enhanced bioactivity of glass ionomer cement by incorporating calcium silicates, Biomatter 6 (2016) e1123842. https://doi.org/10.1080/21592535.2015.1123842 according to STM opt out.

type of additive, the amount of addition, and the time elapsed in SBF solution soaking. Comparing these figures, it can be concluded that GIC can be modified in a manner such that the formation of the apatite layer can be spread at the surface of the cement, which signifies osteoconductivity.

The foregoing examples may serve when evaluating bioactivity via SEM and the expectation of osteoconduction. Energy-dispersive X-ray spectroscopy (EDX) analysis is complementary to confirm the precipitation of Ca and P ions. These examples may also help in the course of materials selection for designing new scaffolds or other bone substitutes. The design of new products in general, and specifically for the bone substitutes, includes both material and process selection. The details of the processes that are used to build the porous scaffolds or other applications are described in the original articles of the figures.

Review questions

If the reader of this chapter is using it for self-study or as part of an education course, it is recommended that he or she tries to find examples and/or figures from the available library and attach them to the answers.

1. Describe the osteogenesis process.
2. Explain the four types of cells of bone: osteogenic cells, osteoblasts, osteocytes, and osteoclasts.
3. Describe the osteoinduction process.
4. Describe the osteoconduction process.
5. Describe the osseointegration process.
6. Describe the use of soaking of bioceramics in SBF solution.
7. Explain why the scaffolds are made porous.
8. What are the parameters that affect the surface morphology of bioceramics soaked in SBF solution? Try team work to address most of the parameters.
9. What is the vital parameter that osteoblast attachment depends on?
10. What is the vital parameter that osteoblast ingrowth depends on?
11. What are the properties that make PLLA polymer suitable for building scaffolds?
12. Explain why different microstructures are obtained with the PLLA/BGC scaffolds in Fig. 3.4.
13. Explain the reasons for different morphologies of the porous PLLA/BGC composites shown in Fig. 3.5.
14. Explain the benefits of the utilization of nanopowders and the surface grafting in the BG/PLLA composites shown in Fig. 3.6.
15. Describe the scaffold morphologies shown in Fig. 3.7 and the reason for the different morphologies.
16. What are the benefits of using commercial open-cell polyurethane sponges as polymer templates?
17. Why is the utilization of polymer templates of different pore densities reasonable?
18. Why the fabricated scaffolds should have analogous structure to the living bone?
19. Why should the polymer template be of narrow size distribution?
20. Why is presintering performed on the porous scaffold before final sintering?
21. Why is SEM observation necessary after final sintering of the porous scaffold?
22. A denser structure of the porous scaffold is preferable. Explain.
23. How can strut thickness ranges be altered via the process parameters?
24. Pore strut thickness may be varied according to what?
25. What is the condition that seeded osteoblasts depend on? What is expected in optimum conditions?
26. Explain part (c) of Fig. 3.13.
27. Explain why a denser microstructure of the GIC/wollastonite composite, Fig. 3.14, is obtained with increasing wollastonite content before and after soaking in SBF solution.

28. Explain why a denser microstructure of the GIC/MTA composite, Fig. 3.15, is obtained with increasing MTA content before and after soaking in SBF solution. What differentiates wollastonite from MTA in this case?

29. Referring to Fig. 3.16, what material shows promising osteoconductivity? Explain.

30. Why is EDX analysis a necessary complementary to SEM in some cases of examining bioactivity?

References

[1] T. Albrektsson, C. Johansson, Osteoinduction, osteoconduction and osseointegration, European Spine Journal 10 (2001) S96–S101, https://doi.org/10.1007/s005860100282.

[2] C. Wu, J. Chang, A review of bioactive silicate ceramics, Biomedical Materials 8 (2013) 032001, https://doi.org/10.1088/1748-6041/8/3/032001.

[3] Z. Hong, R.L. Reis, J.F. Mano, Preparation and in vitro characterization of scaffolds of poly(l-lactic acid) containing bioactive glass ceramic nanoparticles, Acta Biomaterialia 4 (2008) 1297–1306, https://doi.org/10.1016/j.actbio.2008.03.007.

[4] A. Liu, Z. Hong, X. Zhuang, X. Chen, Y. Cui, Y. Liu, X. Jing, Surface modification of bioactive glass nanoparticles and the mechanical and biological properties of poly(l-lactide) composites, Acta Biomaterialia 4 (2008) 1005–1015, https://doi.org/10.1016/j.actbio.2008.02.013.

[5] F. Baino, S. Caddeo, G. Novajra, C. Vitale-Brovarone, Using porous bioceramic scaffolds to model healthy and osteoporotic bone, Journal of the European Ceramic Society 36 (2016) 2175–2182, https://doi.org/10.1016/j.jeurceramsoc.2016.01.011.

[6] C. Vitale-Brovarone, E. Verné, L. Robiglio, P. Appendino, F. Bassi, G. Martinasso, G. Muzio, R. Canuto, Development of glass–ceramic scaffolds for bone tissue engineering: characterisation, proliferation of human osteoblasts and nodule formation, Acta Biomaterialia 3 (2007) 199–208, https://doi.org/10.1016/j.actbio.2006.07.012.

[7] S. Chen, Y. Cai, H. Engqvist, W. Xia, Enhanced bioactivity of glass ionomer cement by incorporating calcium silicates, Biomatter 6 (2016) e1123842, https://doi.org/10.1080/21592535.2015.1123842.

Orthopedic and dental applications 4

As seen in Chapter 1, bioceramics can be classified into three categories: bioinert, bioactive, and bioresorbable. Historically, bioceramics are also classified as first, second, and third generation. The first generation is mostly bioinert (or nearly bioinert) oxide ceramics such as alumina and zirconia. Also, carbons are an important subset of bioinert ceramics. The second generation is bioactive ceramics such as bioactive glasses, bioactive glass-ceramics, and calcium phosphates. The third generation is bioactive ceramics that are made bioresorbable by chemical and microstructure engineering means such as the wide range of porous bioactive ceramics and versatile types of bone cements.

Introductory knowledge of the applications of bioceramics is presented in the first three chapters of this book and represents "stage one" in introducing the applications of bioceramics. The applications of bioceramics are very broad, need extensive background, and thus need dedicated volumes for each area of interest. Accordingly, this chapter does not aim to cover the entire application spectrum, but represents "stage two" in the process of introducing the subject within the framework of a textbook. Different application aspects of the subject, which is thought to be closer to materials scientist approaches, are presented. The plan is to present a number of published articles that are relevant to the subject. Other stages of introducing the applications of bioceramics are among the goals of the remaining chapters.

4.1 Orthopedic applications

The products related to total knee prostheses (TKPs) are also given the names first, second, and third generation and are shown in Fig. 4.1 [1]. The first generation is an alumina femoral and tibial component with an ultrahigh molecular weight polyethylene (UHMWPE) insert. The second generation is that which replaces alumina with a titanium alloy tibial component. The titanium alloy tibial component was used because it is thinner and ductile. In addition, the alumina tibial component has shown a high incidence of sinking and an appearance of radiolucent (X-ray transparent) lines for cementless fixation. A high-purity hot isostatic pressing (HIP) alumina femoral component is introduced with the third generation, which produces components with higher strengths reduce the design limitations. In addition, cement fixation of the femoral component is improved via applying a porous coating of ceramic beads on the surface of the femoral component. A further later improvement of the alumina part is performed by introducing the tetragonal zirconia polycrystal (TZP) that produces components with better toughness. Fig. 4.1 shows X-ray radiographs for TKP after years of implantation for second- and third-generation TKP. This is not the end of the story because research activities are continuing to improve bioceramic properties and performance.

Bioceramics: For Materials Science and Engineering. https://doi.org/10.1016/B978-0-08-102233-7.00004-5

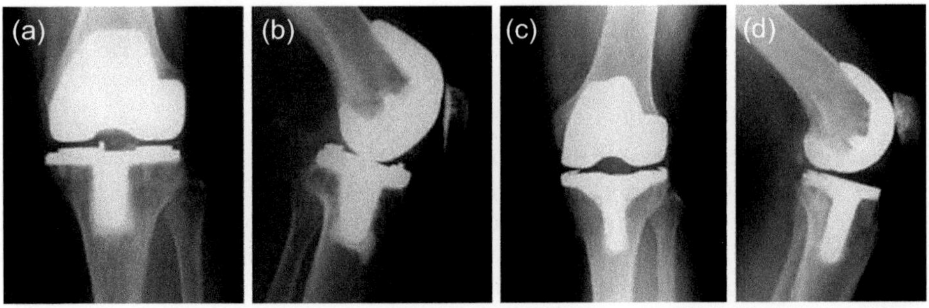

Figure 4.1 X-ray radiographs for total knee prostheses (TKPs). (a) Anteroposterior, (b) lateral second-generation TKP after 14 years of implantation, (c) anteroposterior, and (d) lateral third-generation TKP after 6 years of implantation.
Reused from H. Oonishi, S.-C. Kim, M. Kyomoto, M. Iwamoto, M. Ueno, Comparison of in-vivo wear between polyethylene inserts articulating against ceramic and cobalt-chrome femoral components in total knee prostheses, in: Bioceramics and Alternative Bearings in Joint Arthroplasty, Steinkopff, 2007, pp. 149–159. https://doi.org/10.1007/978-3-7985-1783-7_20 after license via (copyright.com) number 4225830297111.

Alumina found wide application in total hip arthroplasty (THA), where a ceramic-on-ceramic articulating surface design is included. An expression of "third-generation alumina-on-alumina" may be found in the literature in connection with THA, not to be confused with "third-generation" bioactive ceramics. Third-generation alumina-on-alumina denotes a careful process design of HIP of pure alumina that results in a fully dense alumina with small final grain size (<2 μm). This process may include techniques such as "laser marking" on the outer surface of the alumina to improve fixation without the need for cementation, called cementless THA. As expected, clinical results [2], see Fig. 4.2, show no detectible wear or osteolysis (osteolysis: the pathological destruction or disappearance of bone tissue, see https://en.oxforddictionaries.com/). The materials scientist therefore should be aware of the manufacturing process that enhances the performance of the product; in this case, the performance is related to the wear rate that should be brought to the lowest possible value.

The main motivation for utilizing alumina-on-alumina articulating surfaces is caused by the problem of aseptic loosening caused by the polyethylene (PE) wear debris and the accompanying induced osteolysis. The wear debris originates from the acetabular cup that is made of UHMWPE. Patients experiencing debris-induced osteolysis have received THA revision surgeries [3]. An alumina-on-alumina bearing is included in cementless revision implants. Fig. 4.3 shows a radiograph for a patient after THA that reveals osteolysis, and another radiograph after revision using an alumina-on-alumina bearing surface with clearly improved results.

Design consideration is always imperative in THA. The acetabular component, for example, may have different shapes and thicknesses according to specific cases. A study of THA for small-physique patients [4] shows that a deviation from hemispherical geometry of the acetabular cup system (ACS) may lead to catastrophic results. Excessive wear of the acetabular PE component takes place and leaves an empty space

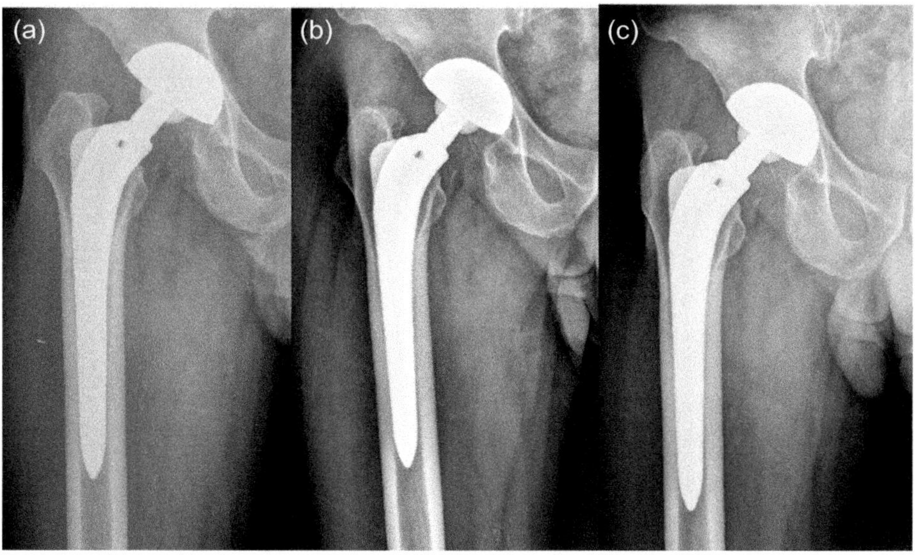

Figure 4.2 Serial radiographs of total hip arthroplasty for a 61-year-old man show no detectible wear or osteolysis in addition to bone-ingrown stability of the prostheses. (a) 1 year postoperation, (b) 10 years postoperation, and (c) 15 years postoperation.
Reused from B.-J. Kang, Y.-C. Ha, D-W. Ham, S.-C. Hwang, Y.-K. Lee, K.-H. Koo, Third-generation alumina-on-alumina total hip arthroplasty: 14 to 16-year follow-up study, The Journal of Arthroplasty 30 (2015) 411–415. https://doi.org/10.1016/j.arth.2014.09.020 after license via (copyright.com) number 4225231361777.

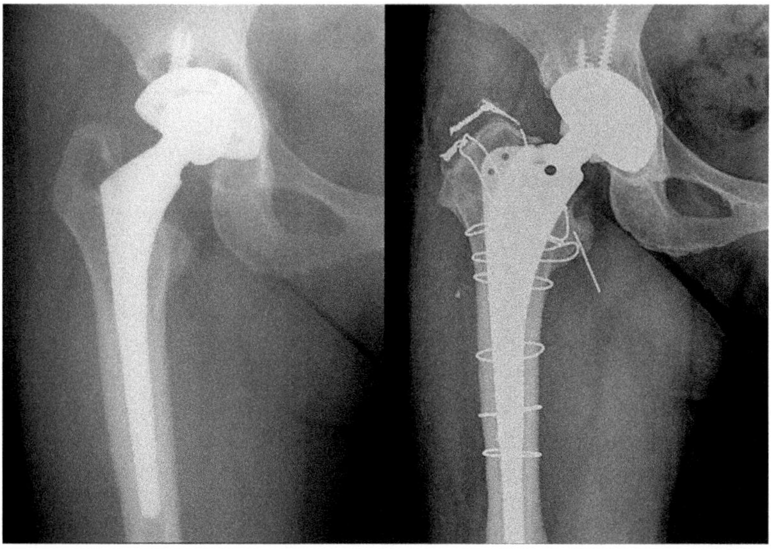

Figure 4.3 Anteroposterior radiograph after 5 years of total hip arthroplasty (THA) of the right hip in a 37-year-old woman. *Left*: osteolysis is shown around a loosened acetabular component and the proximal femur. *Right*: THA revision using alumina-on-alumina bearing surface after 11.9 years.
Reused from J.J. Yoo, P.W. Yoon, Y.-K. Lee, K.-H. Koo, K.S. Yoon, H.J. Kim, Revision total hip arthroplasty using an alumina-on-alumina bearing surface in patients with osteolysis, The Journal of Arthroplasty 28 (2013) 132–138. https://doi.org/10.1016/j.arth.2012.04.030 after license via (copyright.com) number 4225900800899.

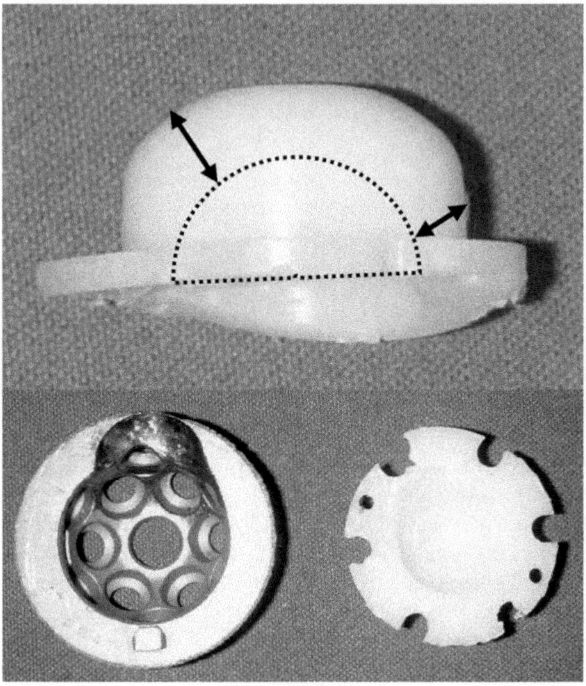

Figure 4.4 Design problems of the acetabular component lead to insufficient congruity between the polyethylene (PE) liner and the metal shell and accelerates wear of the PE. The inefficient locking mechanism results in a distortion of the superior rim.
Reused from Y. Nakamura, H. Mitsui, A. Kikuchi, S. Toh, H. Katano, Total hip arthroplasty using a cylindrical cementless stem in patients with a small physique, The Journal of Arthroplasty 26 (2011) 77–81. https://doi.org/10.1016/j.arth.2009.10.014 after license via (copyright.com) number 4240040502200.

behind it. This situation leads to penetration of the femoral head into the space left by the missing PE and applies stress at the superior rim that leads to its failure, as shown in Fig. 4.4. The situation is improved via the use of porous-coated fixation surfaces and advanced bearing materials.

Another design problem of the same case is the combination of small ball head diameter and large diameter of the neck of the stem. This situation prompts dislocation of the joints. Thus a newly designed anatomic medullary locking cementless stem with PE liner, which benefits from improved material properties, is used, as seen in Fig. 4.5.

In truth, the activities of materials science and engineering are the nonstop research and development of materials properties in response to the need to improve product performance. An example is the ceramic-on-ceramic THA, namely, alumina-on-alumina THA, which has been improved to address better properties of wear and fracture toughness. An alumina delta ceramic-on-alumina delta ceramic (BIOLOX Delta; CeramTec AG, Plochingen, Germany) has a grain size of <0.8 mm, which is smaller than the grain size of alumina forte ceramic (1–5 mm) from the same company. As mentioned earlier,

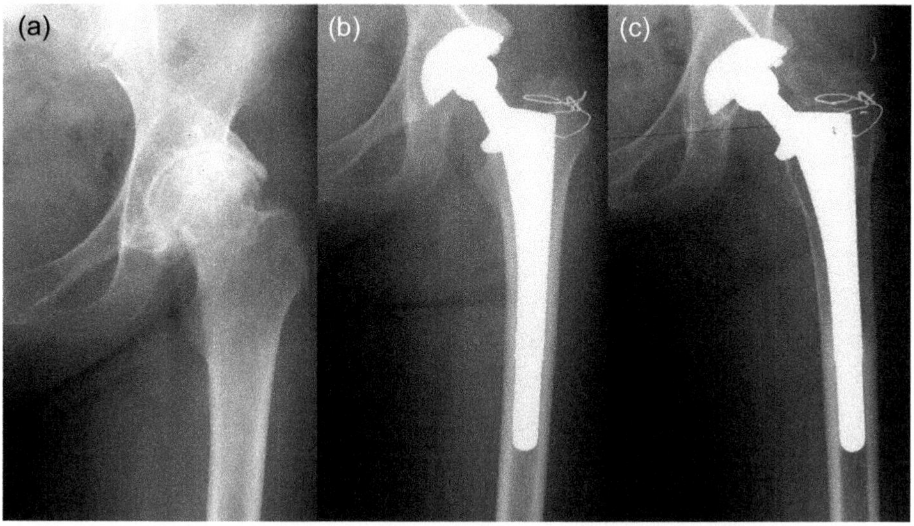

Figure 4.5 (a) Total hip arthroplasty after osteoarthritis for a 55-year-old woman. (b) Improved design of the implant with 48-mm metal shell coupling with acetabular cup system polyethylene liner. (c) After 16 years of surgery, a typical bone ingrowth with the femur. Reused from Reused from Y. Nakamura, H. Mitsui, A. Kikuchi, S. Toh, H. Katano, Total hip arthroplasty using a cylindrical cementless stem in patients with a small physique, The Journal of Arthroplasty 26 (2011) 77–81. https://doi.org/10.1016/j.arth.2009.10.014 after license via (copyright.com) number 4240040502200.

the smaller grain size of the final product could be attainable via higher purity level, introducing new additives, and utilization of the HIP technique in the manufacturing process. The enhanced properties of the new alumina product make it possible to successfully utilize cementless ultrashort metaphyseal-fitting anatomic THA. The midterm results show that thigh pain and aseptic loosening are largely reduced. Besides, no osteolysis has been detected via the radiographs and CT (computed tomography) scans, i.e., a computer-assisted build of cross-sectional images of the X-ray scanned area.

Fig. 4.6 shows ultrashort metaphyseal-fitting anatomic cementless stems. The implant is designed to fit the case. The acetabular components are embedded in a position of 50 degrees inclination in the right hip and 25 degrees inclination in the left hip. The anteroposterior view is for a 36-year-old woman with osteonecrosis after 7 days and 9 years of hip arthroplasty. The acetabular components and the stem fixes are stable and no evidence of osteolysis is observed.

In fact, we use the word "design" with two different meanings in materials science and engineering. The previous case is an example of "product design." Product design includes the selection of materials, based on their properties, and structural design of the product. The designed structure of the product depends on stress distribution considerations, which are obvious in the previous case. The second meaning of design is somehow hidden for some students and is called "materials design." Materials design makes the most of the success stories in materials science and engineering.

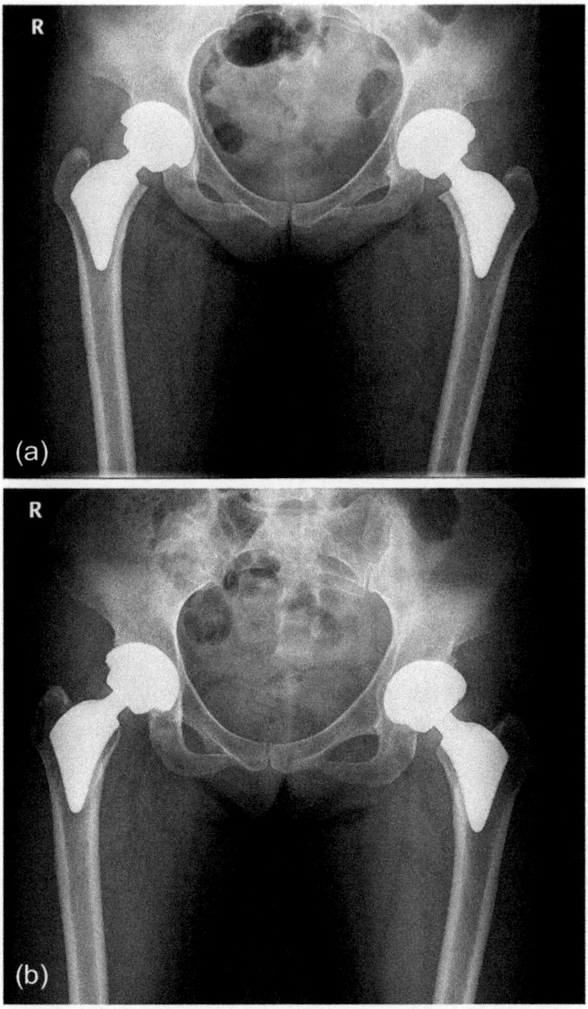

Figure 4.6 An anteroposterior radiograph after arthroplasty of both hips for a 36-year-old woman with osteonecrosis. (a) 7 days after hip arthroplasty, (b) 9 years after hip arthroplasty with neither hip displaying femoral or acetabular osteolysis.
Reused from Y.-H. Kim, J.-W. Park, J.-S. Kim, Alumina delta-on-alumina delta bearing in cementless total hip arthroplasty in patients aged <50 years, The Journal of Arthroplasty 31 (2016) 2209–2214. https://doi.org/10.1016/j.arth.2016.03.016 after license via (copyright.com) number 4241260066205.

Recognition of biocompatible and bioactive materials is an essential stage of materials design; in addition, developing materials with better wear properties is a highlight of materials design. Certainly, materials design depends on deep recognition of materials properties based on structure, microstructure, and the type of the material. A good example of materials design is that for BIOLOX Delta, which was introduced in 2004 by CeramTec AG and called the fourth generation of ceramic bearings. The material

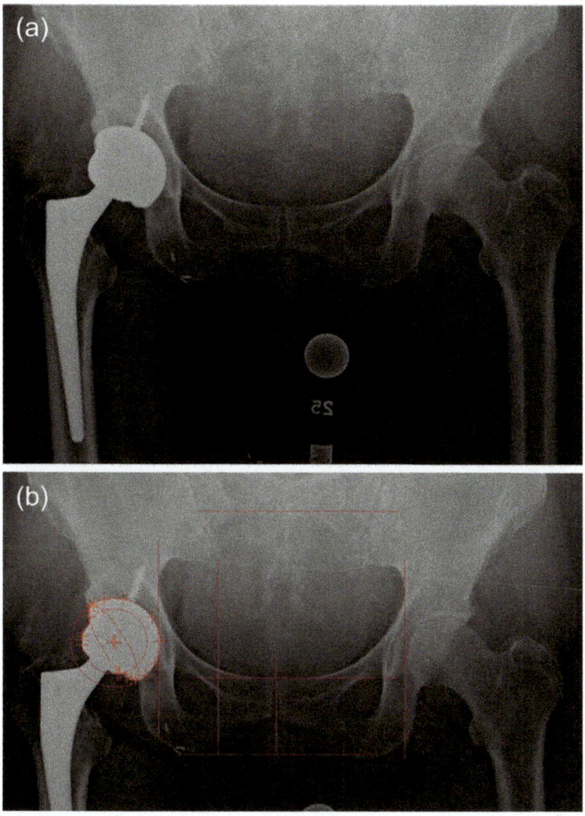

Figure 4.7 (a) An anteroposterior X-ray radiograph of the patient with audible hip squeaking after a fall. (b) An Ein Bild Röntgen Analyse (digital software for monitoring implant migration) analysis revealed cup inclination of 59.65 degrees and anteversion of 19.98 degrees. Reused from A.A. Aoude, J. Antoniou, L.M. Epure, O.L. Huk, D.J. Zukor, M. Tanzer, Midterm outcomes of the recently FDA approved ceramic on ceramic bearing in total hip arthroplasty patients under 65 years of age, The Journal of Arthroplasty 30 (2015) 1388–1392. https://doi.org/10.1016/j.arth.2015.03.028 after license via (copyright.com) number 4246950235550.

is a 17% TZP-toughened alumina with traces of chromium dioxide and strontium as strontium aluminates. Both types of trace develop very hard elongated grains in the microstructure that contribute to the enhancement of the toughness, mainly through a crack-deflection mechanism.

The improved toughness and wear resistance of the fourth generation of ceramic bearings allow the synthesis of better and safer bearings for THA for young, active patients [6]. An example of the achievement of such a ceramic is the case of a 50-year-old female patient. She underwent THA and fourth-generation alumina parts were used. After 2 years of operation, she fell and had the implanted cup displaced by 59.7 degrees of inclination and 20.0 degrees of anteversion, as seen in Fig. 4.7. Accordingly, the implant causes audible hip squeaking but causes no pain and thus she was refused revision surgery. The improved strength and fracture toughness of this type of alumina maintain the integrity of the implant and show no complication after surgery.

4.2 Dental applications

Because of the esthetic properties of porcelain coats, porcelain-fused-to-metal restorations have been used for dental prostheses for some time. To overcome the problem of brittleness of porcelain coats and chipping of veneering porcelain, all-ceramic fixed dental prostheses (FDPs) systems are proposed. Carefully sintered polycrystalline zirconia has an improved translucency and has been used in the molar region. On the other hand, better combination of mechanical and esthetics properties has been achieved with composites of high-strength ceramic matrices with fillers of porcelain and other glassy materials to enhance esthetics.

Microstructures of newly designed dental ceramic composites for the foregoing purpose and available in the market are shown in Fig. 4.8 [7]. Cercon is an yttria-stabilized zirconia (Y-TZP), which after sintering at 1350°C has high sintered density and grain size of 0.3 μm. The higher density improves translucency and the lower grain size improves mechanical and wear properties. Another type shown in the figure

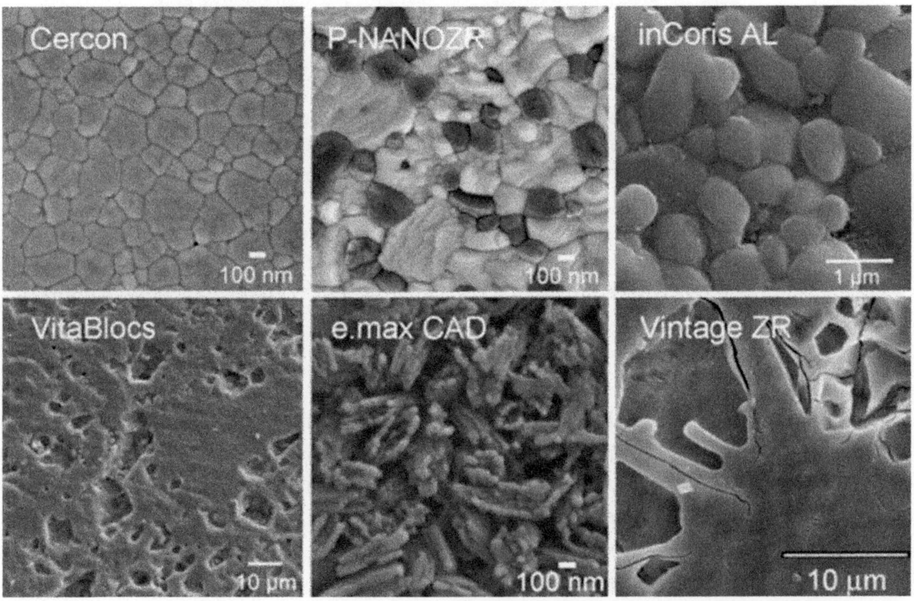

Figure 4.8 Scanning electron microscope micrographs for six types of dental ceramics. Adapted from T. Miyazaki, T. Nakamura, H. Matsumura, S. Ban, T. Kobayashi, Current status of zirconia restoration, Journal of Prosthodontic Research 57 (2013) 236–261. https://doi.org/10.1016/j.jpor.2013.09.001 via (CC BY NC ND) license.

is P-NANOZR, which has an interpenetrated intragranular nanostructure. The submicron-sized Al_2O_3 and ceria-stabilized zirconia (Ce-TZP) are shown in the microstructure with dispersions of nanometer-sized Al_2O_3 and Ce-TZP. Dense microstructure is shown with an average grain size of about 0.5 μm. The third microstructure, inCoris AL, is for carefully sintered bodies at 1500°C with an average grain size of 1 μm. The high-temperature form of potassium feldspar, called Sanidine, is included by 30 vol% of 2–10 μm grains with the fourth type, Vitablocs. The microstructure is for compacts before sintering. These compacts are often called computer-aided design/computer-aided manufacturing (CAD/CAM) blocks because they are machined via a CAD/CAM machine before sintering, so that the final solid dental implant is attained. Another CAD/CAM block, e.max CAD, contains about 70 vol% elongated lithium disilicate grains, which should greatly enhance the mechanical properties of the block. The lithium disilicate grains have an average grain size of about 1.5 μm and are dispersed in glass medium. Finally, Vintage ZR is designed as a veneering porcelain for zirconia that consists of 4.5 wt% of leucite dispersed in glass medium. The microstructure shows 5–10 μm-sized leucite crystals.

Y-TZP is currently the most used ceramic for dental implants. Zirconia stabilized with 3 mol% yttria is commonly found as CAD/CAM blocks. However, the condition of the surface of the implant significantly affects bioactivity. Implant attachment, proliferation, and differentiation of osteoblast-like cells determine the efficiency of the implant attachment to the host tissue. Surface topographical influences on osteoblast attachment and development are studied [8]. As-sintered, abraded, polished, and porous surfaces of Y-TZP are examined. The prepared surfaces were seeded with cell-line human osteosarcoma (a type of cell that shows noticeable proliferation of osteoblasts) following the procedure detailed in [8].

Fig. 4.9 shows that after 48 h of incubation, the cells are clustered on the rough surface and do not completely cover the zirconia surface because of clustering. On the

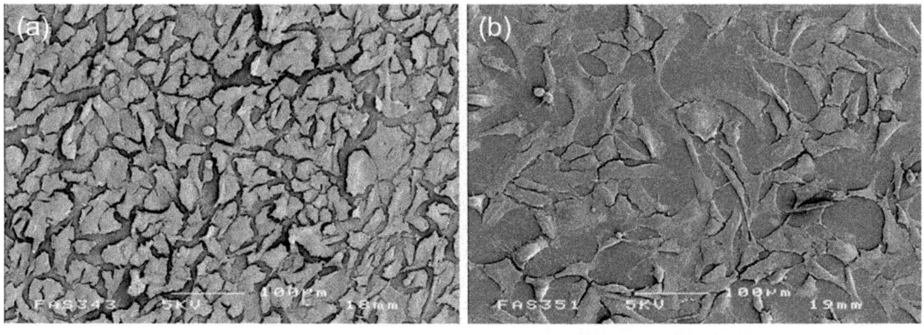

Figure 4.9 Scanning electron microscope micrographs of human osteosarcoma cell attachment to surfaces of zirconia after 48 h of incubation. (a) Abraded surface and (b) polished surface. (Scale bars represent 100 μm.)

Reused from H.M.T.U. Herath, L. Di Silvio, J.R.G. Evans, Osteoblast response to zirconia surfaces with different topographies, Materials Science and Engineering: C 57 (2015) 363–370. https://doi.org/10.1016/j.msec.2015.07.052 after license via (copyright.com) number 4254310828091.

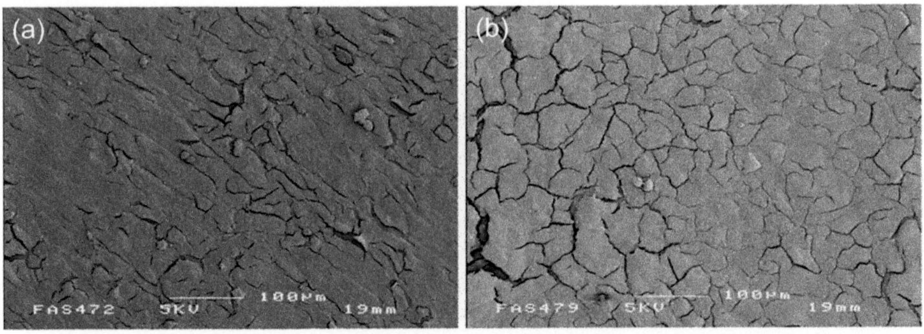

Figure 4.10 Scanning electron microscope micrographs of human osteosarcoma cell attachment to surfaces of zirconia after 168 h of incubation. (a) Abraded surface and (b) polished surface. (Scale bars represent 100 µm.)
Reused from H.M.T.U. Herath, L. Di Silvio, J.R.G. Evans, Osteoblast response to zirconia surfaces with different topographies, Materials Science and Engineering: C 57 (2015) 363–370. https://doi.org/10.1016/j.msec.2015.07.052 after license via (copyright.com) number 4254310828091.

other hand, the cells on the smooth surface are spreading and randomly oriented, and there is a spare space for further proliferation. After 168 h of incubation, see Fig. 4.10, growth of cell clustering that made a continuous sheath over the abraded surfaces is observed. In addition, the cells were oriented along the grooves. On the polished surface, the cell population just compensates for the initial lower density and reaches confluence. Explicitly, surface roughness helps in early cell attachment and proliferation. While on the smooth surface of zirconia, the lower initial cell density is compensated for after 168 h via subsequent proliferation.

For the materials scientist to understand Figs. 4.11 and 4.12 a simple explanation of the term "filopodia" is necessary. When the living cell is trying to attach to a surface or adhere to a matrix, it generates long, slender, tapering extensions to facilitate attachment. Filopodia also facilitate cell generation and spreading. Fig. 4.11 shows that the abraded surfaces inhibit the extension of filopodia and limit them along the discontinuities. On the other hand, Fig. 4.12 shows that the dense polished surface allows the filopodia to extend and have more flattened and elongated morphology that gives a better chance for cell attachment and proliferation.

A common trend in the research and development of dental materials is to introduce bioactivity to dental materials that proves good mechanical and wear properties. This research trend is expected to continue to be active. A good example is that utilizing the sol–gel preparation method for the synthesis of zirconia–hydroxyapatite composites [9]. The effect of hydroxyapatite content and heat treatment is studied via Fourier-transform infrared spectroscopy (FTIR) analysis. Bioactivity is first examined by soaking in a solution containing bovine serum albumin (BSA) followed by monitoring FTIR after 24 h of exposure. This was to detect that the composite can adsorb the blood protein, resembling the trend of cell adhesion. Bioactivity is next examined via immersion in simulated body fluid (SBF) solution for 21 days to monitor the formation

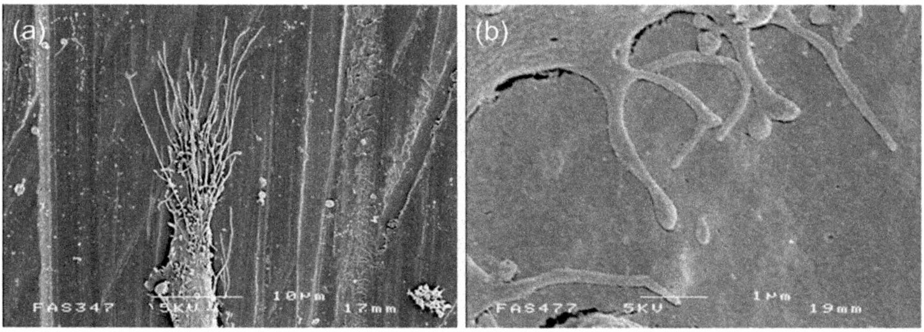

Figure 4.11 Scanning electron microscope micrographs of human osteosarcoma cells on abraded zirconia. (a) Cells tend to align along grooves and (b) terminal ends of filopodia enlarge. Reused from H.M.T.U. Herath, L. Di Silvio, J.R.G. Evans, Osteoblast response to zirconia surfaces with different topographies, Materials Science and Engineering: C 57 (2015) 363–370. https://doi.org/10.1016/j.msec.2015.07.052 after license via (copyright.com) number 4254310828091.

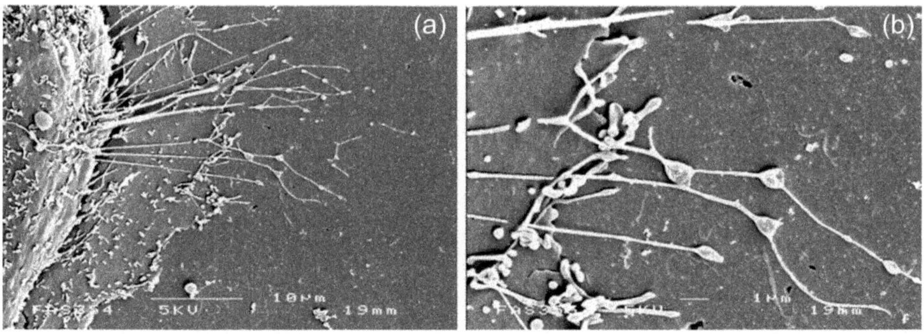

Figure 4.12 Scanning electron microscope micrographs of cells on polished zirconia. (a) Cells were spread closely to the surface and (b) extensions of filopodia terminal ends. Reused from H.M.T.U. Herath, L. Di Silvio, J.R.G. Evans, Osteoblast response to zirconia surfaces with different topographies, Materials Science and Engineering: C 57 (2015) 363–370. https://doi.org/10.1016/j.msec.2015.07.052 after license via (copyright.com) number 4254310828091.

of hydroxyapatite at the surface indicating initiation of osseointegration. Scanning electron microscope (SEM) micrographs conform to the formation of the hydroxyapatite, and energy-dispersive X-ray spectroscopy analysis shows that the Ca/P ratio indicates calcium-deficient hydroxyapatite particles (HAp).

Fig. 4.13 shows the FTIR of ZrO_2 and HAp and their composites heated at 1000°C. The intense peak at 748 cm^{-1} indicates crystalline monoclinic zirconia. The other FTIR band belongs to HAp and its derivatives, as detailed in [9]. The FTIR of BSA and the materials of the previous figure after exposure to BSA for

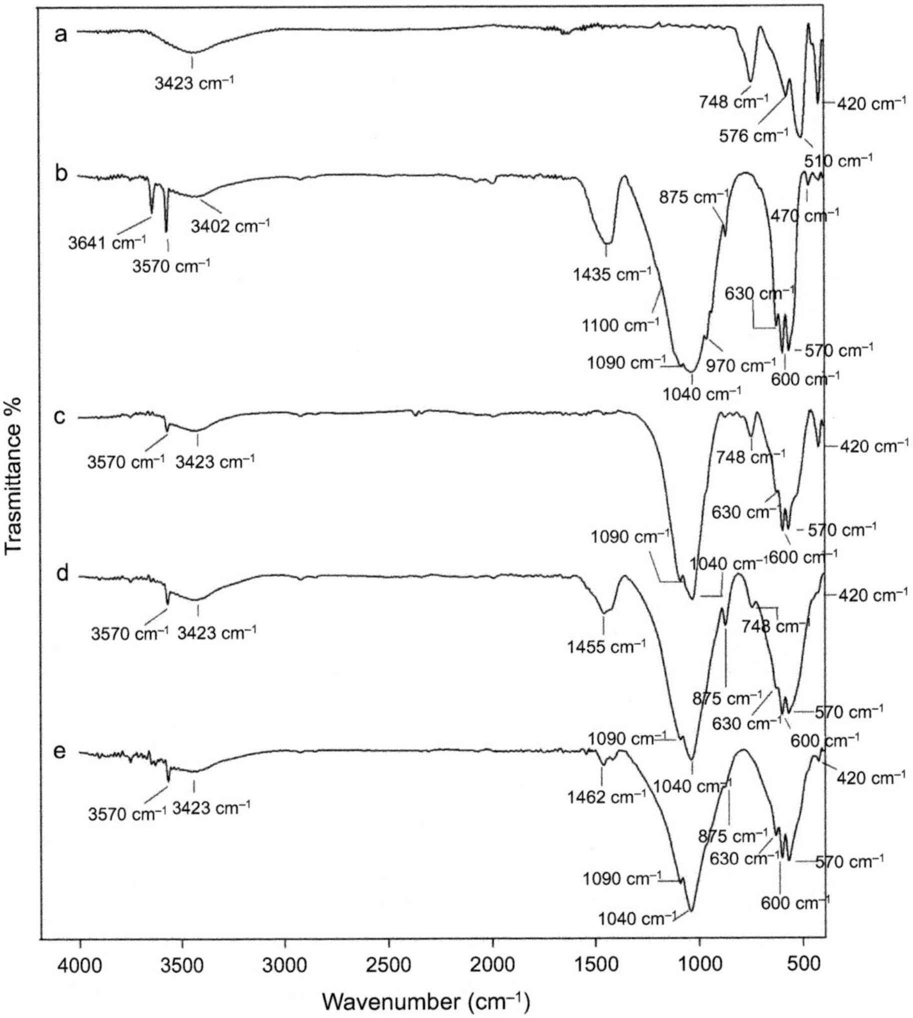

Figure 4.13 FTIR of (a) ZrO_2; (b) HAp; (c) $9ZrO_2 \cdot 1HAp$; (d) $7ZrO_2 \cdot 3HAp$; and (e) $5ZrO_2 \cdot 5HAp$ gels, heated to 1000°C. *FTIR*, Fourier-transform infrared spectroscopy; *HAp*, hydroxyapatite particles.
Adapted from F. Bollino, E. Armenia, E. Tranquillo, Zirconia/hydroxyapatite composites synthesized via sol-gel: influence of hydroxyapatite content and heating on their biological properties, Materials 10 (2017) 757. https://doi.org/10.3390/ma10070757 via (CC BY 4.0) license.

24 h are shown in Fig. 4.14. The FTIR bands of the albumin band at 1654 cm^{-1} and 1543 cm^{-1} are clear, indicating the absorption of the albumin at the surface of the sample confirming the first step that initiates cell adhesion and proliferation. In Fig. 4.15, the newly appeared strong band at 1040 cm^{-1} indicates the formation of HAp after soaking in SBF solution for 21 days. It is advised to read the full article [9] to gain

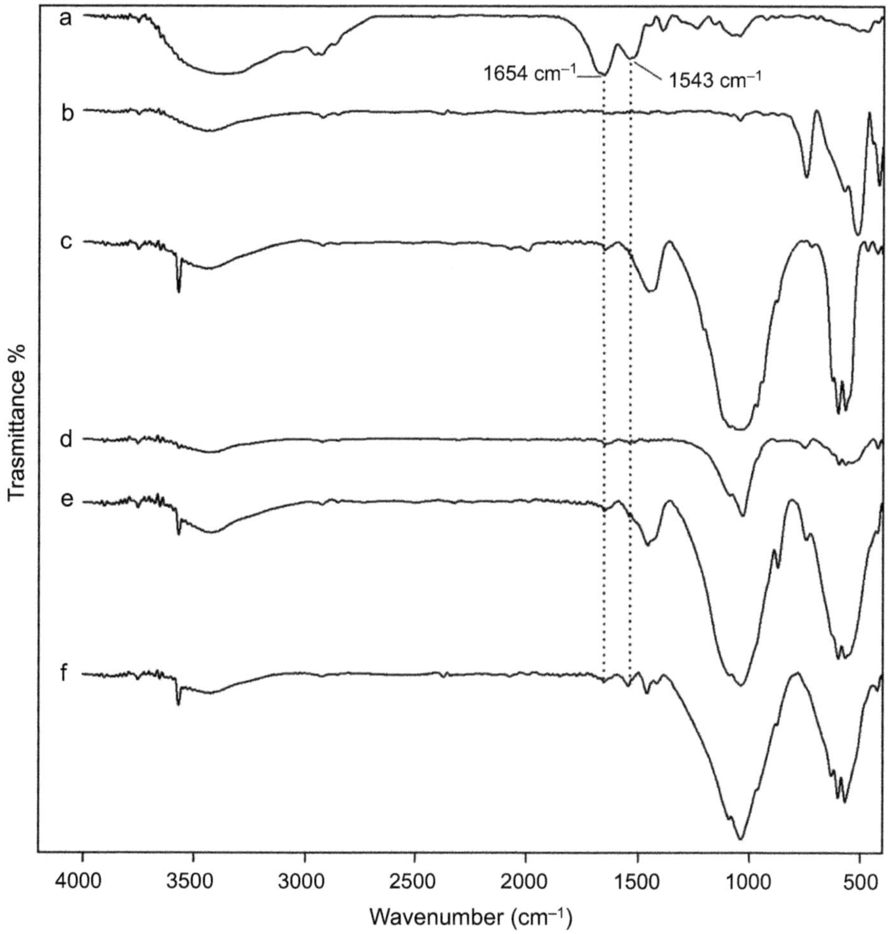

Figure 4.14 FTIR of (a) BSA; (b) ZrO_2; (c) HAp; (d) $9ZrO_2 \cdot 1HAp$; (e) $7ZrO_2 \cdot 3HAp$; and (f) $5ZrO_2 \cdot 5HAp$ gels, heated to 1000°C, after 24 h of exposure to BSA solution. *BSA*, bovine serum albumin; *FTIR*, Fourier-transform infrared spectroscopy; *HAp*, hydroxyapatite particles. Adapted from F. Bollino, E. Armenia, E. Tranquillo, Zirconia/hydroxyapatite composites synthesized via sol-gel: influence of hydroxyapatite content and heating on their biological properties, Materials 10 (2017) 757. https://doi.org/10.3390/ma10070757 via (CC BY 4.0) license.

more experience in FTIR analysis and discussion. SEM micrographs of the same samples of Fig. 4.15 are shown in Fig. 4.16. The formation of globular-shaped particles is a typical indication of the formation of HAp, and much research finds that SEM results are adequate to prove the formation of HAp. Finally, Fig. 4.17 shows that the Ca/P ratio of 1.41 (i.e., <1.67) clearly identifies that the formed HAp at the surface of the samples of Figs. 4.15 and 4.16 are of the type of calcium-deficient HAp frequently found to grow on the surface of bioactive materials after in vitro tests.

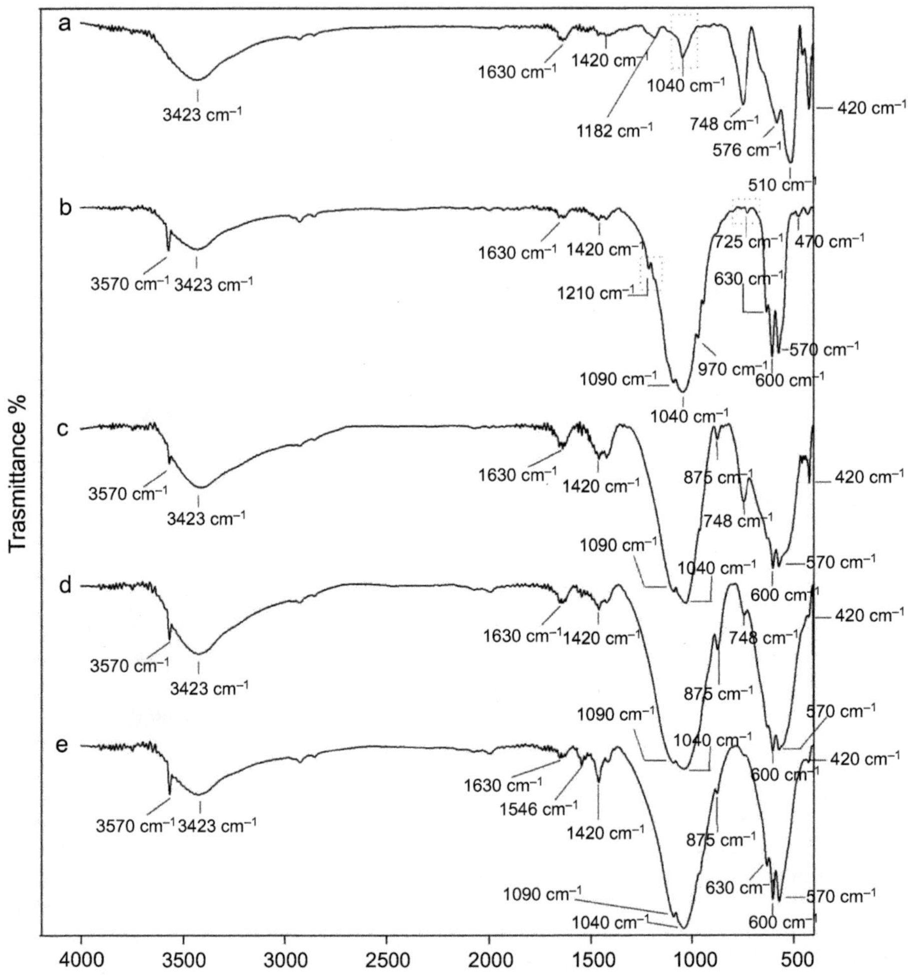

Figure 4.15 FTIR of (a) ZrO_2; (b) HAp; (c) $9ZrO_2 \cdot 1HAp$; (d) $7ZrO_2 \cdot 3HAp$; and (e) $5ZrO_2 \cdot 5HAp$ gels, heated to 1000°C, after 21 days of exposure to SBF. *FTIR*, Fourier-transform infrared spectroscopy; *HAp*, hydroxyapatite particles; *SBF*, simulated body fluid. Adapted from F. Bollino, E. Armenia, E. Tranquillo, Zirconia/hydroxyapatite composites synthesized via sol-gel: influence of hydroxyapatite content and heating on their biological properties, Materials 10 (2017) 757. https://doi.org/10.3390/ma10070757 via (CC BY 4.0) license.

The trend to introduce bioactivity to dental materials is not only limited to dental implants but also includes restorations. An example is the excellent work that appears in [10] that studies the addition of bioactive glass to glass ionomer cements. The study includes X-ray diffraction (XRD), FTIR, SEM, and other characterizations, which are worth careful reading and only some of the results are abbreviated here.

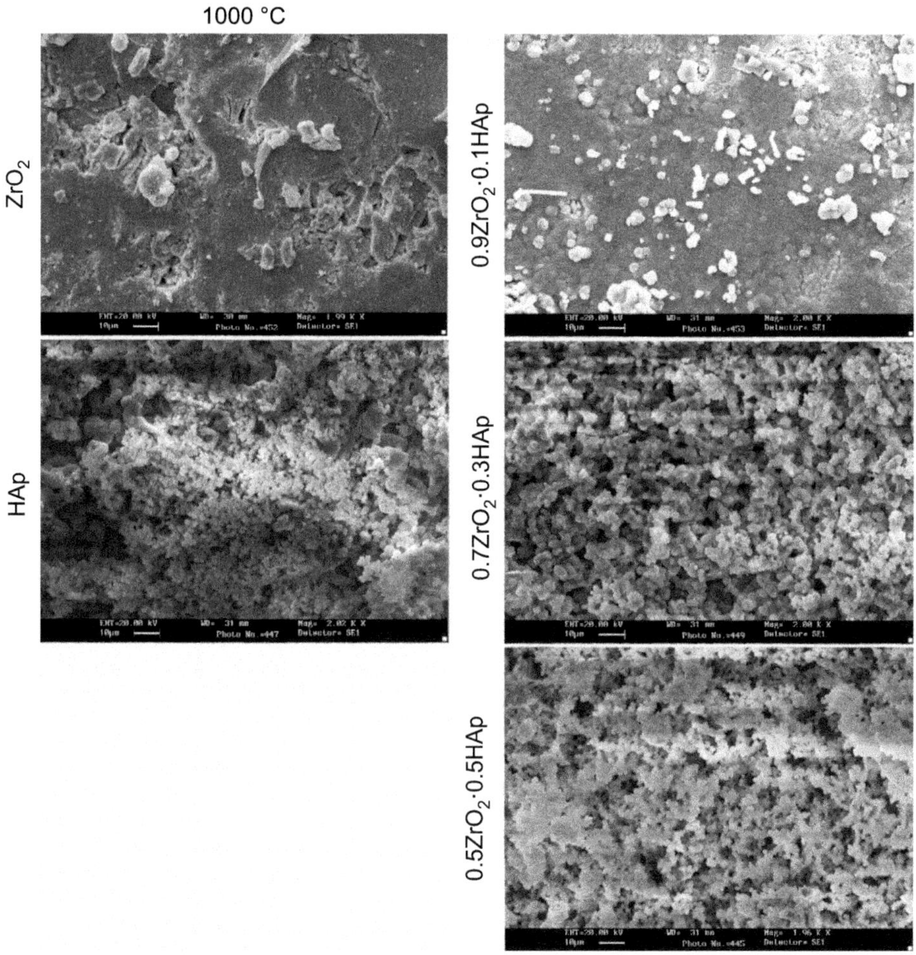

Figure 4.16 Scanning electron microscope micrographs of samples heated at 1000°C after 21 days of exposure to simulated body fluid.
Adapted from F. Bollino, E. Armenia, E. Tranquillo, Zirconia/hydroxyapatite composites synthesized via sol-gel: influence of hydroxyapatite content and heating on their biological properties, Materials 10 (2017) 757. https://doi.org/10.3390/ma10070757 via (CC BY 4.0) license.

Table 4.1 shows the synthesized glasses in this study with the symbols that will be used in the captions of the next three figures.

The development of the apatite layer is clear after incubation in SBF for both 45S5F-containing cements (Fig. 4.18) and CF9-containing cements (Fig. 4.19). The amount of apatite formation increases the increase in bioactive glass content. However, the authors of the original article [10] have some concerns about the high amounts of apatite that formed at the surface of the CF9-containing cements. They found that the

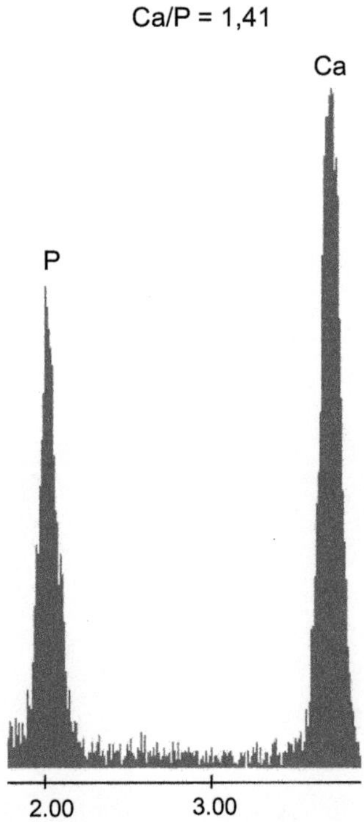

Figure 4.17 Energy-dispersive X-ray spectroscopy analysis of the globular precipitate on the surface of the samples heated at 1000°C after 21 days of exposure to simulated body fluid. Adapted from F. Bollino, E. Armenia, E. Tranquillo, Zirconia/hydroxyapatite composites synthesized via sol-gel: influence of hydroxyapatite content and heating on their biological properties, Materials 10 (2017) 757. https://doi.org/10.3390/ma10070757 via (CC BY 4.0) license.

Table 4.1 Glass compositions in mol% and synthesis conditions in °C and hours

	ASG	45S5F-0Al	45S5F-10Al	45S5F-20Al	CF9-0Al	CF9-10Al	CF9-20Al
SiO_2	32.1	48	38	28	34.6	24.6	14.6
Al_2O_3	21.4	0	5	10	0	5	10
Na_2O	0	25.4	25.4	25.4	0	0	0
CaO	21.4	14	14	14	50.38	50.38	50.38
CaF_2	14.3	10	10	10	9.28	9.28	9.28
P_2O_5	10.7	2.6	2.6	2	5.74	5.74	5.74
Temperature	1450	1430	1430	1500	1430	1430	1430
Time	2	1.5	1.5	3	1	1	1.5

ASG is conventional aluminosilicate glass; 45S5F and CF9 are fluoride-containing modified bioactive glasses [11–14]; and xAl indicates the glass contains 0.5× mol% of alumina.
Reused from T. De Caluwé, C.W.J. Vercruysse, I. Ladik, R. Convents, H. Declercq, L.C. Martens, R.M.H. Verbeeck, Addition of bioactive glass to glass ionomer cements: effect on the physico-chemical properties and biocompatibility, Dental Materials 33 (2017) e186–e203. https://doi.org/10.1016/j.dental.2017.01.007 after license via (copyright.com) number 4255270064488.

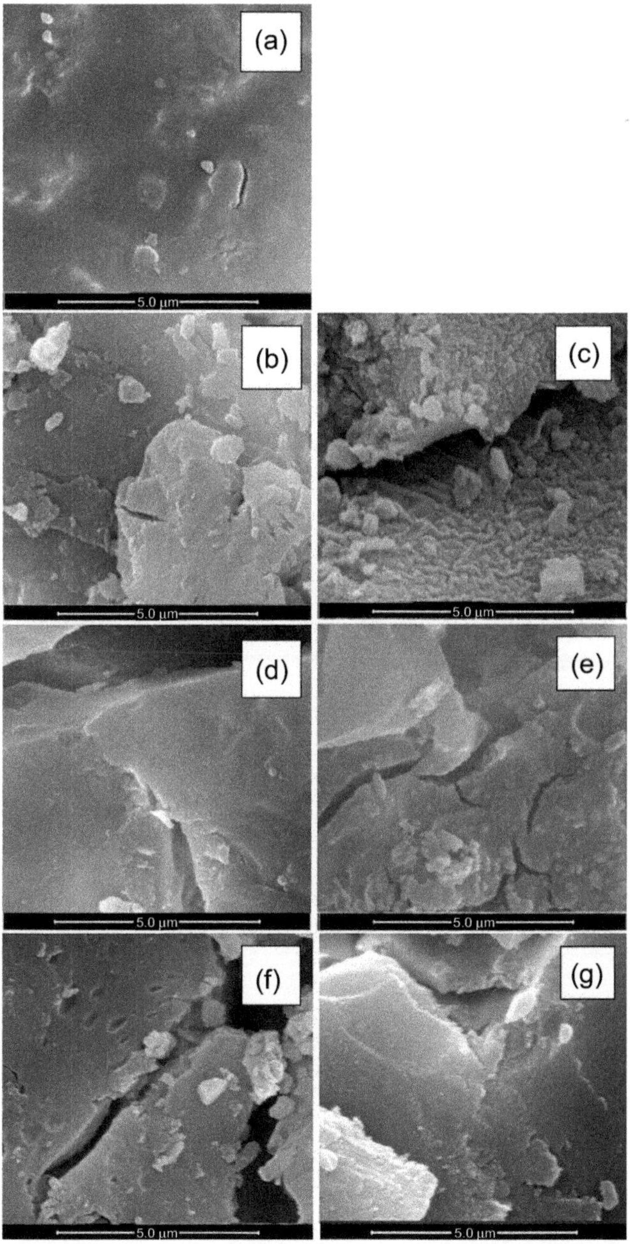

Figure 4.18 Scanning electron microscope micrographs of the surfaces of the 45S5F-containing cements. (a) 20-45S5F-0Al before incubation in simulated body fluid (SBF), (b and c) 10- and 20-45S5F-0Al after 28 days of incubation in SBF, (d and e) 10- and 20-45S5F-10Al after 28 days of incubation in SBF, and (f and g) 10- and 20-45S5F-20Al after 28 days of incubation in SBF. Reused from T. De Caluwé, C.W.J. Vercruysse, I. Ladik, R. Convents, H. Declercq, L.C. Martens, R.M.H. Verbeeck, Addition of bioactive glass to glass ionomer cements: effect on the physico-chemical properties and biocompatibility, Dental Materials 33 (2017) e186–e203. https://doi.org/10.1016/j.dental.2017.01.007 after license via (copyright.com) number 4255270064488.

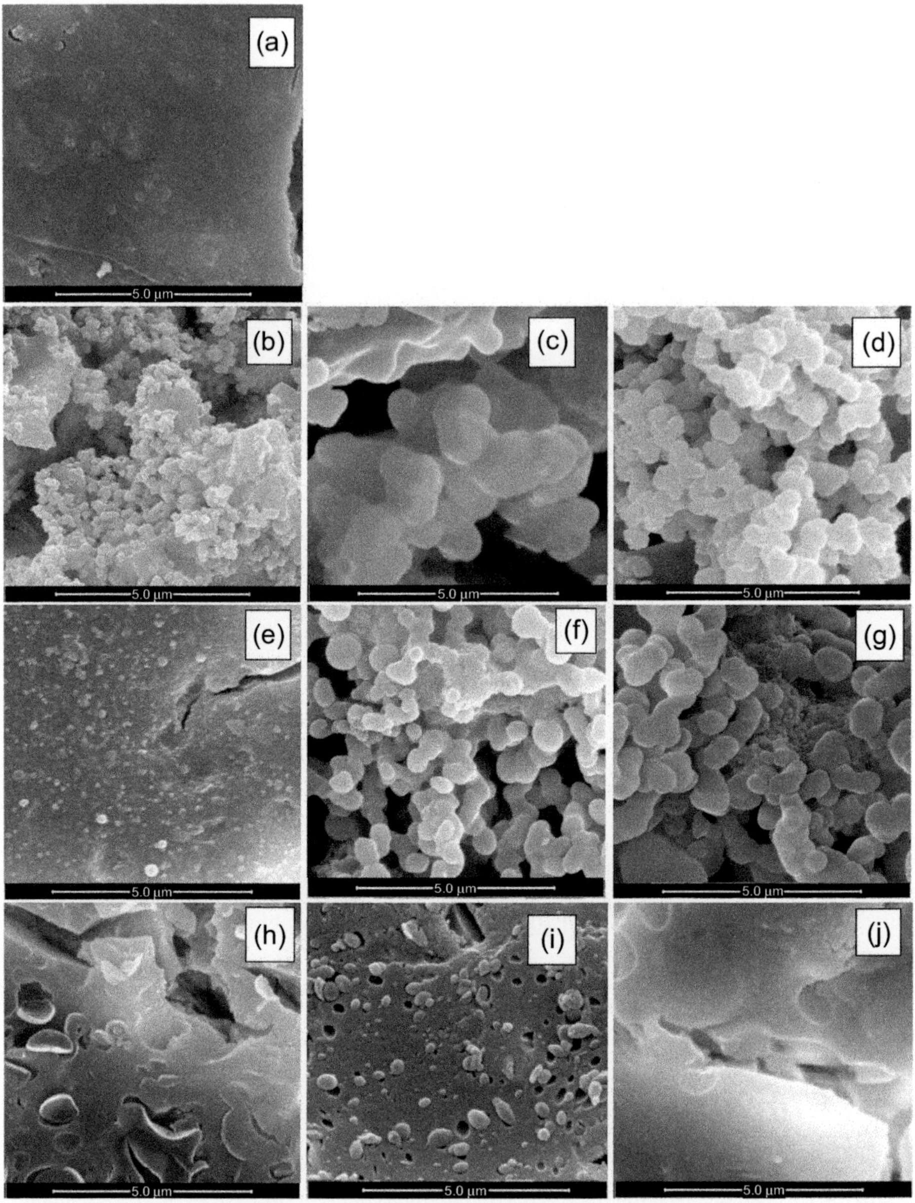

Figure 4.19 Scanning electron microscope micrographs of the surfaces of CF9-containing cements. (a) 30-CF9-0Al before incubation in simulated body fluid (SBF), (b–d) 10-, 20-, and 30-CF9-0Al, respectively, after 28 days of incubation in SBF, (e–g) 10-, 20-, and 30-CF9-10Al, respectively, after 28 days of incubation in SBF, and (h–j) 10-, 20-, and 30-CF9-20Al, respectively, after 28 days of incubation in SBF.
Reused from T. De Caluwé, C.W.J. Vercruysse, I. Ladik, R. Convents, H. Declercq, L.C. Martens, R.M.H. Verbeeck, Addition of bioactive glass to glass ionomer cements: effect on the physico-chemical properties and biocompatibility, Dental Materials 33 (2017) e186–e203. https://doi.org/10.1016/j.dental.2017.01.007 after license via (copyright.com) number 4255270064488.

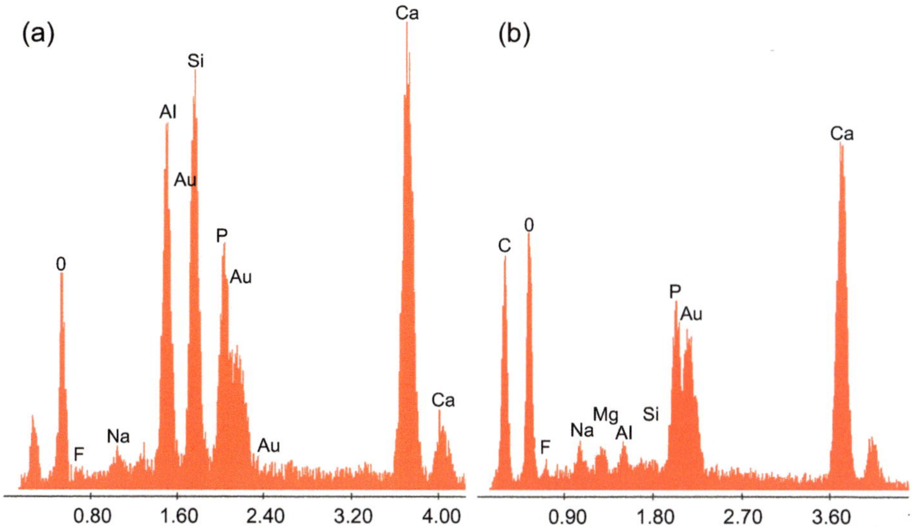

Figure 4.20 Energy-dispersive X-ray spectroscopy of the plain surface (a) of 30-CF9-0Al and of the spherical structures (b) on the surface of 30-CF9-0Al after incubation in simulated body fluid.
Reused from T. De Caluwé, C.W.J. Vercruysse, I. Ladik, R. Convents, H. Declercq, L.C. Martens, R.M.H. Verbeeck, Addition of bioactive glass to glass ionomer cements: effect on the physico-chemical properties and biocompatibility, Dental Materials 33 (2017) e186–e203. https://doi.org/10.1016/j.dental.2017.01.007 after license via (copyright.com) number 4255270064488.

high amounts of apatite, as seen in Fig. 4.20, impede cell proliferation, especially in the early stages after implantation.

In conclusion, in spite of the success stories of bioceramics in orthopedics and dentistry, demineralized bone matrix, an acid-extracted organic matrix from human bone sources, continues to be the subject of various research because of its long clinical history. A good review appears in Ref. [11].

Review questions

1. Make a table that includes examples of the first, second, and third generations of bioceramics.
2. Distinguish between the first, second, and third generations of the materials used in TKPs.
3. Write a short assay about the problem of radiolucent lines in alumina prostheses.
4. Try to find out why ceria further improves TZP-reinforced alumina.
5. Working as a group, go through the literature, learn about ductile ceramics, and suggest candidate ductile ceramics for orthopedic applications.
6. Briefly discuss the synthesis of third-generation alumina-on-alumina for THA and their advantages versus cost.

7. Find an example in the literature that shows the importance of the design consideration in THA and briefly present it.
8. Do the first, second, and third generations of bioceramics resemble examples of materials design? On what basis?
9. How does BIOLOX Delta resemble advanced materials design? What are the outcomes?
10. Draw a sketch that shows the correlations between structure, microstructure, characterization, properties, and performance of materials.
11. Compare your sketch with those of your colleagues and discuss the differences. How do these types of discussion enrich your knowledge?
12. Distinguish between the role of strength and fracture toughness of bioceramics in orthopedic implants. You can use the case of Fig. 4.7 as an example.
13. State the advantages of using zirconia for all-ceramic fixed dental prostheses.
14. State the advantages of materials designs shown in Fig. 4.8.
15. Briefly state the effect of surface properties of Y-TZP on the bioactivity of dental implants based on a discussion of Figs. 4.9–4.12.
16. Distinguish between the utilization of SBF and BSA in the course of in vitro tests.
17. In Figs. 4.13–4.15, how are FTIR measurements utilized? Refer to the references of these figures.
18. Briefly discuss why the role of EDX is to complete the conception of SEM in many cases. Use Figs. 4.16 and 4.17 or choose another article related to bioceramics.
19. Refer to the original article of Figs. 4.18–4.20 and try to find a numerical relation between the XRD and FTIR peak intensities with bioactive glass content. Then try finding a relation with the alumina content of the composites.
20. What lesson is extracted from the foregoing relations? Does EDX help in completing the picture?

References

[1] H. Oonishi, S.-C. Kim, M. Kyomoto, M. Iwamoto, M. Ueno, Comparison of in-vivo wear between polyethylene inserts articulating against ceramic and cobalt-chrome femoral components in total knee prostheses, in: Bioceramics and Alternative Bearings in Joint Arthroplasty, Steinkopff, 2007, pp. 149–159, https://doi.org/10.1007/978-3-7985-1783-7_20.

[2] B.-J. Kang, Y.-C. Ha, D.-W. Ham, S.-C. Hwang, Y.-K. Lee, K.-H. Koo, Third-generation alumina-on-alumina total hip arthroplasty: 14 to 16-year follow-up study, The Journal of Arthroplasty 30 (2015) 411–415, https://doi.org/10.1016/j.arth.2014.09.020.

[3] J.J. Yoo, P.W. Yoon, Y.-K. Lee, K.-H. Koo, K.S. Yoon, H.J. Kim, Revision total hip arthroplasty using an alumina-on-alumina bearing surface in patients with osteolysis, The Journal of Arthroplasty 28 (2013) 132–138, https://doi.org/10.1016/j.arth.2012.04.030.

[4] Y. Nakamura, H. Mitsui, A. Kikuchi, S. Toh, H. Katano, Total hip arthroplasty using a cylindrical cementless stem in patients with a small physique, The Journal of Arthroplasty 26 (2011) 77–81, https://doi.org/10.1016/j.arth.2009.10.014.

[5] Y.-H. Kim, J.-W. Park, J.-S. Kim, Alumina delta-on-alumina delta bearing in cementless total hip arthroplasty in patients aged <50 years, The Journal of Arthroplasty 31 (2016) 2209–2214, https://doi.org/10.1016/j.arth.2016.03.016.

[6] A.A. Aoude, J. Antoniou, L.M. Epure, O.L. Huk, D.J. Zukor, M. Tanzer, Midterm outcomes of the recently FDA approved ceramic on ceramic bearing in total hip arthroplasty patients under 65 years of age, The Journal of Arthroplasty 30 (2015) 1388–1392, https://doi.org/10.1016/j.arth.2015.03.028.

[7] T. Miyazaki, T. Nakamura, H. Matsumura, S. Ban, T. Kobayashi, Current status of zirconia restoration, Journal of Prosthodontic Research 57 (2013) 236–261, https://doi.org/10.1016/j.jpor.2013.09.001.
[8] H.M.T.U. Herath, L. Di Silvio, J.R.G. Evans, Osteoblast response to zirconia surfaces with different topographies, Materials Science and Engineering: C 57 (2015) 363–370, https://doi.org/10.1016/j.msec.2015.07.052.
[9] F. Bollino, E. Armenia, E. Tranquillo, Zirconia/hydroxyapatite composites synthesized via sol-gel: influence of hydroxyapatite content and heating on their biological properties, Materials 10 (2017) 757, https://doi.org/10.3390/ma10070757.
[10] T. De Caluwé, C.W.J. Vercruysse, I. Ladik, R. Convents, H. Declercq, L.C. Martens, R.M.H. Verbeeck, Addition of bioactive glass to glass ionomer cements: effect on the physico-chemical properties and biocompatibility, Dental Materials 33 (2017) e186–e203, https://doi.org/10.1016/j.dental.2017.01.007.
[11] E. Gruskin, B.A. Doll, F.W. Futrell, J.P. Schmitz, J.O. Hollinger, Demineralized bone matrix in bone repair: history and use, Advanced Drug Delivery Reviews 64 (2012) 1063–1077, https://doi.org/10.1016/j.addr.2012.06.008.
[12] G. Lusvardi, G. Malavasi, L. Menabue, V. Aina, C. Morterra, Fluoride-containing bioactive glasses: surface reactivity in simulated body fluids solutions, Acta Biomaterialia 5 (2009) 3548–3562, https://doi.org/10.1016/j.actbio.2009.06.009.
[13] D.S. Brauer, M.N. Anjum, M. Mneimne, R.M. Wilson, H. Doweidar, R.G. Hill, Fluoride-containing bioactive glass-ceramics, Journal of Non-Crystalline Solids 358 (2012) 1438–1442, https://doi.org/10.1016/j.jnoncrysol.2012.03.014.
[14] M. Mneimne, R.G. Hill, A.J. Bushby, D.S. Brauer, High phosphate content significantly increases apatite formation of fluoride-containing bioactive glasses, Acta Biomaterialia 7 (2011) 1827–1834, https://doi.org/10.1016/j.actbio.2010.11.037.

Hard tissue engineering applications

5

Tissue engineering is a treatment concept that aims to recover or replace damaged or missing tissue. Tissue engineering has a different strategy to replacing the missing organ by an implant. Nevertheless, tissue engineering relies on biodegradable and/or biosorbable materials that provide an in vivo chemical environment suitable for the growth of new tissue. A lot of research work has been performed for this rather new discipline, but it needs further efforts for development and maturity. Hard tissue engineering is at a better development stage compared with that of soft tissue. The discovery of bioactive glass may assign the benchmark toward hard tissue engineering. Calcium phosphate bioceramics show outstanding biocompatibility with bone and teeth because of the chemical similarity with hard tissues in mammals. The controlled dissociation of bioceramic implants in vivo injects the host environment with the necessary ions that enhance the growth of natural tissue. The success stories of calcium phosphate bioceramics extend to skin and muscle tissue replacement, but this chapter is limited to hard tissue engineering.

To be closer to materials science, tissue engineering may be defined as guided cell growth and tissue regeneration. To accomplish this, materials and microstructural design factors should be fulfilled. Design factors are discussed in Ref. [1] and a brief description will be given here of the case of hard tissue engineering. Materials selection and design for hard tissue engineering begin with the selection procedure of bioactive materials to encourage cell attachment. Another factor is that the selected material is bioresorbable to provide a suitable chemical environment that encourages cell propagation (proliferation). Examples of these bioceramics have already been mentioned in previous chapters. The shape-forming process may acquire suitable binders that make polymers, including natural or synthetic polymers, necessary. The included polymers are ordinarily biodegradable. In other words, in most cases the materials used for hard tissue engineering are composites of bioresorbable ceramics and biodegradable polymers. The microstructural design factors are the porosity, pore size, and interconnection of the porosity. Total porosity affects the speed of tissue regeneration in favor of large surface area, choice of a sufficiently large pore size helps to provide enough space for cell growth, and interconnected porosity is mandatory to ensure efficient material transport and cell migration. It may be useful to expand our knowledge by careful reading of parts I and II of the aforementioned study [1,2].

Typically, cells are seeded on a porous scaffold to enhance new tissue generation. The process is a complicated mechanism of cell growth, proliferation, and apoptosis (programmed cell death by a physiological process). These mechanisms are outside the scope of materials science. Adaptation between the experience of the materials scientist and that of the surgeon needs huge efforts from both sides. In addition, tissue engineering is considered to be in its early development stages because it needs further work to explore cell–scaffold (cell–material) interactions [3].

Bioceramics: For Materials Science and Engineering. https://doi.org/10.1016/B978-0-08-102233-7.00005-7

Degradable materials were previously called bioresorbable materials, as seen previously in this book. However, the degradation–resorption process should be controlled for successful tissue regeneration. Normally, this starts with the selection of the proper materials. Table 5.1 shows a number of biodegradable materials used in hard tissue engineering together with their degradation times. The mechanical properties of these materials (polymers and ceramics) are also shown and compared with those of human cortical and cancellous bone. Bioglass is not included in the table because it is generally not degradable and is usually used for bone defect fillers. On the other hand, other types of bioactive glasses and glass-ceramics used for degradable scaffolds can be found in the literature and the following examples.

The first example is that bioactive glass type 13-93 and polyurethane foam were used to prepare porous scaffolds via a polymer foam replication technique; details can be found in Ref. [108]. The resultant microstructure had a porosity of $85 \pm 2\%$ and pore size of 100–500 μm, analogous to that of human trabecular bone, as seen in Fig. 5.1. It is always necessary to check for bioactivity by, e.g., soaking in simulated body fluid (SBF) solution. Bioactivity is confirmed by the observation of a porous network of nanometer-sized, needle-like crystals at the surface (Fig. 5.2) that is shown smooth before the bioactivity test in Fig. 5.1.

Fig. 5.3 shows the morphology of MC3T3-E1 cell growth on the surface of the 13-93 glass scaffolds for various times. A simple description of MC3T3-E1 is that they are osteoblast precursor cells that can be grown for prolonged periods in vitro and thus are widely used as model systems in bone biology. Cell growth and spread are increased with time along the dense struts of the scaffold. The high-magnification part of Fig. 5.3(c) reveals that the cells grow into pores of size less than 100 μm.

We can find a lot of accomplishments for bioactive glass 13-93 in the literature. This type of glass, for example, is used to fabricate scaffolds with an oriented microstructure [109] and is implanted in rat calvarial defects. Two types of microstructure are fabricated and inspected. Oriented and trabecular microstructures of the scaffolds are fabricated according to the methods described in Refs. [108,110]. The properties of the fabricated scaffolds are shown in Table 5.2, and the cross-sections of these scaffolds are shown in Fig. 5.4.

The scaffolds are implanted in rat calvarial defects, and the progress of bone regeneration and integration is observed after 12 and 24 weeks of implantation via the synchrotron microcomputed X-ray tomography (SR microCT or μCT) technique. μCT is a high-resolution CT that allows observation at the micrometer level. In X-rays or ultrasound tomography, the differences in density of the scanned object signify different compositions and serve to read the image. Fig. 5.5 shows μCT for the slice at the middle across the thickness of the implant. The light gray color indicates a calcium-rich area of the unconverted bioactive glass and also indicates partial conversion of the glass into calcium phosphates and mineralized tissue. The dark gray areas show calcium-depleted regions. The figure shows new bone growth after 12 weeks within the oriented scaffold and to lesser degree than that of trabecular scaffolds. Progress of bone regeneration and integration is observed after 24 weeks, especially at the periphery of the scaffolds.

Table 5.1 **Physical properties of natural bone tissue compared with other degradable materials and their applications [4–13]**

Material type	Compressive strength (MPa)	Tensile strength (MPa)	Young's modulus (GPA)	Elongation (%)	Degradation time (months)	Loss of total strength (months)	Applications for bone repair and regeneration
A. Bone							
Human cortical	131–224	35–283	17–20	1.07–2.10	NBR	None	Autograft and allograft used for defect filling, alveolar ridge augmentation, sinus
Human cancellous	5–10	1.5–38	0.05–0.1	0.5–3	NBR	0.5–1	Augmentation, dental ridge preservation [15–24]
B. Degradable							
Collagen	0.5–1	50–150	0.002–5	3	2–4	1–4	Carriers (sponges) for BMP [25–27], composite with HA [28], membranes for GBR [29,30], scaffolds [31]
Chitosan	1.7–3.4	35–75	2–18	1–2	4–6	<3	Scaffolds, microgranules, composite materials, VBA, membranes, xerogels [32–36]
PGA	340–920	55–80	5–7	15–20	3–4	1	Internal fixation, graft material, scaffold, composite [37–39]
PLLA	80–500	45–70	2.7	5–10	>24	3	Carrier for BMP, scaffolds, composite with HA [40–46]
D,L(PLA)	15–25	90–103	1.9	3–10	12–16	4	Fracture fixation, interference screws [47–49]
L(PLA)	20–30	100–150	2.7	5–10	>24	3	Fracture fixation, interference screws, scaffolds, bone graft material [38,41,50–53]

Continued

Table 5.1 Continued

Material type	Compressive strength (MPa)	Tensile strength (MPa)	Young's modulus (GPA)	Elongation (%)	Degradation time (months)	Loss of total strength (months)	Applications for bone repair and regeneration
PLGA	40–55	55–80	1.4–2.8	3–10	1–12	1	Interference screws, microspheres, and carriers for BMP, scaffolds, composite [54–57]
PCL	20–40	10–35	0.4–0.6	300–500	>24	>6	Scaffolds and composites with HA fillers [58–63]
HA	500–1000	40–200	80–110	0.5–1	>24	>12	Scaffolds, composites, bone fillers (granules and blocks), pastes, vertebroplasty, drug delivery, coatings [64–75]
TCP	154	25–80	60–75	1–2	>24	1–6	Bone fillers, injectable pastes, cements [76–86]
Brushite	35–60	15–25	40–55	2–3	>24	1–6	Drug delivery, restoration of metaphyseal defects, ligament anchor, reinforcement of
Monetite	15–25	10–15	22–35	3–4	3–6	1–3	Osteosynthesis screws, ridge preservation, vertical bone augmentation, defect filling, vertebroplasty [87–107]

BMP, Bone morphogenetic proteins; *Brushite*, $CaHPO_4 \cdot 2H_2O$; *GBR*, guided bone regeneration; *HA*, hydroxyapatite; *Monetite*, anhydrous Brushite; *NBR*, natural bone remodeling; *PCL*, polycaprolactone; *PEO*, polyethylene oxide; *PGA*, polyglycolic acid; *PLA*, polylactic acid; *PLGA*, polylactic glycolic acid; *PLLA*, poly-L-lactic acid; *TCP*, tricalcium phosphate; *VBA*, vertical bone augmentation.

Reused from Z. Sheikh, S. Najeeb, Z. Khurshid, V. Verma, H. Rashid, M. Glogauer, Biodegradable materials for bone repair and tissue engineering applications, Materials 8 (2015) 5744–5794. https://doi.org/10.3390/ma8095273 after (CC BY 4.0) license.

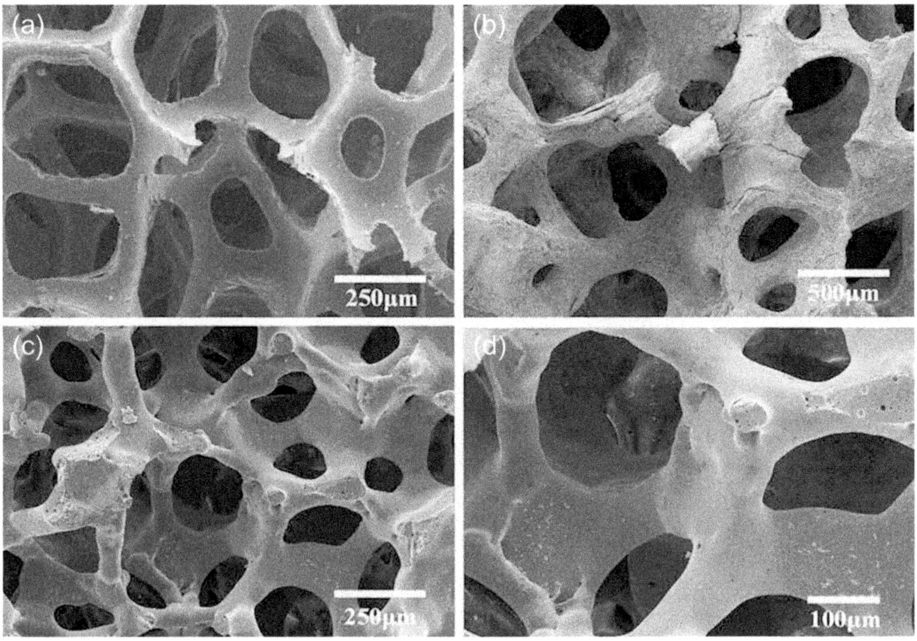

Figure 5.1 Scanning electron microscope micrographs show the microstructures of: (a) polyurethane foam used in the experiments; (b) dry human trabecular bone; and (c and d) 13–93 glass scaffolds fabricated by a polymer foam replication technique.
Reused from Q. Fu, M.N. Rahaman, B. Sonny Bal, R.F. Brown, D.E. Day, Mechanical and in vitro performance of 13–93 bioactive glass scaffolds prepared by a polymer foam replication technique, Acta Biomaterialia 4 (2008) 1854–1864. https://doi.org/10.1016/j.actbio.2008.04.019 after license via (copyright.com) number 4262990987260.

Bioglass-derived glass-ceramic scaffolds have been fabricated via the replication technique using premolded polyurethane sponges [111]. Porosity gradient of the scaffolds has been achieved by modifying mold profile and the mode of performance of the polyurethane. Continuous and stepwise gradient is possible for the same reason. After molding in trapezoidal-shaped aluminum foils and the process of the burning of the polymer, a Bioglass continuous gradient structure accomplished with different porosity levels can be seen, as in Fig. 5.6. In addition, stepwise gradient is achieved by using two polyurethane foams allowing fabrication of stepwise porosity with homogeneous and coherent interconnection (Fig. 5.7). After sintering the green porous glass scaffolds, as appear in Fig. 5.6, at 1100°C for 1 h, glass-ceramic scaffolds are produced with enhanced mechanical properties compared with the green glass scaffolds (Fig. 5.8). Accordingly, glass-ceramic scaffolds with high and graded porosity that mimic bone tissue have been achieved.

To conclude regarding the use of Bioglass in hard tissue engineering, it may be useful to learn from Table 5.3 that the various types of bioactive glasses, matrices, fabrication techniques, and their references may be found useful for students.

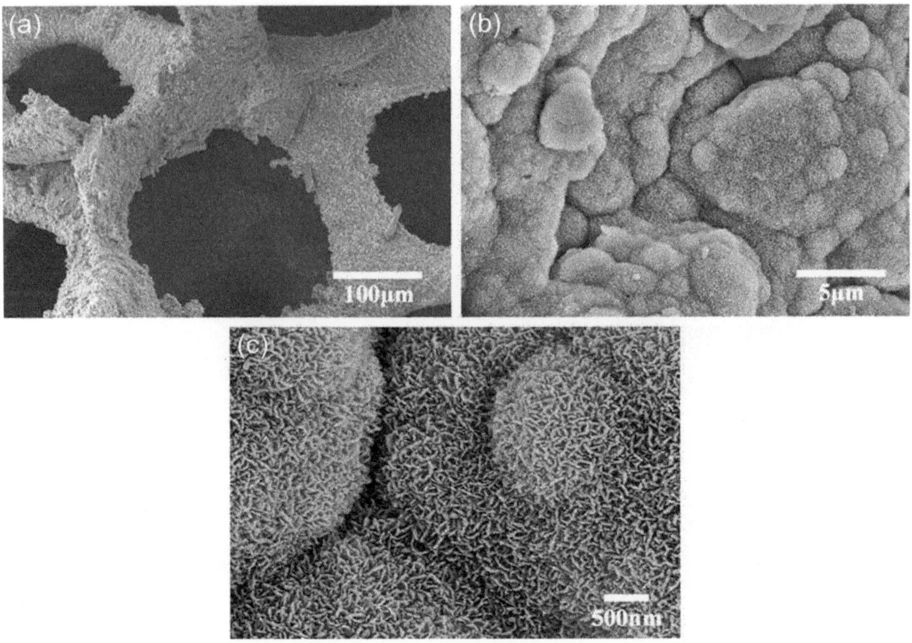

Figure 5.2 Scanning electron microscope micrographs of the surface of a 13–93 glass scaffold after immersion for 7 days in simulated body fluid: (a) lower magnification image; and (b and c) higher magnification image showing fine needle-like hydroxyapatite crystals.
Reused from Q. Fu, M.N. Rahaman, B. Sonny Bal, R.F. Brown, D.E. Day, Mechanical and in vitro performance of 13–93 bioactive glass scaffolds prepared by a polymer foam replication technique, Acta Biomaterialia 4 (2008) 1854–1864. https://doi.org/10.1016/j.actbio.2008.04.019 after license via (copyright.com) number 4262990987260.

Hydroxyapatite (HA) ceramic is also included in the design of scaffolds because of its known bioactivity and biodegradation. The porous ceramic scaffolds have the challenge of reduced mechanical properties with the increase in total porosity. Accordingly, their uses are limited to nonload-bearing applications. On the other hand, the final mechanical properties depend on the type of the process of fabrication of the scaffolds. The following example describes the use of freeze casting for the synthesis of porous scaffolds with compressive strengths. The scaffolds are fabricated via controlled freezing of HA slurries with different concentrations that end with different total porosities [135]. The obtained compressive strengths are 145 MPa for the scaffolds of 47% porosity and 65 MPa for the scaffolds of 56% porosity. The final product has three spatial zones of different porosities, as seen in Fig. 5.9. The figure shows dense zone followed by a zone with cellular morphology, and finally a long zone with pores parallel to the ice front associated with the freeze-casting process. The last zone is shown close to laminar morphology with interconnected macropores, as seen in Fig. 5.10. The concentration of the slurry is reflected in the final total porosity, as seen in Fig. 5.11.

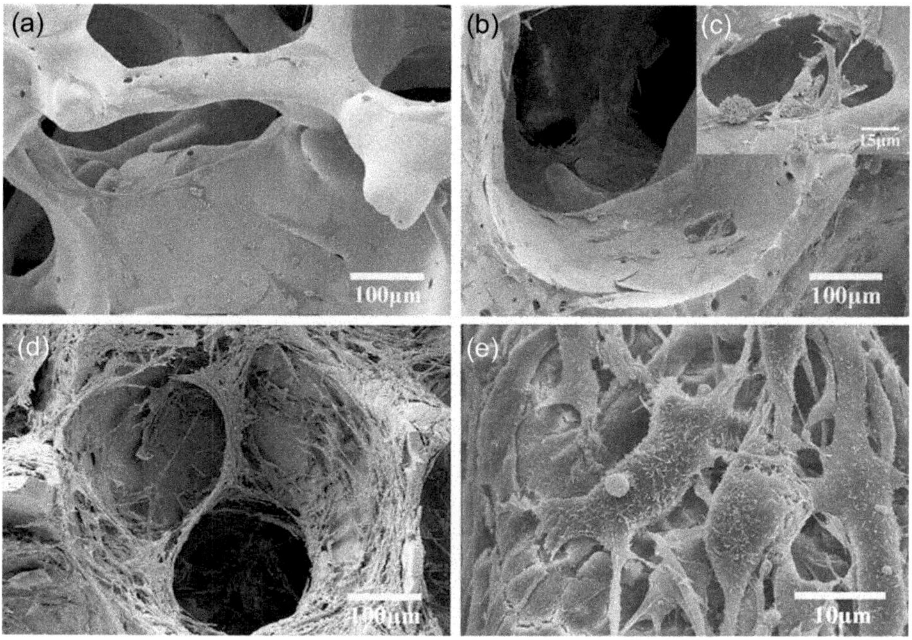

Figure 5.3 Scanning electron microscope micrographs of 13–93 glass scaffolds seeded with MC3T3-E1 cells and cultured for: (a) 2 days; (b and c) 4 days; and (d and e) 6 days.
Reused from Q. Fu, M.N. Rahaman, B. Sonny Bal, R.F. Brown, D.E. Day, Mechanical and in vitro performance of 13–93 bioactive glass scaffolds prepared by a polymer foam replication technique, Acta Biomaterialia 4 (2008) 1854–1864. https://doi.org/10.1016/j.actbio.2008.04.019 after license via (copyright.com) number 4262990987260.

Table 5.2 The properties of 13–93 bioactive glass scaffolds fabricated with oriented and trabecular microstructure

Scaffold	Porosity (%)	Pore size (μm)	Compressive strength (MPa)	Elastic modulus (GPa)	Fabrication method
Oriented	50±4	50–150	47±5	11±3	Unidirectional freezing of suspensions
Trabecular	80±5	100–500	11±1	3±0.5	Polymer foam replication

Reused from X. Liu, M.N. Rahaman, Q. Fu, Bone regeneration in strong porous bioactive glass (13–93) scaffolds with an oriented microstructure implanted in rat calvarial defects, Acta Biomaterialia 9 (2013) 4889–4898. https://doi.org/10.1016/j.actbio.2012.08.029 after license via (copyright.com) number 4264090327830.

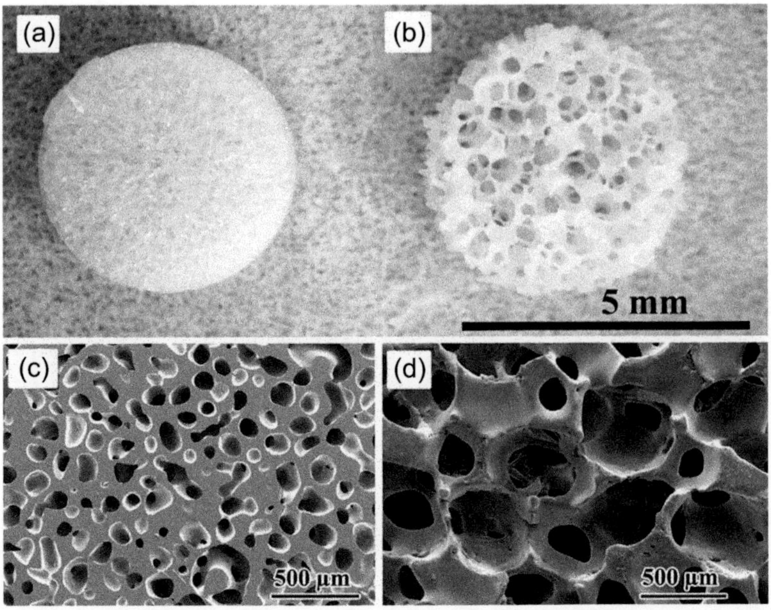

Figure 5.4 Optical micrographs of disc-shaped bioactive glass (13–93) scaffolds with (a) an oriented microstructure and (b) a trabecular microstructure (positive control). Scanning electron microscope micrographs of cross-sections of the (c) oriented scaffolds perpendicular to the pore orientation direction and (d) trabecular scaffolds.
Reused from X. Liu, M.N. Rahaman, Q. Fu, Bone regeneration in strong porous bioactive glass (13–93) scaffolds with an oriented microstructure implanted in rat calvarial defects, Acta Biomaterialia 9 (2013) 4889–4898. https://doi.org/10.1016/j.actbio.2012.08.029 after license via (copyright.com) number 4264090327830.

The wet chemical route is also used for the synthesis of HA [136]. The $(NH_4)_2HPO_4$ solution is added to the $Ca(NO_3)_2{\cdot}4H_2O$ solution in an amount that keeps the Ca/P molar ratio at 1.67 and results in a gel. The gel is dissolved by adding concentrated HNO_3. Finally, NH_4OH is added (pH ~ 10) to precipitate the powder particles. The resulting powder is calcined at 850°C for 2h to produce crystalline HA. The polymeric replica sponge method is utilized to produce scaffolds from solutions of HA and polyvinyl alcohol binder. After drying and sintering at 1250°C for 4h, the produced scaffolds are ready for characterization. Fig. 5.12 shows that there is an optimum solid (HA) loading that has a rigid microstructure with sufficiently open and interconnected pores. In addition, Fig. 5.13 shows new morphology after immersion in SBF, which indicates bioactivity of the scaffold, and the energy-dispersive X-ray spectroscopy and Fourier-transform infrared spectroscopy (FTIR) spectrum indicate the formation of carbonated HA.

The polymeric replica sponge method is also utilized to produce scaffolds from sol-gel–derived HA and polymer slurry, as shown in Fig. 5.14; details in Ref. [137]. This figure should be studied carefully because it is a typical experimental flowchart that presents similar studies. Apparently, the obtained porous body

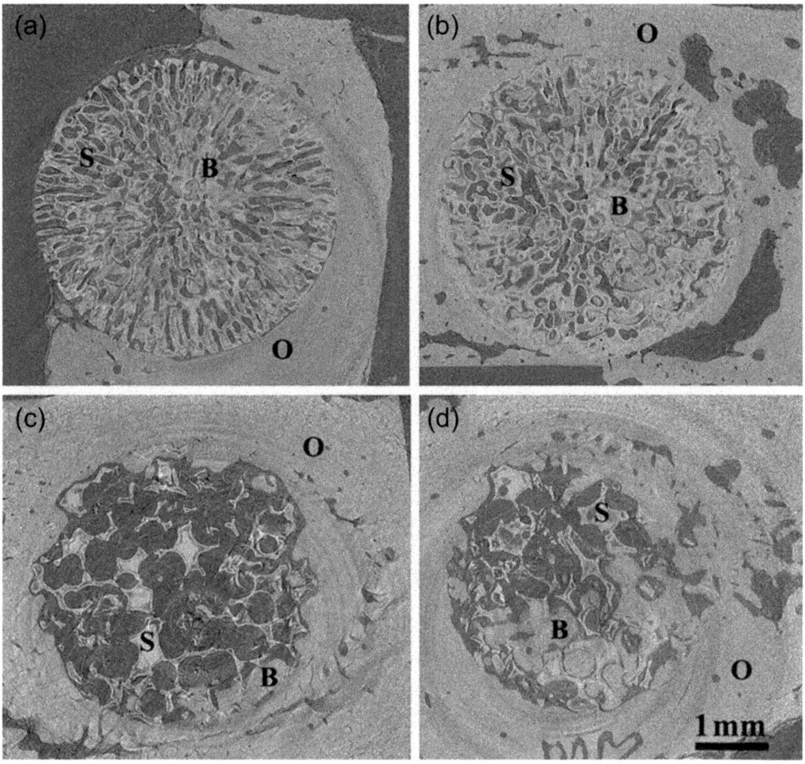

Figure 5.5 Synchrotron microcomputed X-ray tomography images of oriented scaffold after implantation for (a) 12 weeks and (b) 24 weeks, and trabecular scaffold after implantation for (c) 12 weeks and (d) 24 weeks. The distribution of old bone (O), new bone (B), and the bioactive glass scaffold (S) is shown.
Reused from X. Liu, M.N. Rahaman, Q. Fu, Bone regeneration in strong porous bioactive glass (13–93) scaffolds with an oriented microstructure implanted in rat calvarial defects, Acta Biomaterialia 9 (2013) 4889–4898. https://doi.org/10.1016/j.actbio.2012.08.029 after license via (copyright.com) number 4264090327830.

(Fig. 5.15) is more smooth and uniform than that obtained in the previous study, which may be attributed to lower solid loading and/or the absence of binder. Finally, osteoblast cell culturing is performed using SaOS2 cells. SaOS2 cells are originally derived from cancerous tumor in human bone, which can serve as an in vitro model for studying the transition of human osteoblasts to osteocytes. The results of culturing are shown in Fig. 5.16. Obviously, the cultured cells are attached to the scaffold, proliferated, and spread along the pores in a manner that maintains the cellular morphology.

The materials scientist should try to incorporate wollastonite with HA and to fabricate porous scaffolds and examine the mechanical properties, bioactivity, and biodegradation of the resultant scaffolds. In fact, this study has been performed [138] and it was found that the optimum mechanical strength of the sintered scaffolds was

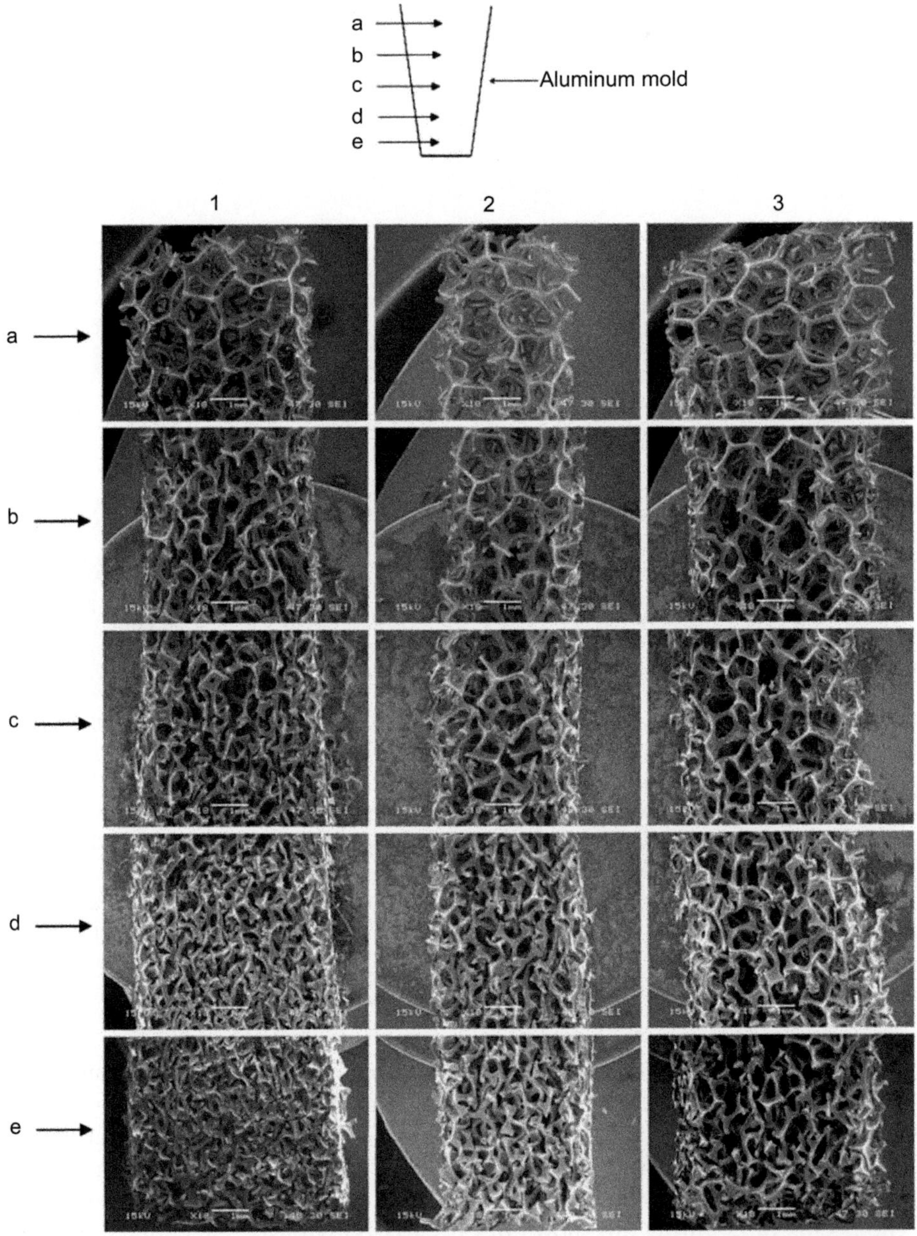

Figure 5.6 Scanning electron microscope micrographs of foams with 3D continuous gradient of porosity before sintering at different degrees of compaction: (1) 75%, (2) 65%, and (3) 50%. Reused from O. Bretcanu, C. Samaille, A.R. Boccaccini, Simple methods to fabricate Bioglass-derived glass–ceramic scaffolds exhibiting porosity gradient, Journal of Materials Science 43 (2008) 4127–4134. https://doi.org/10.1007/s10853-008-2536-y after license via (copyright.com) number 4265550239707.

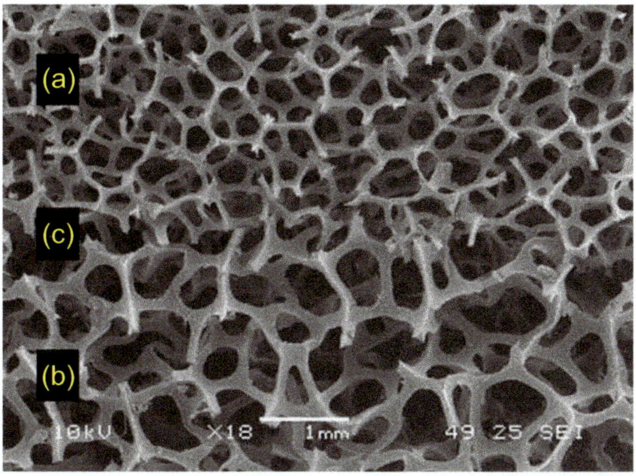

Figure 5.7 Scanning electron microscope micrographs of Bioglass preformed foam with stepwise gradient of porosity before sintering: (a) 65 ppi foam, (b) 45 ppi foam, and (c) interface. Reused from O. Bretcanu, C. Samaille, A.R. Boccaccini, Simple methods to fabricate Bioglass-derived glass–ceramic scaffolds exhibiting porosity gradient, Journal of Materials Science 43 (2008) 4127–4134. https://doi.org/10.1007/s10853-008-2536-y after license via (copyright.com) number 4265550239707.

obtained at 50% HA/50% wollastonite. In addition, bioactivity and biodegradability were also improved when the wollastonite was incorporated with the HA porous scaffolds.

Another worthy suggestion is to utilize calcium silicate as ceramic scaffolds because of its excellent bioactivity and biodegradability. The only barrier to using calcium silicate to fabricate porous scaffolds is its known brittleness. To overcome this difficulty, HA whiskers are used for reinforcing the calcium silicate [139]. The reinforcement contents were 0–30 wt%, but the optimum mechanical properties were obtained at 20 wt% of reinforcement. The compressive and flexural strengths, Young's modulus, and fracture toughness were 27.28 MPa, 15.64 MPa, 156.2 MPa, and 1.43 MPa $m^{1/2}$, respectively, at the optimum condition. The mechanical properties were enhanced in the presence of the HA whiskers via whisker pullout, crack deflection, and crack bridging. On the other hand, the known degradation rate for the composite was lower with the higher HA whisker content but with no serious effect. It is found that MG-63 cells (an osteosarcoma very like SaOS2 cells) are well proliferated and spread along the scaffolds with increasing culture time. It remains to state that the technique of "selective laser sintering" is utilized to fabricate the porous scaffolds. The selective laser sintering technique is a type of additive manufacturing called 3D printing with accompanied sintering by high-power laser.

A triphasic composite of HA, tricalcium phosphate, and calcium silicate (HASi) has been used as a coating for HA [140]. Porous HA scaffold was synthesized first via a freeze-drying technique, sintering at 1100 and 1300°C for 1 h, and dipping in a silica solution. The solution of silica was prepared via hydrolysis of tetraethyl orthosilicate

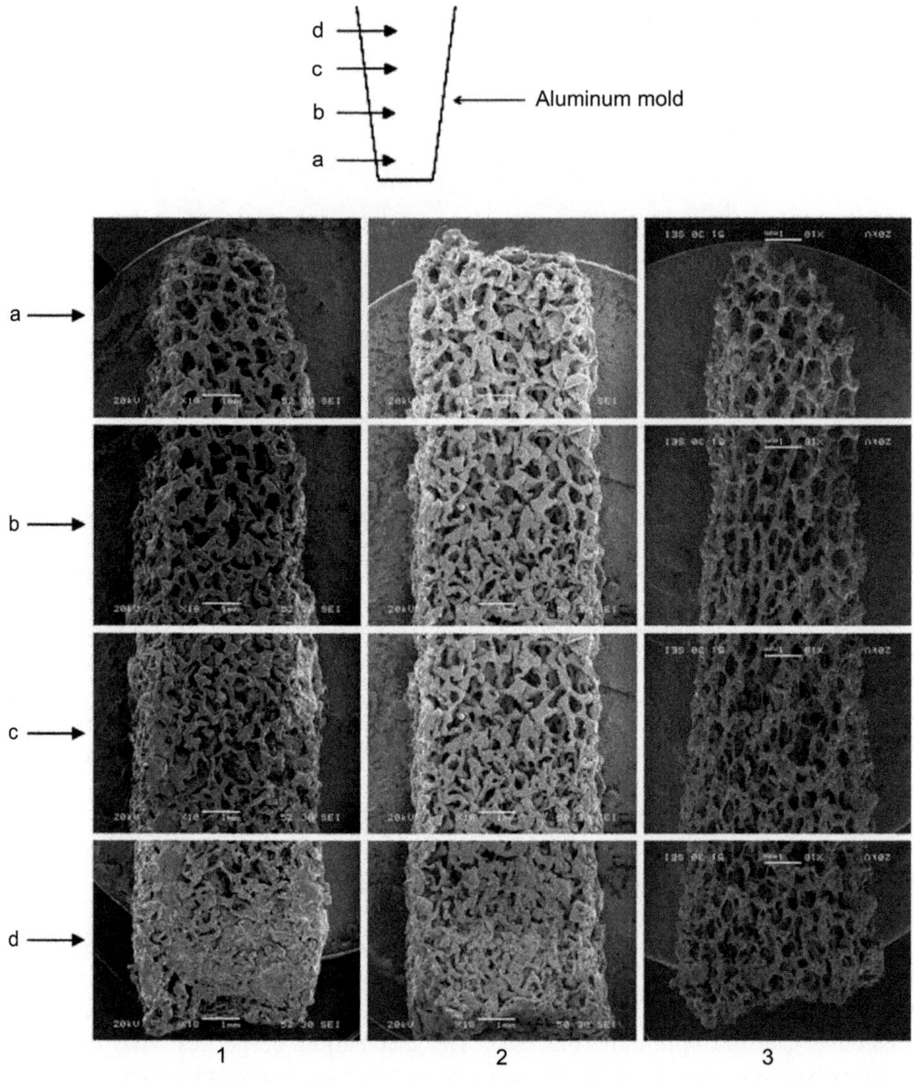

Figure 5.8 Scanning electron microscope micrographs of foams with 3D continuous gradient of porosity after sintering at different degrees of compaction: (1) 75%, (2) 65%, and (3) 50%. Reused from O. Bretcanu, C. Samaille, A.R. Boccaccini, Simple methods to fabricate Bioglass-derived glass–ceramic scaffolds exhibiting porosity gradient, Journal of Materials Science 43 (2008) 4127–4134. https://doi.org/10.1007/s10853-008-2536-y after license via (copyright.com) number 4265550991747.

Table 5.3 Overview of studies performed on bioactive glass containing composite scaffolds for bone tissue engineering

Bioactive glass	wt%	Particle size	Matrix	Fabrication technique/process	References
45S5 m-BG	5, 29, 40	<40 μm	PDLLA	Coextrusion + compaction; TIPS	[113]
45S5 m-BG	4.8, 28.6	5–20 μm	PDLLA	TIPS	[114]
45S5 m-BG	10	<5 μm	P(3HB)	ST/PL	[115]
45S5 n-BG	10	30 nm	P(3HB)	ST/PL	[115]
S53P4 m-BG	20, 50	90–315 μm	P(CL/DLLA)	ST/PL	[116]
S53P4 m-BG	30	<45 μm	P(CL/DLLA)	ST/PL	[117]
45S5 m-BG	10, 30	<40 μm	PLGA	Microsphere emulsification	[118]
45S5 m-BG	10	4 μm	PDLG	TIPS	[119]
45S5 m-BG	25, 50	50–63 μm	PLA	Freeze-extraction technique	[120]
45S5 m-BG	5, 40	>90 μm	PDLLA	Solvent casting	[121]
45S5 m-BG	10, 25, 50	<5 μm	PDLLA	TIPS	[122]
45S5 m-BG	10, 25, 50	<5 μm	PLGA	TIPS	[122]
45S5 m-BG	5, 10, 40	<5 μm	PDLLA	TIPS	[123]
45S5 m-BG	5, 40	<5 μm	PDLLA	TIPS	[124]
45S5 m-BG	10, 25, 50	<5 μm	PLGA	TIPS	[125]
45S5 m-BG	25	<40 μm	PLGA	Solvent casting	[126]
45S5 m-BG	20	<10 μm	P(3HB)	Solvent casting	[127]
45S5 m-BG	20	<5 μm	P(3HB)	Solvent casting	[128]
45S5 n-BG	10, 20	29 nm	P(3HB)	Solvent casting	[129]
45S5 m-BG	10, 20, 30	<5 μm	P(3HB)	Solvent casting	[130]
45S5 n-BG	10, 20, 30	30–50 nm	P(3HB)	Solvent casting	[130]
45S5 m-BG	5, 30	5 μm	PDLLA	TIPS	[131]
45S5 m-BG	5, 30	5 μm	PDLLA	TIPS	[132]
45S5 m-BG	5, 40	<5 μm	PDLLA	TIPS	[133]
SiO_2-3CaO-P_2O_5-MgO	10, 30, 50	10 μm	PLA	TIPS	[134]

m-BG, Micron-sized bioactive glass; *n-BG*, nanosized bioactive glass; *P(3HB)*, poly(3-hydroxybutyrate); *P(CL/DLLA)*, poly(caprolactone/D, L lactide); *PDLG*, poly(D, L lactide-*co*-glycolide); *PLA*, poly(L lactide); *PDLLA*, poly(D, L lactide); *PLGA*, poly(lactic-*co*-glycolic acid); *S53P4*, 53 wt% SiO_2, 23 wt% Na_2O, 20 wt% CaO, 4 wt% P_2O_5; *ST/PL*, sugar template/particulate leaching; *TIPS*, thermally induced phase separation.

Reused from L.-C. Gerhardt, A.R. Boccaccini, Bioactive glass and glass-ceramic scaffolds for bone tissue engineering, Materials (Basel) 3 (2010) 3867–3910. https://doi.org/doi:10.3390/ma3073867 after CC BY 3.0 license.

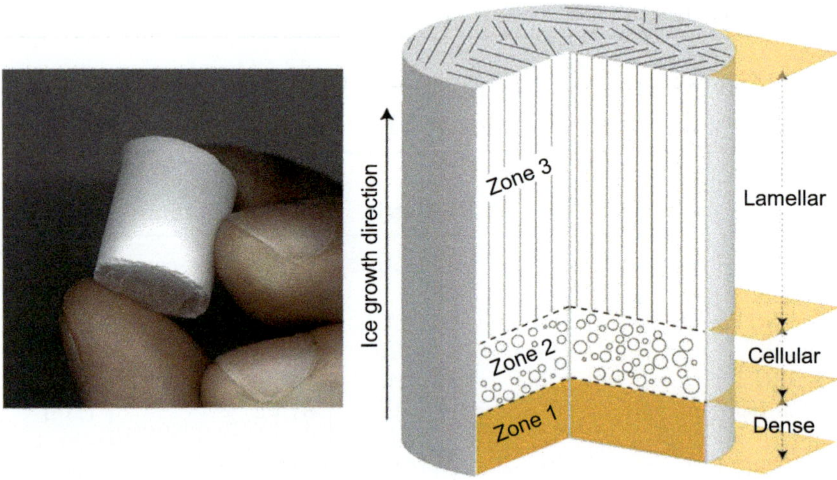

Figure 5.9 Typical sample (*left*) and general microstructure of porosity (*right*). Three distinctive zones are found, their dimensions depending largely on processing conditions.
Reused from S. Deville, E. Saiz, A.P. Tomsia, Freeze casting of hydroxyapatite scaffolds for bone tissue engineering, Biomaterials 27 (2006) 5480–5489. https://doi.org/10.1016/j.biomaterials.2006.06.028 after license via (copyright.com) number 4266921189736.

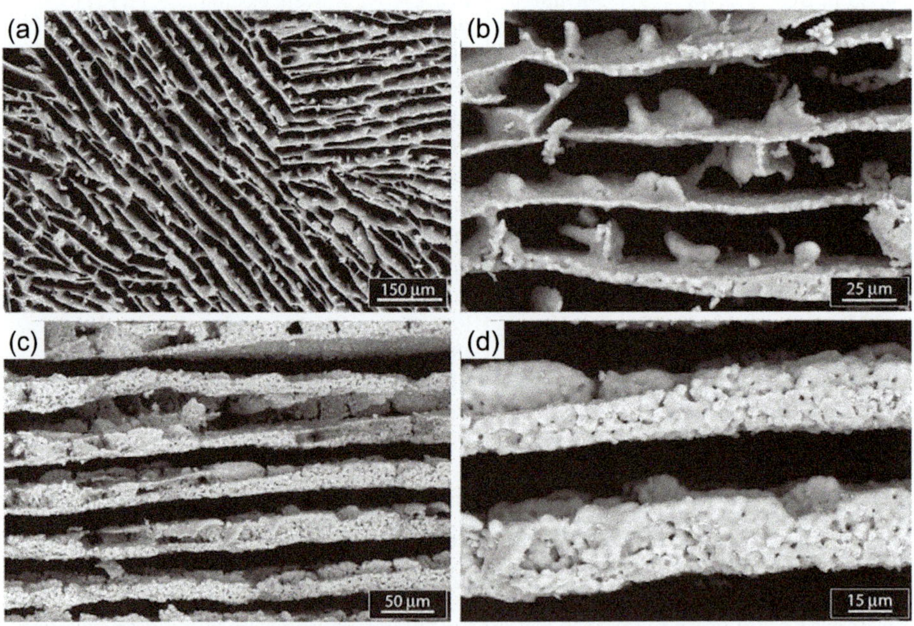

Figure 5.10 Microstructure of porous hydroxyapatite samples with 64% porosity. Cross-sections parallel to the ice front (a) and detail (b), and perpendicular to the ice front (c) and detail (d). The slight difference in wall thickness (b and d) arises from the presence of a small gradient of density at the upper surface of the sample (a and b) caused by particle segregation at the top of the mold during freezing.
Reused from S. Deville, E. Saiz, A.P. Tomsia, Freeze casting of hydroxyapatite scaffolds for bone tissue engineering, Biomaterials 27 (2006) 5480–5489. https://doi.org/10.1016/j.biomaterials.2006.06.028 after license via (copyright.com) number 4266921189736.

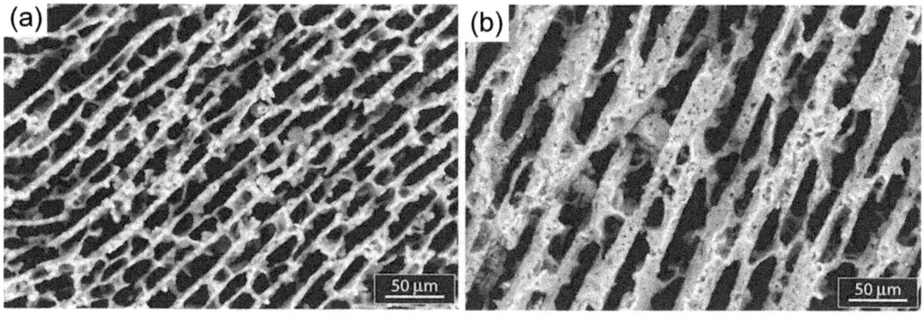

Figure 5.11 Effect of initial slurry concentration. Microstructure of porous hydroxyapatite samples is parallel to the ice front with (a) 64% porosity and (b) 47% porosity.
Reused from S. Deville, E. Saiz, A.P. Tomsia, Freeze casting of hydroxyapatite scaffolds for bone tissue engineering, Biomaterials 27 (2006) 5480–5489. https://doi.org/10.1016/j.biomaterials.2006.06.028 after license via (copyright.com) number 4266921189736.

dissolved in a mixture of ethanol and water for 1 min. The triphasic coat was achieved after sintering at 1200°C for 2 h. After that, a cleaning and sterilization procedure was applied. Goat bone marrow aspiration was utilized to produce bone marrow stromal (connective tissue) cells (BMSCs) to examine bioactivity, proliferation, and the mode of spreading along the interconnected pores of the scaffolds. BMSCs were used because of the ease of harvest from a donor bone marrow and their differentiation ability. Fig. 5.17 shows the interconnected pore morphology of HA before and after performing the coat, and Fig. 5.18 compares the differentiation of BMSCs on both types of HA. The figure clearly shows the advantage of the HASi scaffold in that it enhances adhesion, spreading of the cells, and forming of a cell sheet–like structure.

Introducing piezoelectricity to the bone substitute materials is known to benefit bone growth, remodeling, and fracture healing. A HA/barium titanate suspension is freeze-cast to fabricate an aligned porous piezoelectric composite scaffold [141]. The obtained piezoelectric coefficient of the scaffold is higher than that of natural bone. The presented process methodology and the resultant scaffold properties may fulfill potential customized needs of bone substitutes.

Porous HA scaffolds were prepared via a template method. Then, the scaffolds were coated by impregnation with collagen or with homogeneous collagen–HA slurry [142]. It was found that the mechanical properties were enhanced with both types of coating, especially with higher sintering temperature because of reduced porosity. Thus impregnation of the scaffolds with collagen or with a homogeneous collagen–ceramic mixture before sintering may offer another tool to tailor the properties of the scaffolds. Another work studied the effect of coating with an HA/poly(vinyl alcohol) nanocomposite via a vacuum-assisted impregnation method [143]. The scaffolds were macroporous TiO_2 fabricated via a polyurethane foam replication method with pore sizes of 100–500 μm. Yet again, the coating improved both the mechanical properties and the in vitro bioactivity.

An alternative processing route for producing porous scaffolds is the air pressure-aided deposition (APAD) of polymer ceramic slurry. The methoxypoly(ethylene

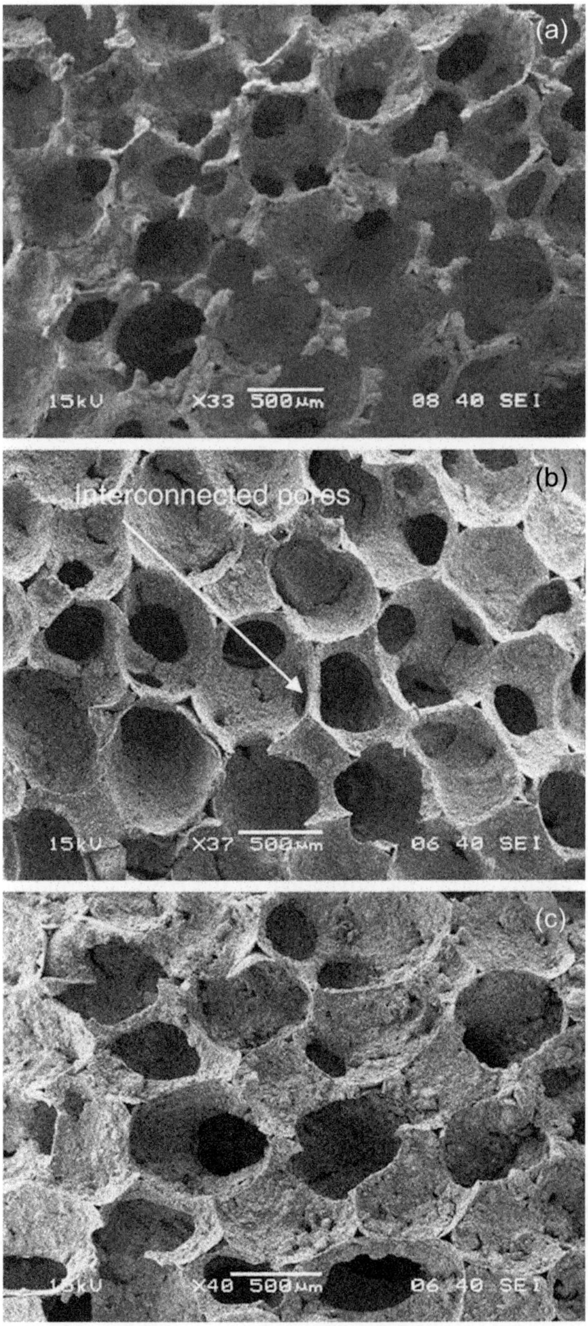

Figure 5.12 Scanning electron microscope micrographs of sintered hydroxyapatite scaffolds at 3 wt% polyvinyl alcohol with varying hydroxyapatite powder loadings: (a) 30 wt%, (b) 40 wt%, and (c) 50 wt%.

Reused from S.K. Swain, S. Bhattacharyya, D. Sarkar, Preparation of porous scaffold from hydroxyapatite powders, Materials Science and Engineering: C 31 (2011) 1240–1244. https://doi.org/10.1016/j.msec.2010.11.014 after license via (copyright.com) number 4267870620576.

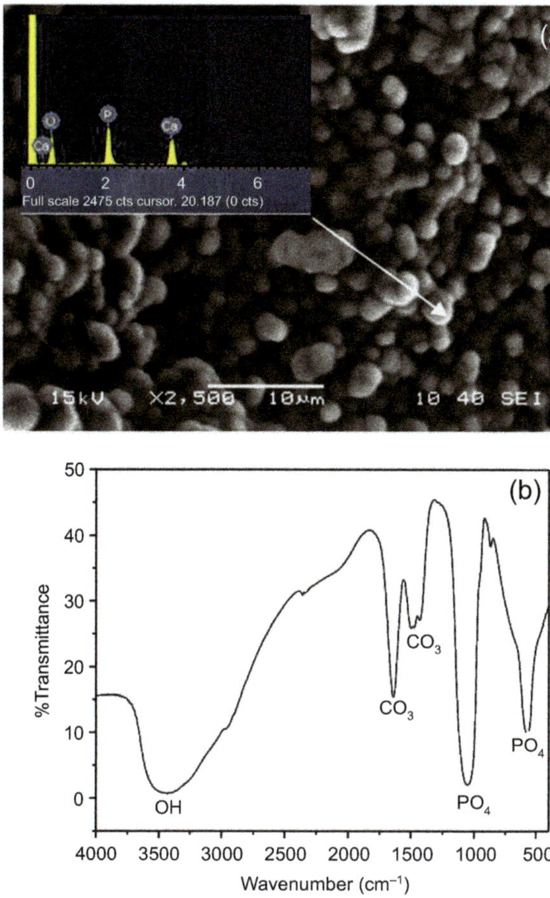

Figure 5.13 (a) Scanning electron microscope micrograph and energy-dispersive X-ray spectroscopy after simulated body fluid treatment of the hydroxyapatite scaffold and (b) their Fourier-transform infrared spectroscopy spectrum behavior.
Reused from S.K. Swain, S. Bhattacharyya, D. Sarkar, Preparation of porous scaffold from hydroxyapatite powders, Materials Science and Engineering: C 31 (2011) 1240–1244. https://doi.org/10.1016/j.msec.2010.11.014 after license via (copyright.com) number 4267870620576.

glycol)–poly(caprolactone) (PCL)–methoxypoly(ethylene glycol) triblock copolymer was used as a biopolymer, and the APAD process was utilized to fabricate scaffolds of the biopolymer–HA composite [144]. The APAD process was shown as a reproducible 3D porous biopolymer and biocomposite bone scaffold fabrication process with controlled pore size. Biocompatibility was examined via MC3T3-E1 cell seeding, and the cell attachment, proliferation, and spread were confirmed.

Materials scientists continue research and development studies to improve the mechanical and bioactivity properties of scaffolds. Developments in both materials and processes are interrelated. Both the materials and the processes are responsible

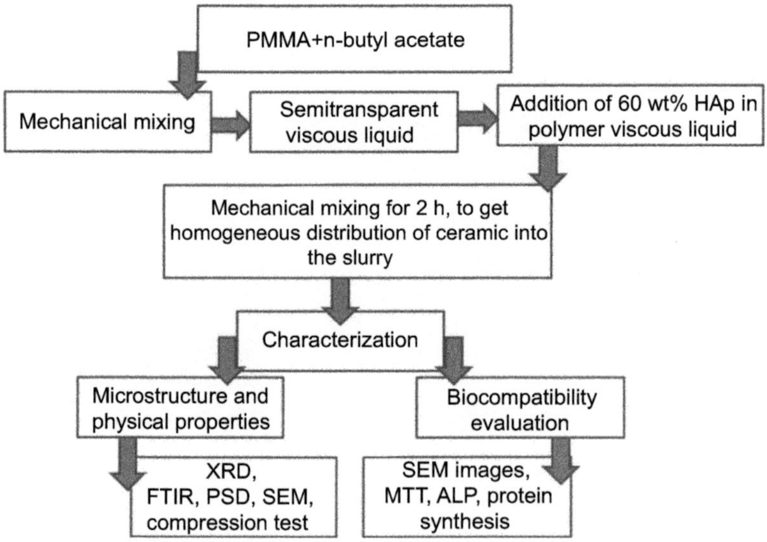

Figure 5.14 Schematic illustration of preparation and characterization of porous scaffold. *FTIR*, Fourier-transform infrared; *HAp*, hydroxyapatite particles; *MTT* and *ALP* are assays used for measuring the functionality of animal and human cells; *PMMA*, polymethyl methacrylate; *PSD*, particle size distribution; *SEM*, scanning electron microscope; *XRD*, X-ray diffraction. Reused from G. Tripathi, B. Basu, A porous hydroxyapatite scaffold for bone tissue engineering: physico-mechanical and biological evaluations, Ceramics International 38 (2012) 341–349. https://doi.org/10.1016/j.ceramint.2011.07.012 after license via (copyright.com) number 4270390649074.

for the final composition and microstructure that determine the final properties of the scaffolds. All the examples shown in this chapter are sample applications that show this connection between materials processes and mechanical bioactivity properties.

Chitosan, a natural biopolymer [145], is invested in greatly in the field of tissue engineering. Hydroxyapatite/chitosan (HA/CS) bilayered scaffolds are fabricated via two steps. The steps are outlined here, and the details are described in the original article. The first is utilizing the polyurethane replica method to obtain porous HA and sintering the scaffolds at 1300°C for 3 h. The second step is obtaining 3 wt% chitosan solution by dissolving in acetic acid. The bilayered scaffolds are fabricated via impregnation of the HA scaffolds by the chitosan solution, left to rest for 1 min, and freeze-dried. Finally, a cartilage-like layer is obtained on the top of a bonelike layer for each scaffold. Fig. 5.19 shows scanning electron microscope micrographs of the obtained HA/CS bilayered scaffolds, and Fig. 5.20 shows a μCT image of the scaffolds. Fig. 5.21 shows that the results of culturing with goat marrow stromal cells (GBMCs) are positive for the obtained scaffolds.

In fact, a lot of research work can be found in the literature that utilizes HA/CS in composites for scaffolds. A nice example is the utilization of the composite of HA/β-TCP/CS for scaffolds, as detailed in Ref. [147]. HA is made from mussel shells and the chitosan from crab shells. The utilized composition mixtures are shown in Table 5.4.

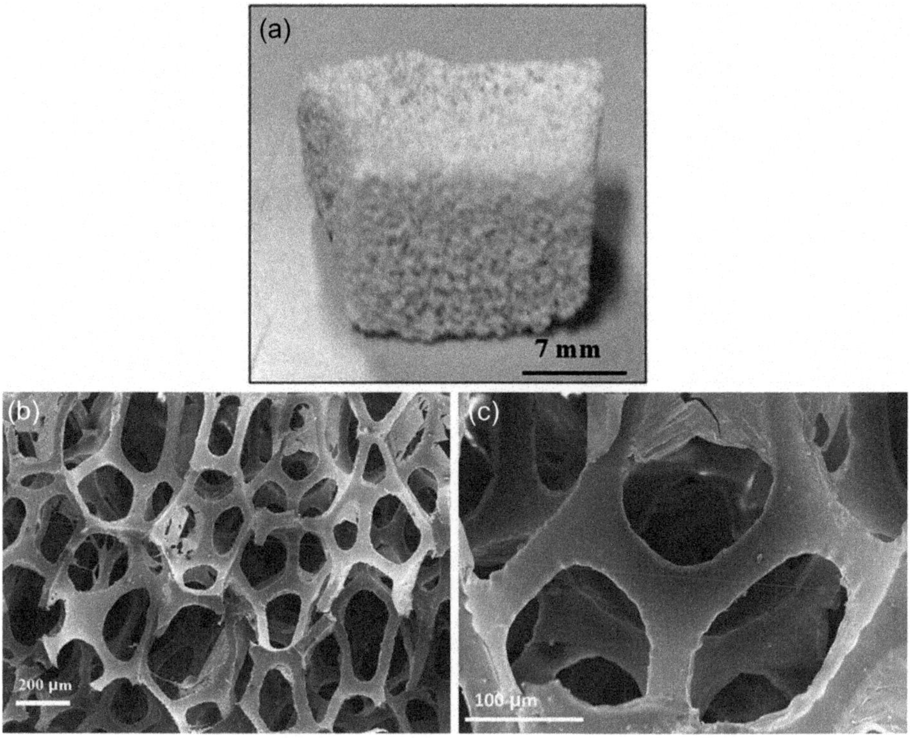

Figure 5.15 (a) Porous hydroxyapatite body of rectangular shape produced via the polymeric sponge method using sol-gel-derived hydroxyapatite powder and polymer slurry (b) and (c) scanning electron microscope of scaffold.
Reused from G. Tripathi, B. Basu, A porous hydroxyapatite scaffold for bone tissue engineering: physico-mechanical and biological evaluations, Ceramics International 38 (2012) 341–349. https://doi.org/10.1016/j.ceramint.2011.07.012 after license via (copyright.com) number 4270390649074.

An ethanol solution (1:10w/v) of the powder mixture is prepared first to make pastes. The pastes are then added to chitosan solution, homogenized, and finally 0%–10% of tripolyphosphate (TPP) ($Na_5P_3O_{10}$) is added to improve the cross-linking of HA/β-TCP/CS composite and accordingly the mechanical properties. The residual TPP is removed, and glycerol is also added (0.5, 1, 2.5, and 5%) because of its known control of chitosan secondary structural transitions and positive influence on the final mechanical properties. The effect of differing TPP and glycerol concentrations on the final microstructure is shown in Fig. 5.22. When the TPP concentration is increased, the pore wall thickness is increased and the pores collapse at a concentration of 5% TPP. Thus 2.5% concentration of TPP was accredited in this study. In addition, Fig. 5.23 shows different final morphologies and pore structures of the scaffolds because of the use of different HA/β-TCP concentrations. Cytocompatibility and cell growth were examined and confirmed utilizing SaOS2 cells and L929 mouse

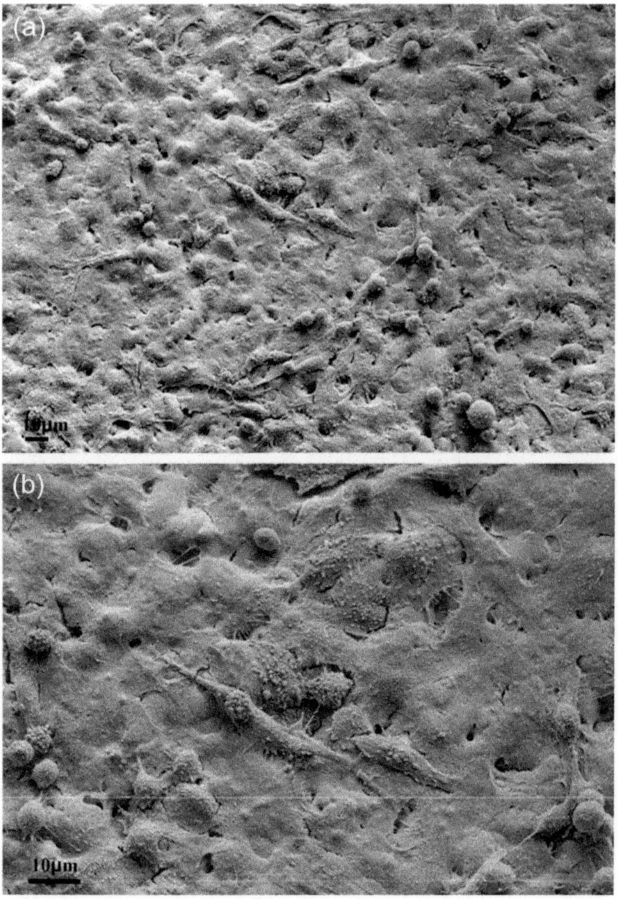

Figure 5.16 Scanning electron microscope image of osteoblast cells cultured on scaffold (a) after 7 days and (b) after 10 days of culture.
Reused from from G. Tripathi, B. Basu, A porous hydroxyapatite scaffold for bone tissue engineering: physico-mechanical and biological evaluations, Ceramics International 38 (2012) 341–349. https://doi.org/10.1016/j.ceramint.2011.07.012 after license via (copyright.com) number 4270390649074.

fibroblastic-like cells. Mostly, the same conclusions were made by the same authors in another publication [148], but the chitosan is extracted from squid pens.

In vivo analysis is attractive and informative. A composite of HA/CS–alginate was utilized to fabricate porous scaffolds via freeze drying, and in vivo analysis was performed as detailed in Ref. [149]. Alginate or alginic acid $(C_6H_8O_6)_n$ is an anionic biocompatible and biodegradable polymer. In vivo examination of the scaffolds was performed on critical-sized calvarial bone defects in severe combined immunodeficient (SCID) mice. The result of the transplantation was evaluated via μCT imaging, as shown in Fig. 5.24. The site implanted with the fabricated scaffold had started

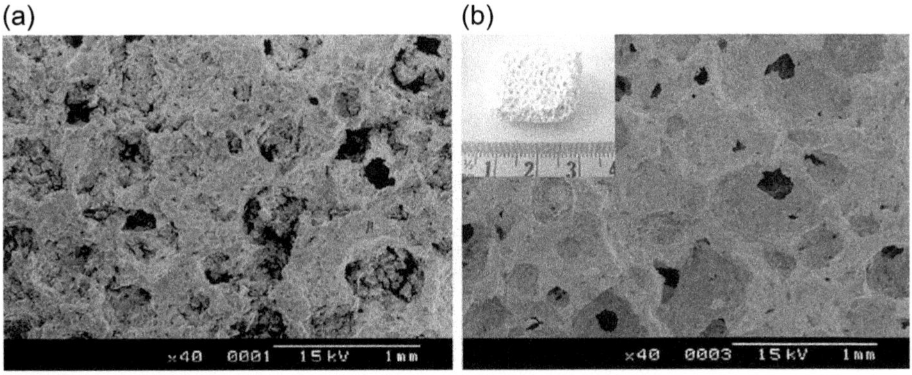

Figure 5.17 Scanning electron microscope micrograph showing interconnected porous nature of the hydroxyapatite with pore size of about 50–500 μm: (a) uncoated; (b) hydroxyapatite, tricalcium phosphate, and calcium silicate (HASi). The inset shows the gross view of HASi. Reused from M.B. Nair, S. Suresh Babu, H.K. Varma, A. John, A triphasic ceramic-coated porous hydroxyapatite for tissue engineering application, Acta Biomaterialia 4 (2008) 173–181. https://doi.org/10.1016/j.actbio.2007.07.004 after license via (copyright.com) number 4271281295364.

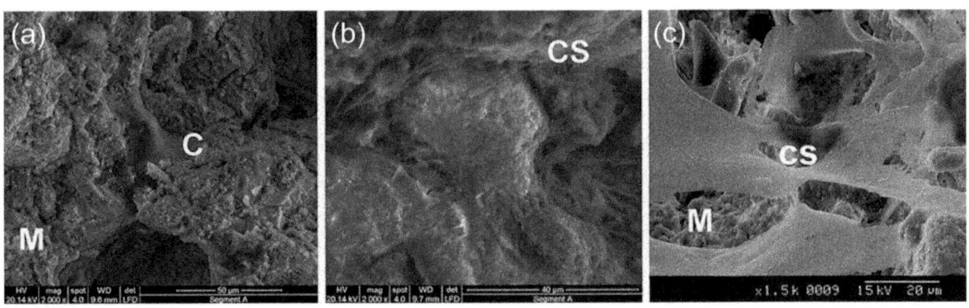

Figure 5.18 Scanning electron microscope micrograph of differentiated bone marrow stromal cells on hydroxyapatite and hydroxyapatite, tricalcium phosphate, and calcium silicate (HASi). The coated material offers a more appropriate platform where cell–cell/cell–material interactions are far better, favoring the formation of a cell sheet–like structure. (a) Hydroxyapatite on day 7, (b) HASi on day 7, and (c) HASi on day 14. *C*, Cell; *CS*, cell sheet; *M*, material.
Reused from M.B. Nair, S. Suresh Babu, H.K. Varma, A. John, A triphasic ceramic-coated porous hydroxyapatite for tissue engineering application, Acta Biomaterialia 4 (2008) 173–181. https://doi.org/10.1016/j.actbio.2007.07.004 after license via (copyright.com) number 4271281295364.

to heal via new generated bone, especially after 8 weeks of surgery. The figure also shows alizarin red analysis of the mouse skull. Alizarin red ($C_{14}H_8O_4$) is an old red dye used for textile fabrics and is also used in biological research because it stains free calcium and certain calcium compounds. The red color at the site implanted with the composite scaffold after 4 weeks (Fig. 5.24(b)) was converted after 8 weeks to a dark red color in vivo, i.e., the calcium was consumed for the generation of new bone.

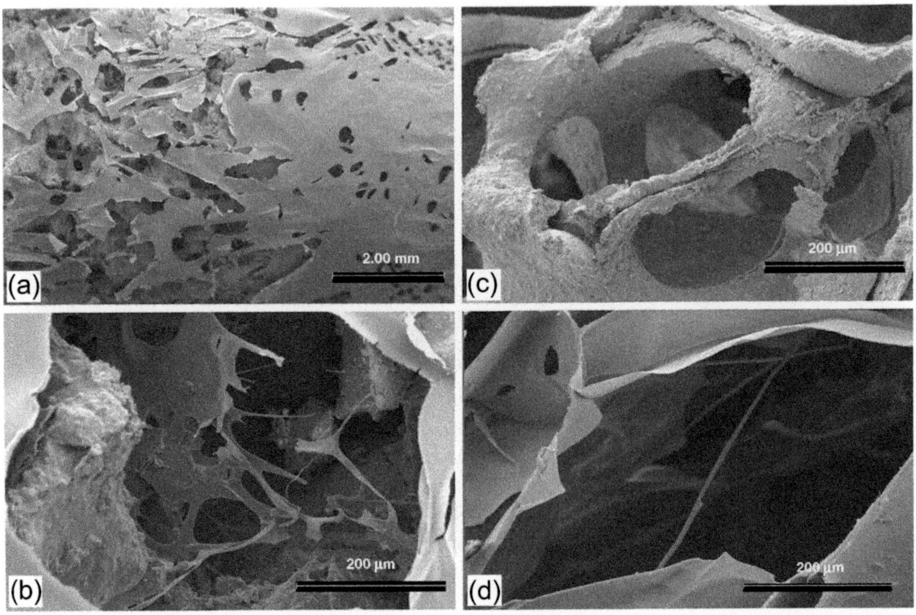

Figure 5.19 Scanning electron microscope micrographs of the hydroxyapatite/chitosan (HA/CS) bilayered scaffolds. (a) interface, (b) typical pore at interface, (c) pore of HA scaffolds, and (d) pore of CS layer.
Reused from J.M. Oliveira, M.T. Rodrigues, S.S. Silva, P.B. Malafaya, M.E. Gomes, C.A. Viegas, I.R. Dias, J.T. Azevedo, J.F. Mano, R.L. Reis, Novel hydroxyapatite/chitosan bilayered scaffold for osteochondral tissue-engineering applications: scaffold design and its performance when seeded with goat bone marrow stromal cells, Biomaterials 27 (2006) 6123–6137. https://doi.org/10.1016/j.biomaterials.2006.07.034 after license via (copyright.com) number 4272121247938.

A different technique to produce porous scaffolds is that used material can be dissolved in water. PCL and PCL/HA mixed with NaCl and water-soluble poly(ethylene oxide) (PEO) are used to produce injection-molded scaffolds. PCL is a biocompatible, biodegradable polyester with slow degradation rate. After leaching of the NaCl and the PEO with deionized water, porous scaffolds with interconnected microstructures were obtained, as detailed in Ref. [150]. Figs. 5.25 and 5.26 show unique morphology of the interconnected small and large pores of the PCL and PCL/HA scaffolds, respectively. The small pores were left after the dissolution of PEO, and the large pores were caused by NaCl particles. There was no obvious difference between the microstructures of PCL and PCL/HA scaffolds, but the latter has larger elastic and loss moduli. Human mesenchymal stem cells (hMSCs) are used to examine biocompatibility. hMSCs are stromal cells with great differentiation capacity originating primarily from bone marrow. One of the research outcomes is that culturing the PCL and PCL/HA scaffolds with hMSCs establishes cell attachment and proliferation.

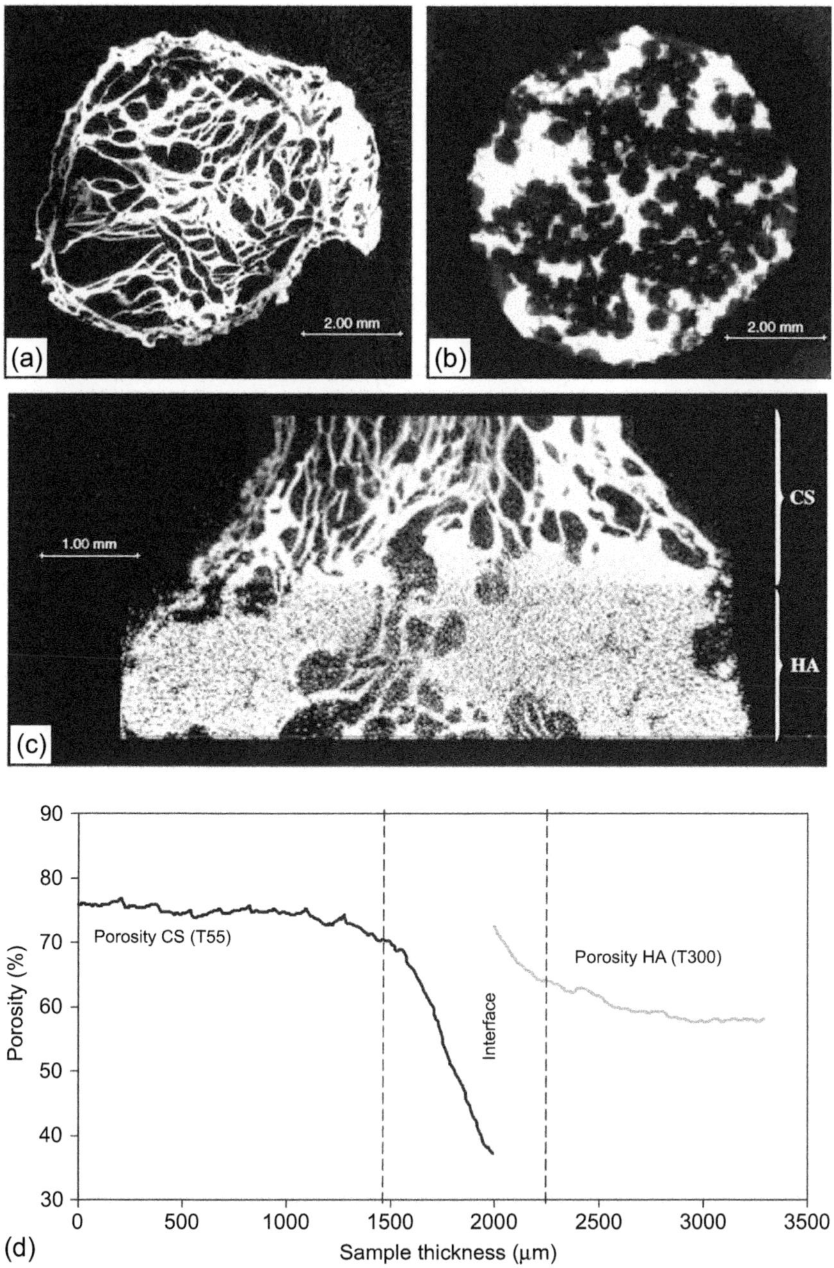

Figure 5.20 Microcomputed X-ray tomography images of the hydroxyapatite/chitosan (HA/CS) bilayered scaffolds. (a) Transversal view of the CS scaffold, (b) transversal view of the HA scaffold, (c) longitudinal view of the interface between HA (*bottom layer*) and CS (*top layer*), and (d) respective percentage of porosity.

Reused from J.M. Oliveira, M.T. Rodrigues, S.S. Silva, P.B. Malafaya, M.E. Gomes, C.A. Viegas, I.R. Dias, J.T. Azevedo, J.F. Mano, R.L. Reis, Novel hydroxyapatite/chitosan bilayered scaffold for osteochondral tissue-engineering applications: scaffold design and its performance when seeded with goat bone marrow stromal cells, Biomaterials 27 (2006) 6123–6137. https://doi.org/10.1016/j.biomaterials.2006.07.034 after license via (copyright.com) number 4272121247938.

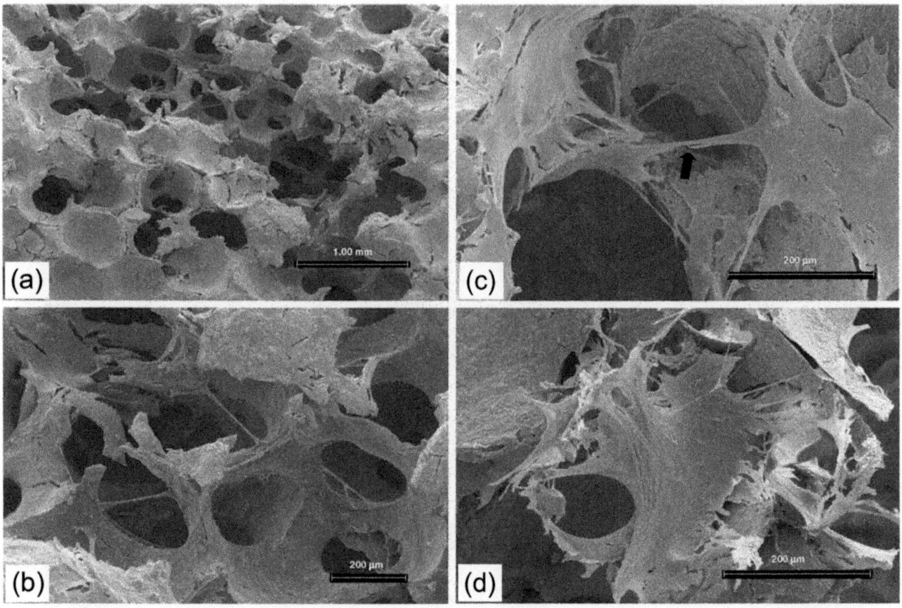

Figure 5.21 Scanning electron microscope micrographs of the hydroxyapatite (HA) scaffold seeded with goat marrow stromal cells (GBMCs) and cultured for 14 days in osteogenic media. (a and b) Surface of the cell–HA constructs, (c) GBMC infiltration into an HA macropore, and (d) GBMCs on the core of the HA scaffolds.
Reused from J.M. Oliveira, M.T. Rodrigues, S.S. Silva, P.B. Malafaya, M.E. Gomes, C.A. Viegas, I.R. Dias, J.T. Azevedo, J.F. Mano, R.L. Reis, Novel hydroxyapatite/chitosan bilayered scaffold for osteochondral tissue-engineering applications: scaffold design and its performance when seeded with goat bone marrow stromal cells, Biomaterials 27 (2006) 6123–6137. https://doi.org/10.1016/j.biomaterials.2006.07.034 after license via (copyright.com) number 4272121247938.

Table 5.4 **Composition of HA/TCP/CS composites**

Compound %	A0	A1	A2	A3
HA	0	20	30	40
β-TCP	0	10	20	30
Chitosan	100	70	50	30

β-TCP, β-Tricalcium phosphate; *CS*, Chitosan; *HA*, hydroxyapatite.
Reused from A. Shavandi, A.E.-D.A. Bekhit, M.A. Ali, Z. Sun, M. Gould, Development and characterization of hydroxyapatite/β-TCP/chitosan composites for tissue engineering applications, Materials Science and Engineering: C 56 (2015) 481–493. https://doi.org/10.1016/j.msec.2015.07.004 after license via (copyright.com) number 4272450125821.

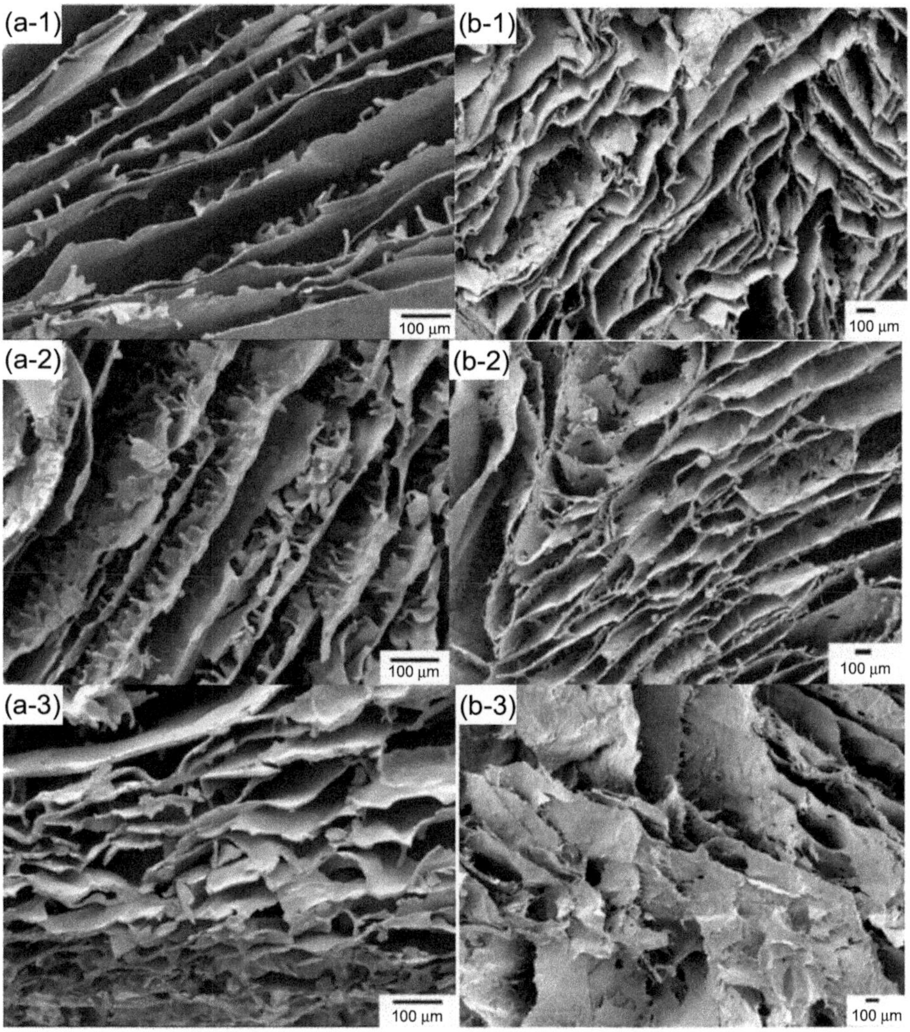

Figure 5.22 The effect of differing tripolyphosphate (TPP) and glycerol concentrations on the scaffold A2 (50% HA/β-TCP, 50% chitosan). Scanning electron microscope micrographs of scaffolds exposed to TTP of (a-1) 0%, (a-2) 2.5%, and (a-3) 5%. The different glycerol concentrations are shown for (b-1) 0.5%, (b-2) 1%, and (b-3) 2.5%.
Reused from A. Shavandi, A.E-D.A. Bekhit, M.A. Ali, Z. Sun, M. Gould, Development and characterization of hydroxyapatite/β-TCP/chitosan composites for tissue engineering applications, Materials Science and Engineering: C 56 (2015) 481–493. https://doi.org/10.1016/j.msec.2015.07.004 after license via (copyright.com) number 4272450125821.

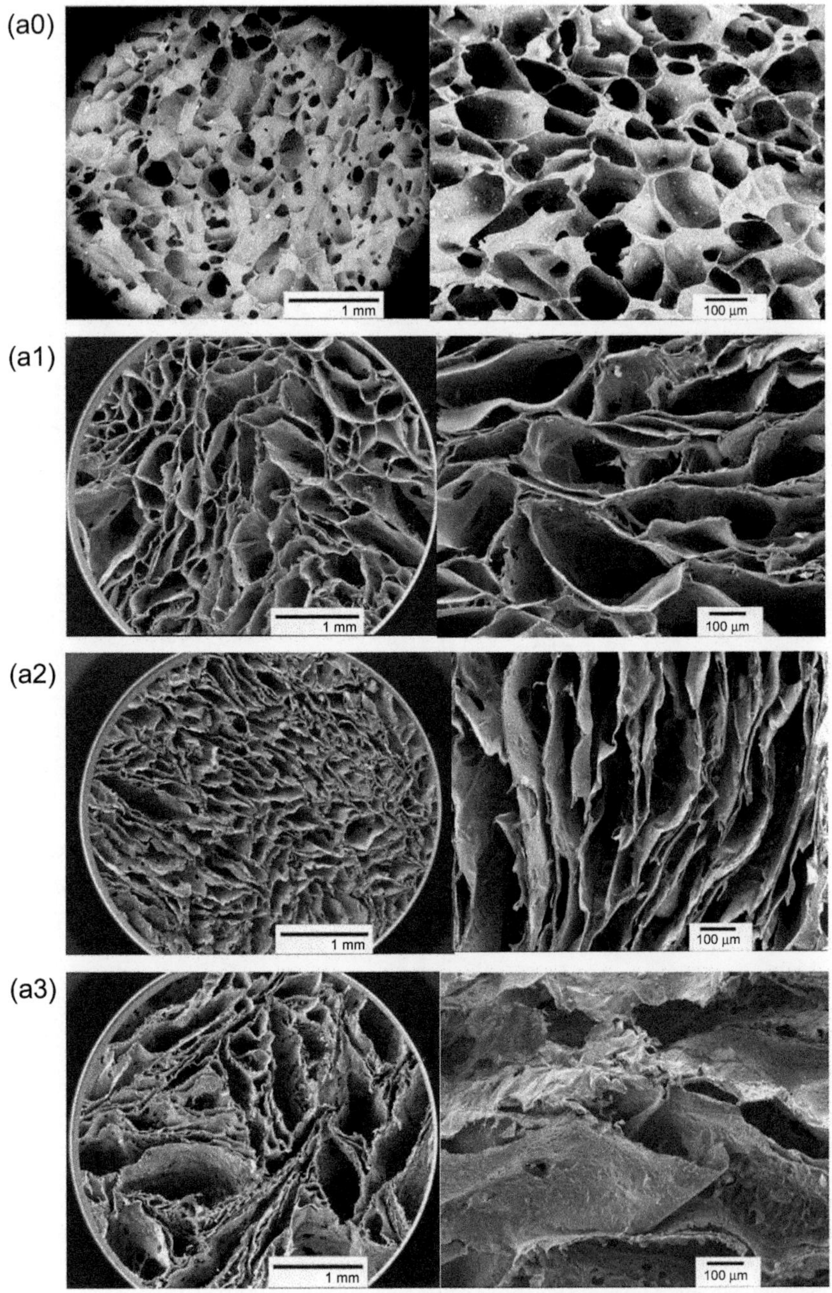

Figure 5.23 The effect of differing hydroxyapatite (HA)/β-tricalcium phosphate (β-TCP) concentrations on the scaffolds. Scanning electron microscope micrographs of scaffolds of (a0) 0% HA/β-TCP, (a1) 30% HA/β-TCP, (a2) 50% HA/β-TCP, and (a3) 70% HA/β-TCP. Reused from A. Shavandi, A.E-D.A. Bekhit, M.A. Ali, Z. Sun, M. Gould, Development and characterization of hydroxyapatite/β-TCP/chitosan composites for tissue engineering applications, Materials Science and Engineering: C 56 (2015) 481–493. https://doi.org/10.1016/j.msec.2015.07.004 after license via (copyright.com) number 4272450125821.

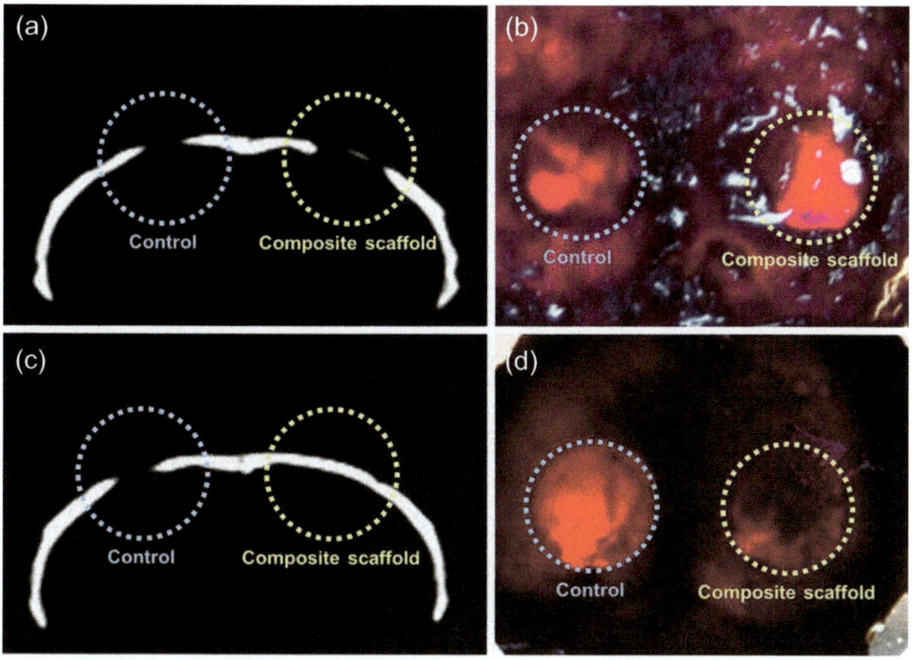

Figure 5.24 Microcomputed X-ray tomography images of the mouse skull after transplantation for (a) 4 and (c) 8 weeks. Photographs of mice skulls stained with alizarin red after transplantation for (b) 4 and (d) 8 weeks (For interpretation of the references to color in this figure legend, the reader is referred to the web version of the original article or the book chapter.)
Reused from H.-H. Jin, D.-H. Kim, T.-W. Kim, K.-K. Shin, J.S. Jung, H.-C. Park, S.-Y. Yoon, In vivo evaluation of porous hydroxyapatite/chitosan–alginate composite scaffolds for bone tissue engineering, International Journal of Biological Macromolecules 51 (2012) 1079–1085. https://doi.org/10.1016/j.ijbiomac.2012.08.027 after license via (copyright.com) number 4272690592938.

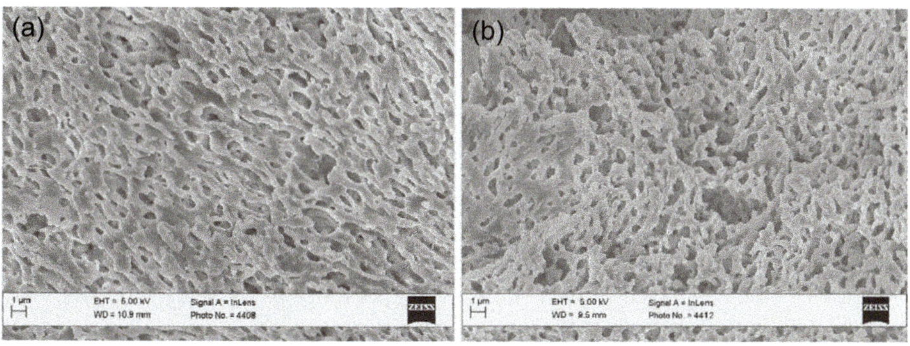

Figure 5.25 Scanning electron microscope micrographs of molded polycaprolactone/polyethylene oxide/NaCl samples after leaching for (a) 6 h and (b) 9 h.
Reused from Z. Cui, B. Nelson, Y. Peng, K. Li, S. Pilla, W.-J. Li, L.-S. Turng, C. Shen, Fabrication and characterization of injection molded poly (ε-caprolactone) and poly (ε-caprolactone)/hydroxyapatite scaffolds for tissue engineering, Materials Science and Engineering: C 32 (2012) 1674–1681. https://doi.org/10.1016/j.msec.2012.04.064 after license via (copyright.com) number 4272940847966.

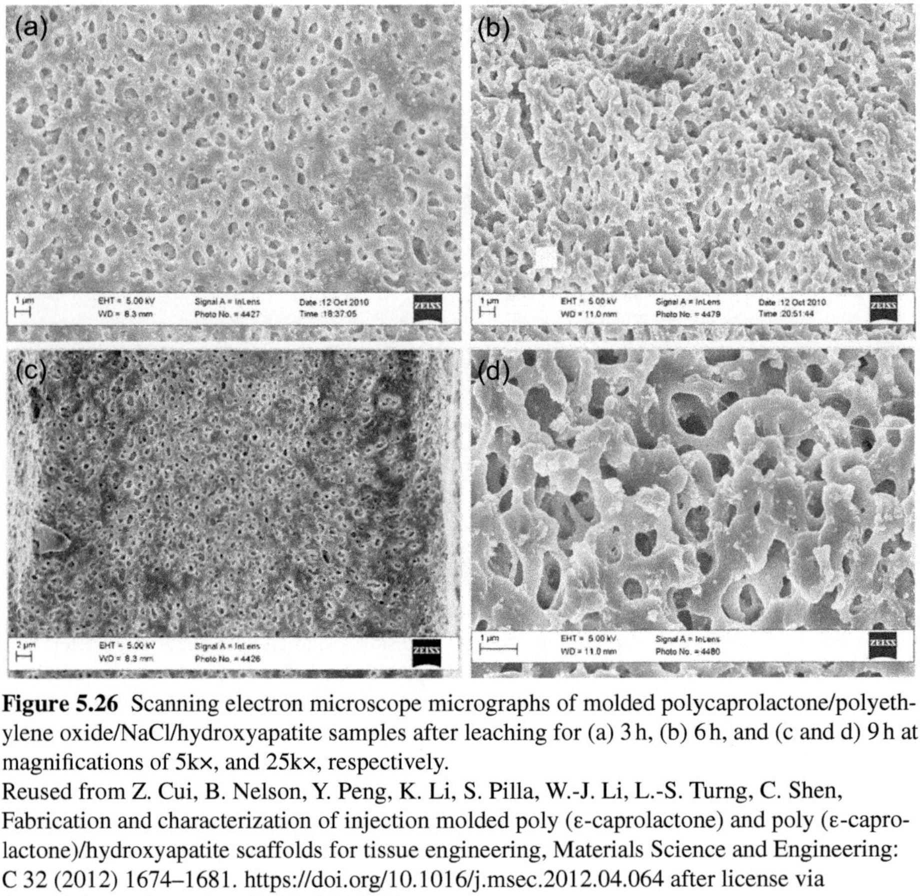

Figure 5.26 Scanning electron microscope micrographs of molded polycaprolactone/polyethylene oxide/NaCl/hydroxyapatite samples after leaching for (a) 3 h, (b) 6 h, and (c and d) 9 h at magnifications of 5k×, and 25k×, respectively.
Reused from Z. Cui, B. Nelson, Y. Peng, K. Li, S. Pilla, W.-J. Li, L.-S. Turng, C. Shen, Fabrication and characterization of injection molded poly (ε-caprolactone) and poly (ε-caprolactone)/hydroxyapatite scaffolds for tissue engineering, Materials Science and Engineering: C 32 (2012) 1674–1681. https://doi.org/10.1016/j.msec.2012.04.064 after license via (copyright.com) number 4272940847966.

To conclude, it is necessary to mention two of the most important parameters that help the surgeon to select the proper scaffold:

1. The target tissue regeneration site, age, and other conditions related to the patient. For example, density and microstructure of the bone are different depending on the site [151], as seen in Fig. 5.27. Also, the mechanical properties of porous ceramic scaffolds depend on the materials used and the processing route as seen in this chapter, in addition to the size, shape, and population of the porosity [152].
2. Histological data associated with the selected scaffolds. Although histological analysis is beyond the scope of this book, discussion of histology can be found with most tissue engineering articles. The references to the figures included in this chapter generally contain histological analysis for the proposed scaffolds. A good place to start learning histology connected to hard tissue engineering is the *Handbook of Histology Methods for Bone and Cartilage* [152], especially "Part Vi: Analysis Techniques."

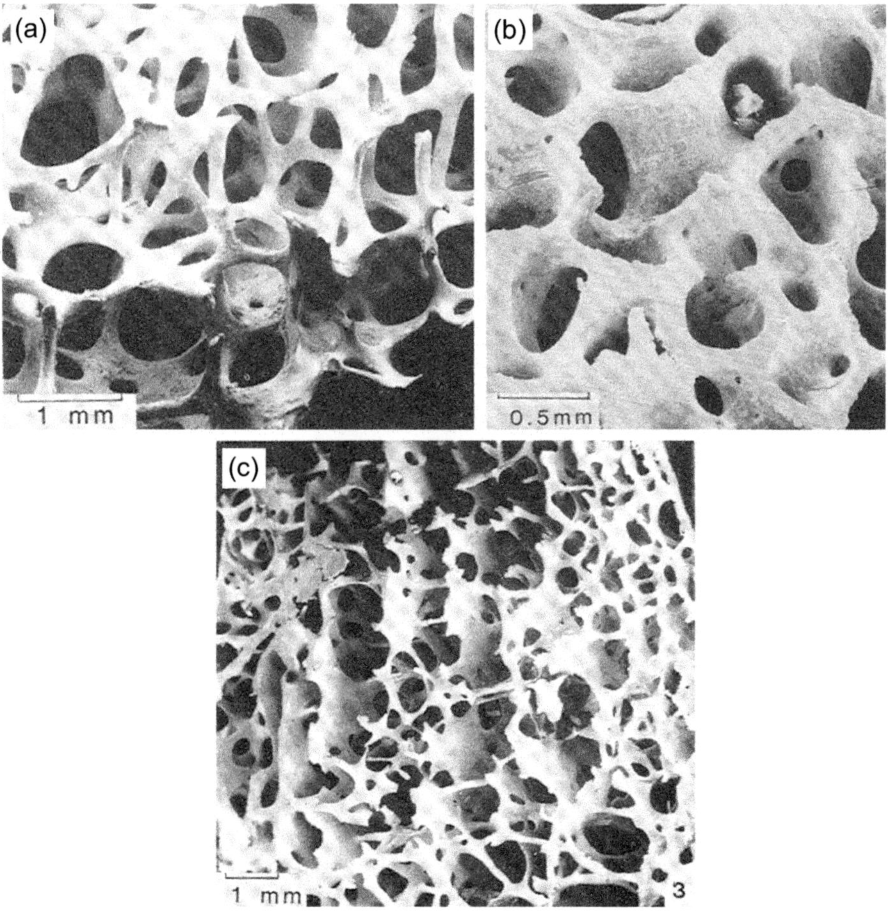

Figure 5.27 Scanning electron microscope micrographs of (a) low-density cancellous bone with an asymmetric rodlike structure. Specimen taken from the femoral head. (b) High-density cancellous bone with an asymmetric plate–like structure. Specimen taken from the femoral head. (c) Platelike cancellous bone with columnar structure. Specimen taken from the femoral condyle.
Reused from L.J. Gibson, The mechanical behaviour of cancellous bone, Journal of Biomechanics 18 (1985) 317–328. https://doi.org/10.1016/0021-9290(85)90287-8 after license via (copyright.com) number 4266361426094.

Review questions

1. Working as a group, make a table of the preparation methods of the scaffolds mentioned in this chapter with brief descriptions. Add extra processing methodologies if found useful.
2. Also working as a group, construct a table of the mechanical properties of the aforementioned scaffolds and compare with those of the target bone.
3. For interested students, attach brief histological results associated with the proposed scaffold.

4. As yet another group, collect all the types of cells used to examine biocompatibility, attachment, and proliferation that are mentioned in this chapter. Add other cell types according to the directions of the instructor.
5. μCT scan emerges as an important technique to monitor the generation of new tissue. A report should be written by another group that contains few example cases.
6. Evaluation of bioactivity via x-ray spectroscopy and FTIR examination should be included in another report.
7. In all aspects of ceramic materials science and engineering, the researcher should learn a great deal about polymers. State and describe the biocompatible and biodegradable polymers used to build scaffolds for hard tissue engineering mentioned in this chapter and add extra information if useful.

References

[1] S. Yang, K.F. Leong, Z. Du, C.K. Chua, The design of scaffolds for use in tissue engineering. Part I. Traditional factors, Tissue Engineering 7 (2001) 679–689, https://doi.org/10.1089/107632701753337645.

[2] S. Yang, K.-F. Leong, Z. Du, C.-K. Chua, The design of scaffolds for use in tissue engineering. Part II. Rapid prototyping techniques, Tissue Engineering 8 (2002) 1–11, https://doi.org/10.1089/107632702753503009.

[3] D. Shi, Introduction to biomaterials, Chp: 15, in: Cells and Biomolecules for Tissue Engineering, Tsinghua University Press and World Scientific Publishing Co. Pte. Ltd., 2006, pp. 227–237.

[4] K.A. Athanasiou, C.-F. Zhu, D.R. Lanctot, C.M. Agrawal, X. Wang, Fundamentals of biomechanics in tissue engineering of bone, Tissue Engineering 6 (2000) 361–381, https://doi.org/10.1089/107632700418083.

[5] M.J. Yaszemski, R.G. Payne, W.C. Hayes, R. Langer, A.G. Mikos, Evolution of bone transplantation: molecular, cellular and tissue strategies to engineer human bone, Biomaterials 17 (1996) 175–185, https://doi.org/10.1016/0142-9612(96)85762-0.

[6] D. Eglin, M. Alini, Degradable polymeric materials for osteosynthesis: tutorial, European Cells and Materials 16 (2008) 80–91.

[7] F. Tamimi, Z. Sheikh, J. Barralet, Dicalcium phosphate cements: brushite and monetite, Acta Biomaterialia 8 (2012) 474–487, https://doi.org/10.1016/j.actbio.2011.08.005.

[8] L.E. Claes, Mechanical characterization of biodegradable implants, Clinical Materials 10 (1992) 41–46, https://doi.org/10.1016/0267-6605(92)90083-6.

[9] J. Blackburn, R. Hodgskinson, J.D. Currey, J.E. Mason, Mechanical properties of microcallus in human cancellous bone, Journal of Orthopaedic Research 10 (1992) 237–246, https://doi.org/10.1002/jor.1100100211.

[10] L. Tan, X. Yu, P. Wan, K. Yang, Biodegradable materials for bone repairs: a review, Journal of Materials Science and Technology 29 (2013) 503–513, https://doi.org/10.1016/j.jmst.2013.03.002.

[11] I. Armentano, M. Dottori, E. Fortunati, S. Mattioli, J.M. Kenny, Biodegradable polymer matrix nanocomposites for tissue engineering: a review, Polymer Degradation and Stability 95 (2010) 2126–2146, https://doi.org/10.1016/j.polymdegradstab.2010.06.007.

[12] F. Witte, N. Hort, C. Vogt, S. Cohen, K.U. Kainer, R. Willumeit, F. Feyerabend, Degradable biomaterials based on magnesium corrosion, Current Opinion in Solid State and Materials Science 12 (2008) 63–72, https://doi.org/10.1016/j.cossms.2009.04.001.

[13] P.V. Giannoudis, H. Dinopoulos, E. Tsiridis, Bone substitutes: an update, Injury 36 (2005) S20–S27, https://doi.org/10.1016/j.injury.2005.07.029.
[14] Z. Sheikh, S. Najeeb, Z. Khurshid, V. Verma, H. Rashid, M. Glogauer, Biodegradable materials for bone repair and tissue engineering applications, Materials 8 (2015) 5744–5794, https://doi.org/10.3390/ma8095273.
[15] F. Khoury, Augmentation of the sinus floor with mandibular bone block and simultaneous implantation: a 6-year clinical investigation, The International Journal of Oral and Maxillofacial Implants 14 (1999) 557–564.
[16] M.S. Block, M. Degen, Horizontal ridge augmentation using human mineralized particulate bone: preliminary results, Journal of Oral and Maxillofacial Surgery 62 (2004) 67–72, https://doi.org/10.1016/j.joms.2004.05.209.
[17] M.E. Bolander, G. Balian, The use of demineralized bone matrix in the repair of segmental defects. Augmentation with extracted matrix proteins and a comparison with autologous grafts, Journal of Bone and Joint Surgery American Volume 68 (1986) 1264–1274.
[18] P.P.T. Araújo, K.P. Oliveira, S.C.L. Montenegro, A.F.P. Carreiro, J.S.P. Silva, A.R. Germano, Block allograft for reconstruction of alveolar bone ridge in implantology: a systematic review, Implant Dentistry 22 (2013) 304–308, https://doi.org/10.1097/ID.0b013e318289e311.
[19] T.W. Sterio, J.A. Katancik, S.B. Blanchard, P. Xenoudi, B.L. Mealey, A Prospective, Multicenter study of bovine pericardium membrane with cancellous particulate allograft for localized alveolar ridge augmentation, The International Journal of Periodontics and Restorative Dentistry 33 (2013) 499–507, https://doi.org/10.11607/prd.1704.
[20] J.M. Whittaker, R.A. James, J. Lozada, C. Cordova, D.J. GaRey, Histological response and clinical evaluation of heterograft and allograft materials in the elevation of the maxillary sinus for the preparation of endosteal dental implant sites. Simultaneous sinus elevation and root form implantation: an eight-month autopsy report, Journal of Oral Implantology 15 (1989) 141–144.
[21] P. Valentini, D. Abensur, Maxillary sinus floor elevation for implant placement with demineralized freeze-dried bone and bovine bone (Bio-Oss): a clinical study of 20 patients, The International Journal of Periodontics and Restorative Dentistry 17 (1997) 232–241.
[22] J.S. Guerrero, B.A. Al-Jandan, Allograft for maxillary sinus floor augmentation: a retrospective study of 90 cases, Implant Dentistry 21 (2012) 136–140, https://doi.org/10.1097/ID.0b013e31824a023b.
[23] G. Avila, R. Neiva, C.E. Misch, P. Galindo-Moreno, E. Benavides, I. Rudek, H.-L. Wang, Clinical and histologic outcomes after the use of a novel allograft for maxillary sinus augmentation: a case series, Implant Dentistry 19 (2010) 330–341, https://doi.org/10.1097/ID.0b013e3181e59b32.
[24] D.-S. Sohn, J.-K. Lee, K.-M. An, H.-I. Shin, Histomorphometric evaluation of mineralized cancellous allograft in the maxillary sinus augmentation: a 4 case report, Implant Dentistry 18 (2009) 172–181, https://doi.org/10.1097/ID.0b013e318199045d.
[25] J.-Y. Jo, S.-I. Jeong, Y.-M. Shin, S.-S. Kang, S.-E. Kim, C.-M. Jeong, J.-B. Huh, Sequential delivery of BMP-2 and BMP-7 for bone regeneration using a heparinized collagen membrane, International Journal of Oral and Maxillofacial Surgery 44 (2015) 921–928, https://doi.org/10.1016/j.ijom.2015.02.015.
[26] J.-K. Cha, J.-S. Lee, M.-S. Kim, S.-H. Choi, K.-S. Cho, U.-W. Jung, Sinus augmentation using BMP-2 in a bovine hydroxyapatite/collagen carrier in dogs, Journal of Clinical Periodontology 41 (2014) 86–93, https://doi.org/10.1111/jcpe.12174.

[27] M. Geiger, R.H. Li, W. Friess, Collagen sponges for bone regeneration with rhBMP-2, Advanced Drug Delivery Reviews 55 (2003) 1613–1629, https://doi.org/10.1016/j.addr.2003.08.010.
[28] A. John, L. Hong, Y. Ikada, Y. Tabata, A trial to prepare biodegradable collagen–hydroxy-apatite composites for bone repair, Journal of Biomaterials Science, Polymer Edition 12 (2001) 689–705, https://doi.org/10.1163/156856201316883485.
[29] K.M. Chung, L.M. Salkin, M.D. Stein, A.L. Freedman, Clinical evaluation of a biodegradable collagen membrane in guided tissue regeneration, Journal of Periodontology 61 (1990) 732–736, https://doi.org/10.1902/jop.1990.61.12.732.
[30] Z. Sheikh, M.-N. Abdallah, N. Hamdan, M.A. Javaid, Z. Khurshid, Barrier membranes for periodontal guided tissue regeneration applications, in: Handbook of Oral Biomaterials, first ed., Taylor & Francis Group, New York, 2014, p. 636. https://www.taylorfrancis.com/books/9789814463133/chapters/10.1201%2Fb15644-19.
[31] X. Liu, P.X. Ma, Polymeric scaffolds for bone tissue engineering, Annals of Biomedical Engineering 32 (2004) 477–486.
[32] G.A. Silva, P. Ducheyne, R.L. Reis, Materials in particulate form for tissue engineering. 1. Basic concepts, Journal of Tissue Engineering and Regenerative Medicine 1 (2007) 4–24, https://doi.org/10.1002/term.2.
[33] J.-Y. Lee, K.-H. Kim, S.-Y. Shin, I.-C. Rhyu, Y.-M. Lee, Y.-J. Park, C.-P. Chung, S.-J. Lee, Enhanced bone formation by transforming growth factor-β1-releasing collagen/chitosan microgranules, Journal of Biomedical Materials Research 76A (2006) 530–539, https://doi.org/10.1002/jbm.a.30434.
[34] H. Zhao, L. Ma, C. Gao, J. Shen, Fabrication and properties of mineralized collagen-chitosan/hydroxyapatite scaffolds, Polymers for Advanced Technologies 19 (2008) 1590–1596, https://doi.org/10.1002/pat.1174.
[35] E.-J. Lee, S.-H. Jun, H.-E. Kim, H.-W. Kim, Y.-H. Koh, J.-H. Jang, Silica xerogel-chitosan nano-hybrids for use as drug eluting bone replacement, Journal of Materials Science: Materials in Medicine 21 (2010) 207–214, https://doi.org/10.1007/s10856-009-3835-9.
[36] C.G. Ambrose, B.E. Hartline, T.O. Clanton, W.R. Lowe, W.C. McGarvey, Polymers in orthopaedic surgery, in: Advanced Polymers in Medicine, Springer, Cham, 2015, pp. 129–145, https://doi.org/10.1007/978-3-319-12478-0_5.
[37] P. Törmälä, Biodegradable self-reinforced composite materials; manufacturing structure and mechanical properties, Clinical Materials 10 (1992) 29–34, https://doi.org/10.1016/0267-6605(92)90081-4.
[38] P. Christel, Biodegradable composites for internal fixation, Biomaterials 1 (1980) 271–280.
[39] W. Linhart, F. Peters, W. Lehmann, K. Schwarz, A.F. Schilling, M. Amling, J.M. Rueger, M. Epple, Biologically and chemically optimized composites of carbonated apatite and polyglycolide as bone substitution materials, Journal of Biomedical Materials Research 54 (2001) 162–171, https://doi.org/10.1002/1097-4636(200102)54.2<162::AID-JBM2>3.0.CO;2-3.
[40] X. Niu, Q. Feng, M. Wang, X. Guo, Q. Zheng, Porous nano-HA/collagen/PLLA scaffold containing chitosan microspheres for controlled delivery of synthetic peptide derived from BMP-2, Journal of Controlled Release 134 (2009) 111–117, https://doi.org/10.1016/j.jconrel.2008.11.020.
[41] Z. Xiong, Y. Yan, R. Zhang, L. Sun, Fabrication of porous poly(l-lactic acid) scaffolds for bone tissue engineering via precise extrusion, Scripta Materialia 45 (2001) 773–779, https://doi.org/10.1016/S1359-6462(01)01094-6.

[42] S. Higashi, T. Yamamuro, T. Nakamura, Y. Ikada, S.-H. Hyon, K. Jamshidi, Polymer-hydroxyapatite composites for biodegradable bone fillers, Biomaterials 7 (1986) 183–187, https://doi.org/10.1016/0142-9612(86)90099-2.

[43] S. Izwan, A. Razak, N. Fadzliana, A. Sharif, W. Aizan, W.A. Rahman, Biodegradable polymers and their bone applications: a review, International Journal of Basic and Applied Sciences and International Journal of Engineering and Sciences 12 (2012) 31–49.

[44] M. Vert, Aliphatic polyesters: great degradable polymers that cannot do everything, Biomacromolecules 6 (2004) 538–546, https://doi.org/10.1021/bm0494702.

[45] E. Nejati, H. Mirzadeh, M. Zandi, Synthesis and characterization of nano-hydroxy-apatite rods/poly(l-lactide acid) composite scaffolds for bone tissue engineering, Composites Part A: Applied Science and Manufacturing 39 (2008) 1589–1596, https://doi.org/10.1016/j.compositesa.2008.05.018.

[46] A.L.C. Lagoa, C. Wedemeyer, M. von Knoch, F. Löer, M. Epple, A strut graft substitute consisting of a metal core and a polymer surface, Journal of Materials Science: Materials in Medicine 19 (2008) 417–424, https://doi.org/10.1007/s10856-006-0022-0.

[47] W.H. Warden, R. Friedman, L.M. Teresi, D.W. Jackson, Magnetic resonance imaging of bioabsorbable polylactic acid interference screws during the first 2 years after anterior cruciate ligament reconstruction, Arthroscopy 15 (1999) 474–480, https://doi.org/10.1053/ar.1999.v15.015047.

[48] K.J. Bozic, L.E. Perez, D.R. Wilson, P.G. Fitzgibbons, J.B. Jupiter, Mechanical testing of bioresorbable implants for use in metacarpal fracture fixation, The Journal of Hand Surgery 26 (2001) 755–761, https://doi.org/10.1053/jhsu.2001.24145.

[49] A.A. Ignatius, L.E. Claes, In vitro biocompatibility of bioresorbable polymers: poly(L, DL-lactide) and poly(L-lactide-co-glycolide), Biomaterials 17 (1996) 831–839, https://doi.org/10.1016/0142-9612(96)81421-9.

[50] J.W. Leenslag, A.J. Pennings, R.R.M. Bos, F.R. Rozema, G. Boering, Resorbable materials of poly(L-lactide): VII. In vivo and in vitro degradation, Biomaterials 8 (1987) 311–314, https://doi.org/10.1016/0142-9612(87)90121-9.

[51] S. Vainionpää, J. Kilpikari, J. Laiho, P. Helevirta, P. Rokkanen, P. Törmälä, Strength and strength retention vitro, of absorbable, self-reinforced polyglycolide (PGA) rods for fracture fixation, Biomaterials 8 (1987) 46–48, https://doi.org/10.1016/0142-9612(87)90028-7.

[52] Y.S. Nam, T.G. Park, Porous biodegradable polymeric scaffolds prepared by thermally induced phase separation, Journal of Biomedical Materials Research 47 (1999) 8–17, https://doi.org/10.1002/(SICI)1097-4636(199910)47. 1<8::AID-JBM2>3.0.CO;2-L.

[53] L. Nie, D. Chen, J. Fu, S. Yang, R. Hou, J. Suo, Macroporous biphasic calcium phosphate scaffolds reinforced by poly-L-lactic acid/hydroxyapatite nanocomposite coatings for bone regeneration, Biochemical Engineering Journal 98 (2015) 29–37, https://doi.org/10.1016/j.bej.2015.02.026.

[54] Y. Ji, G. ping Xu, Z. peng Zhang, J. jun Xia, J. long Yan, S. ha Pan, BMP-2/PLGA delayed-release microspheres composite graft, selection of bone particulate diameters, and prevention of aseptic inflammation for bone tissue engineering, Annals of Biomedical Engineering 38 (2010) 632–639, https://doi.org/10.1007/s10439-009-9888-6.

[55] K. Gavenis, U. Schneider, J. Groll, B. Schmidt-Rohlfing, BMP-7-loaded PGLA microspheres as a new delivery system for the cultivation of human chondrocytes in a collagen type I gel: the common nude mouse model, The International Journal of Artificial Organs 33 (2010) 45–53.

[56] Z. Fei, Y. Hu, D. Wu, H. Wu, R. Lu, J. Bai, H. Song, Preparation and property of a novel bone graft composite consisting of rhBMP-2 loaded PLGA microspheres and calcium phosphate cement, Journal of Materials Science: Materials in Medicine 19 (2008) 1109–1116, https://doi.org/10.1007/s10856-007-3050-5.

[57] F.A. Sheikh, H.W. Ju, B.M. Moon, O.J. Lee, J.-H. Kim, H.J. Park, D.W. Kim, D.-K. Kim, J.E. Jang, G. Khang, C.H. Park, Hybrid scaffolds based on PLGA and silk for bone tissue engineering, Journal of Tissue Engineering and Regenerative Medicine 10 (2016) 209–221, https://doi.org/10.1002/term.1989.
[58] B. Chen, K. Sun, Poly (ε-caprolactone)/hydroxyapatite composites: effects of particle size, molecular weight distribution and irradiation on interfacial interaction and properties, Polymer Testing 24 (2005) 64–70, https://doi.org/10.1016/j.polymertesting.2004.07.010.
[59] F.E. Wiria, K.F. Leong, C.K. Chua, Y. Liu, Poly-ε-caprolactone/hydroxyapatite for tissue engineering scaffold fabrication via selective laser sintering, Acta Biomaterialia 3 (2007) 1–12, https://doi.org/10.1016/j.actbio.2006.07.008.
[60] H. Yu, H.W. Matthew, P.H. Wooley, S.-Y. Yang, Effect of porosity and pore size on microstructures and mechanical properties of poly-ε-caprolactone- hydroxyapatite composites, Journal of Biomedical Materials Research 86B (2008) 541–547, https://doi.org/10.1002/jbm.b.31054.
[61] J.R. Porter, A. Henson, K.C. Popat, Biodegradable poly(ε-caprolactone) nanowires for bone tissue engineering applications, Biomaterials 30 (2009) 780–788, https://doi.org/10.1016/j.biomaterials.2008.10.022.
[62] G.G. Pitt, M.M. Gratzl, G.L. Kimmel, J. Surles, A. Sohindler, Aliphatic polyesters II. The degradation of poly (DL-lactide), poly (ε-caprolactone), and their copolymers in vivo, Biomaterials 2 (1981) 215–220, https://doi.org/10.1016/0142-9612(81)90060-0.
[63] E. Prosecká, M. Rampichová, A. Litvinec, Z. Tonar, M. Králíčková, L. Vojtová, P. Kochová, M. Plencner, M. Buzgo, A. Míčková, J. Jančář, E. Amler, Collagen/hydroxyapatite scaffold enriched with polycaprolactone nanofibers, thrombocyte-rich solution and mesenchymal stem cells promotes regeneration in large bone defect in vivo, Journal of Biomedical Materials Research 103 (2015) 671–682, https://doi.org/10.1002/jbm.a.35216.
[64] C. Balçik, T. Tokdemir, A. Şenköylü, N. Koç, M. Timuçin, S. Akin, P. Korkusuz, F. Korkusuz, Early weight bearing of porous HA/TCP (60/40) ceramics in vivo: a longitudinal study in a segmental bone defect model of rabbit, Acta Biomaterialia 3 (2007) 985–996, https://doi.org/10.1016/j.actbio.2007.04.004.
[65] R. Quarto, M. Mastrogiacomo, R. Cancedda, S.M. Kutepov, V. Mukhachev, A. Lavroukov, E. Kon, M. Marcacci, Repair of large bone defects with the use of autologous bone marrow stromal cells, New England Journal of Medicine 344 (2001) 385–386, https://doi.org/10.1056/NEJM200102013440516.
[66] C.M. Mardziah, I. Sopyan, S. Ramesh, Strontium-doped hydroxyapatite nanopowder via sol-gel method: effect of strontium concentration and calcination temperature on phase behavior, Trends in Biomaterials and Artificial Organs 23 (2009) 105–113.
[67] E.S. Thian, J. Huang, S.M. Best, Z.H. Barber, W. Bonfield, Novel silicon-doped hydroxyapatite (Si-HA) for biomedical coatings: an in vitro study using acellular simulated body fluid, Journal of Biomedical Materials Research 76B (2006) 326–333, https://doi.org/10.1002/jbm.b.30368.
[68] T. Noshi, T. Yoshikawa, M. Ikeuchi, Y. Dohi, H. Ohgushi, K. Horiuchi, M. Sugimura, K. Ichijima, K. Yonemasu, Enhancement of the in vivo osteogenic potential of marrow/hydroxyapatite composites by bovine bone morphogenetic protein, Journal of Biomedical Materials Research 52 (2000) 621–630, https://doi.org/10.1002/1097-4636(20001215)52.
[69] H. Oonishi, Orthopaedic applications of hydroxyapatite, Biomaterials 12 (1991) 171–178, https://doi.org/10.1016/0142-9612(91)90196-H.
[70] S.D. Cook, K.A. Thomas, J.F. Kay, M. Jarcho, Hydroxyapatite-coated titanium for orthopedic implant applications, Clinical Orthopaedics and Related Research (1988) 225–243.

[71] I. Sopyan, M. Mel, S. Ramesh, K.A. Khalid, Porous hydroxyapatite for artificial bone applications, Science and Technology of Advanced Materials 8 (2007) 116–123, https://doi.org/10.1016/j.stam.2006.11.017.
[72] U. Heise, J.F. Osborn, F. Duwe, Hydroxyapatite ceramic as a bone substitute, International Orthopaedics 14 (1990) 329–338, https://doi.org/10.1007/BF00178768.
[73] A. Kumar, K. Biswas, B. Basu, Hydroxyapatite-titanium bulk composites for bone tissue engineering applications, Journal of Biomedical Materials Research 103 (2015) 791–806, https://doi.org/10.1002/jbm.a.35198.
[74] I. Dumic-Cule, M. Pecina, M. Jelic, M. Jankolija, I. Popek, L. Grgurevic, S. Vukicevic, Biological aspects of segmental bone defects management, International Orthopaedics 39 (2015) 1005–1011, https://doi.org/10.1007/s00264-015-2728-4.
[75] A.B. Singh, S. Majumdar, The composite of hydroxyapatite with collagen as a bone grafting material, Journal of Advanced Medical and Dental Sciences Research 2 (2014) 53–55.
[76] K.A. Hing, L.F. Wilson, T. Buckland, Comparative performance of three ceramic bone graft substitutes, The Spine Journal 7 (2007) 475–490, https://doi.org/10.1016/j.spinee.2006.07.017.
[77] S.K. Nandi, S.K. Ghosh, B. Kundu, D.K. De, D. Basu, Evaluation of new porous β-tri-calcium phosphate ceramic as bone substitute in goat model, Small Ruminant Research 75 (2008) 144–153, https://doi.org/10.1016/j.smallrumres.2007.09.006.
[78] S.K. Ghosh, S.K. Nandi, B. Kundu, S. Datta, D.K. De, S.K. Roy, D. Basu, In vivo response of porous hydroxyapatite and β-tricalcium phosphate prepared by aqueous solution combustion method and comparison with bioglass scaffolds, Journal of Biomedical Materials Research 86B (2008) 217–227, https://doi.org/10.1002/jbm.b.31009.
[79] D.E. Cutright, S.N. Bhaskar, J.M. Brady, L. Getter, W.R. Posey, Reaction of bone to tricalcium phosphate ceramic pellets, Oral Surgery, Oral Medicine, Oral Pathology 33 (1972) 850–856, https://doi.org/10.1016/0030-4220(72)90457-4.
[80] M. Bohner, Physical and chemical aspects of calcium phosphates used in spinal surgery, European Spine Journal 10 (2001) S114–S121, https://doi.org/10.1007/s005860100276.
[81] S.J. Peter, P. Kim, A.W. Yasko, M.J. Yaszemski, A.G. Mikos, Crosslinking characteristics of an injectable poly(propylene fumarate)/β-tricalcium phosphate paste and mechanical properties of the crosslinked composite for use as a biodegradable bone cement, Journal of Biomedical Materials Research 44 (1999) 314–321, https://doi.org/10.1002/(SICI)1097-4636(19990305)44.
[82] P. Miranda, E. Saiz, K. Gryn, A.P. Tomsia, Sintering and robocasting of β-tricalcium phosphate scaffolds for orthopaedic applications, Acta Biomaterialia 2 (2006) 457–466, https://doi.org/10.1016/j.actbio.2006.02.004.
[83] L. Galois, D. Mainard, J. Delagoutte, Beta-tricalcium phosphate ceramic as a bone substitute in orthopaedic surgery, International Orthopaedics 26 (2002) 109–115, https://doi.org/10.1007/s00264-001-0329-x.
[84] X. Zhang, S. Meng, Y. Huang, M. Xu, Y. He, H. Lin, J. Han, Y. Chai, Y. Wei, X. Deng, Electrospun gelatin/-TCP composite nanofibers enhance osteogenic differentiation of BMSCs and in vivo bone formation by activating Ca2, Stem Cells International (2015) https://doi.org/10.1155/2015/507154.
[85] B. Liu, D. Lun, Current application of β-tricalcium phosphate composites in orthopaedics, Orthopaedic Surgery 4 (2012) 139–144, https://doi.org/10.1111/j.1757-7861.2012.00189.x.
[86] S. Shadanbaz, G.J. Dias, Calcium phosphate coatings on magnesium alloys for biomedical applications: a review, Acta Biomaterialia 8 (2012) 20–30, https://doi.org/10.1016/j.actbio.2011.10.016.

[87] F. Tamimi, B. Kumarasami, C. Doillon, U. Gbureck, D.L. Nihouannen, E.L. Cabarcos, J.E. Barralet, Brushite–collagen composites for bone regeneration, Acta Biomaterialia 4 (2008) 1315–1321, https://doi.org/10.1016/j.actbio.2008.04.003.

[88] F. Tamimi, J. Torres, K. Al-Abedalla, E. Lopez-Cabarcos, M.H. Alkhraisat, D.C. Bassett, U. Gbureck, J.E. Barralet, Osseointegration of dental implants in 3D-printed synthetic onlay grafts customized according to bone metabolic activity in recipient site, Biomaterials 35 (2014) 5436–5445, https://doi.org/10.1016/j.biomaterials.2014.03.050.

[89] F. Tamimi, J. Torres, D. Bassett, J. Barralet, E.L. Cabarcos, Resorption of monetite granules in alveolar bone defects in human patients, Biomaterials 31 (2010) 2762–2769, https://doi.org/10.1016/j.biomaterials.2009.12.039.

[90] F. Tamimi, J. Torres, R. Bettini, F. Ruggera, C. Rueda, M. López-Ponce, E. Lopez-Cabarcos, Doxycycline sustained release from brushite cements for the treatment of periodontal diseases, Journal of Biomedical Materials Research 85A (2008) 707–714, https://doi.org/10.1002/jbm.a.31610.

[91] F. Tamimi, J. Torres, U. Gbureck, E. Lopez-Cabarcos, D.C. Bassett, M.H. Alkhraisat, J.E. Barralet, Craniofacial vertical bone augmentation: a comparison between 3D printed monolithic monetite blocks and autologous onlay grafts in the rabbit, Biomaterials 30 (2009) 6318–6326, https://doi.org/10.1016/j.biomaterials.2009.07.049.

[92] F. Tamimi, J. Torres, E. Lopez-Cabarcos, D.C. Bassett, P. Habibovic, E. Luceron, J.E. Barralet, Minimally invasive maxillofacial vertical bone augmentation using brushite based cements, Biomaterials 30 (2009) 208–216, https://doi.org/10.1016/j.biomaterials.2008.09.032.

[93] K. Tamura, S. Sato, M. Kishida, S. Asano, M. Murai, K. Ito, The use of porous β-tricalcium phosphate blocks with platelet-rich plasma as an onlay bone graft biomaterial, Journal of Periodontology 78 (2007) 315–321, https://doi.org/10.1902/jop.2007.060228.

[94] F.T. Mariño, J. Torres, I. Tresguerres, L.B. Jerez, E.L. Cabarcos, Vertical bone augmentation with granulated brushite cement set in glycolic acid, Journal of Biomedical Materials Research 81A (2007) 93–102, https://doi.org/10.1002/jbm.a.31014.

[95] P. Van Landuyt, B. Peter, L. Beluze, J. Lemaître, Reinforcement of osteosynthesis screws with brushite cement, Bone 25 (1999) 95S–98S, https://doi.org/10.1016/S8756-3282(99)00142-8.

[96] S.A. Gehrke, G.M. Fama', Buccal dehiscence and sinus lift cases – predictable bone augmentation with synthetic bone material, Implants 11 (2010) 1–14.

[97] J.Z. Paxton, K. Donnelly, R.P. Keatch, K. Baar, L.M. Grover, Factors affecting the longevity and strength in an in vitro model of the bone–ligament interface, Annals of Biomedical Engineering 38 (2010) 2155–2166, https://doi.org/10.1007/s10439-010-0044-0.

[98] J.Z. Paxton, L.M. Grover, K. Baar, Engineering an in vitro model of a functional ligament from bone to bone, Tissue Engineering Part A 16 (2010) 3515–3525, https://doi.org/10.1089/ten.TEA.2010.0039.

[99] N. Mehrban, J.Z. Paxton, J. Bowen, A. Bolarinwa, E. Vorndran, U. Gbureck, L.M. Grover, Comparing physicochemical properties of printed and hand cast biocements designed for ligament replacement, Advances in Applied Ceramics 110 (2011) 162–167, https://doi.org/10.1179/1743676110Y.0000000012.

[100] F. Theiss, D. Apelt, B. Brand, A. Kutter, K. Zlinszky, M. Bohner, S. Matter, C. Frei, J.A. Auer, B. von Rechenberg, Biocompatibility and resorption of a brushite calcium phosphate cement, Biomaterials 26 (2005) 4383–4394, https://doi.org/10.1016/j.biomaterials.2004.11.056.

[101] H. Zhou, T.J.F. Luchini, A.K. Agarwal, V.K. Goel, S.B. Bhaduri, Development of monetite–nanosilica bone cement: a preliminary study, Journal of Biomedical Materials Research 102 (2014) 1620–1626, https://doi.org/10.1002/jbm.b.33149.

[102] S. Saska, L.S. Mendes, A.M.M. Gaspar, T.S. de O. Capote, Bone substitute materials in implant dentistry, Current Concepts in Dental Implantology (2015) https://doi.org/10.5772/59487.
[103] E. Hughes, T. Yanni, P. Jamshidi, L.M. Grover, Inorganic cements for biomedical application: calcium phosphate, calcium sulphate and calcium silicate, Advances in Applied Ceramics 114 (2015) 65–76, https://doi.org/10.1179/1743676114Y.0000000219.
[104] G. Mestres, C.F. Santos, L. Engman, C. Persson, M. Karlsson Ott, Scavenging effect of trolox released from brushite cements, Acta Biomaterialia 11 (2015) 459–466, https://doi.org/10.1016/j.actbio.2014.09.007.
[105] L.C. Rodriguez, J. Chari, S. Aghyarian, I.M. Gindri, V. Kosmopoulos, D.C. Rodrigues, Preparation and characterization of injectable brushite filled-poly (methyl methacrylate) bone cement, Materials 7 (2014) 6779–6795, https://doi.org/10.3390/ma7096779.
[106] S. Zhang, W. Wan, K. Xu, Q. Yuan, M. Xing, Dual-functional biomaterials for bone regeneration and infection control, Journal of Biomaterials and Tissue Engineering 4 (2014) 875–885, https://doi.org/10.1166/jbt.2014.1269.
[107] J.P. Moseley, M.E. Carroll, J.D. McCanless, Composite Bone Graft Substitute Cement and Articles Produced Therefrom, 2006. https://patents.google.com/patent/US7754246B2/en.
[108] Q. Fu, M.N. Rahaman, B. Sonny Bal, R.F. Brown, D.E. Day, Mechanical and in vitro performance of 13–93 bioactive glass scaffolds prepared by a polymer foam replication technique, Acta Biomaterialia 4 (2008) 1854–1864, https://doi.org/10.1016/j.actbio.2008.04.019.
[109] X. Liu, M.N. Rahaman, Q. Fu, Bone regeneration in strong porous bioactive glass (13-93) scaffolds with an oriented microstructure implanted in rat calvarial defects, Acta Biomaterialia 9 (2013) 4889–4898, https://doi.org/10.1016/j.actbio.2012.08.029.
[110] X. Liu, M.N. Rahaman, Q. Fu, A.P. Tomsia, Porous and strong bioactive glass (13-93) scaffolds prepared by unidirectional freezing of camphene-based suspensions, Acta Biomaterialia 8 (2012) 415–423, https://doi.org/10.1016/j.actbio.2011.07.034.
[111] O. Bretcanu, C. Samaille, A.R. Boccaccini, Simple methods to fabricate Bioglass®-derived glass–ceramic scaffolds exhibiting porosity gradient, Journal of Materials Science 43 (2008) 4127–4134, https://doi.org/10.1007/s10853-008-2536-y.
[112] L.-C. Gerhardt, A.R. Boccaccini, Bioactive glass and glass-ceramic scaffolds for bone tissue engineering, Materials (Basel) 3 (2010) 3867–3910, https://doi.org/10.3390/ma3073867.
[113] J.J. Blaker, A. Bismarck, A.R. Boccaccini, A.M. Young, S.N. Nazhat, Premature degradation of poly(α-hydroxyesters) during thermal processing of Bioglass®-containing composites, Acta Biomaterialia 6 (2010) 756–762, https://doi.org/10.1016/j.actbio.2009.08.020.
[114] J.J. Blaker, V. Maquet, R. Jérôme, A.R. Boccaccini, S.N. Nazhat, Mechanical properties of highly porous PDLLA/Bioglass® composite foams as scaffolds for bone tissue engineering, Acta Biomaterialia 1 (2005) 643–652, https://doi.org/10.1016/j.actbio.2005.07.003.
[115] S.K. Misra, T.I. Ansari, S.P. Valappil, D. Mohn, S.E. Philip, W.J. Stark, I. Roy, J.C. Knowles, V. Salih, A.R. Boccaccini, Poly(3-hydroxybutyrate) multifunctional composite scaffolds for tissue engineering applications, Biomaterials 31 (2010) 2806–2815, https://doi.org/10.1016/j.biomaterials.2009.12.045.
[116] V. v. Meretoja, A. o. Helminen, J. j. Korventausta, V. Haapa-aho, J.v. Seppälä, T.o. Närhi, Crosslinked poly(ε-caprolactone/D,L-lactide)/bioactive glass composite scaffolds for bone tissue engineering, Journal of Biomedical Materials Research 77A (2006) 261–268, https://doi.org/10.1002/jbm.a.30630.
[117] V.V. Meretoja, M. Malin, J.V. Seppälä, T.O. Närhi, Osteoblast response to continuous phase macroporous scaffolds under static and dynamic culture conditions, Journal of Biomedical Materials Research 89A (2009) 317–325, https://doi.org/10.1002/jbm.a.31980.

[118] J. Yao, S. Radin, P.S. Leboy, P. Ducheyne, The effect of bioactive glass content on synthesis and bioactivity of composite poly (lactic-co-glycolic acid)/bioactive glass substrate for tissue engineering, Biomaterials 26 (2005) 1935–1943, https://doi.org/10.1016/j.biomaterials.2004.06.027.
[119] H. Keshaw, G. Georgiou, J.J. Blaker, A. Forbes, J.C. Knowles, R.M. Day, Assessment of polymer/bioactive glass-composite microporous spheres for tissue regeneration applications, Tissue Engineering Part a 15 (2008) 1451–1461, https://doi.org/10.1089/ten.tea.2008.0203.
[120] A.M. El-Kady, E.A. Saad, B.M.A. El-Hady, M.M. Farag, Synthesis of silicate glass/poly(L-lactide) composite scaffolds by freeze-extraction technique: characterization and in vitro bioactivity evaluation, Ceramics International 36 (2010) 995–1009, https://doi.org/10.1016/j.ceramint.2009.11.012.
[121] O. Tsigkou, L.L. Hench, A.R. Boccaccini, J.M. Polak, M.M. Stevens, Enhanced differentiation and mineralization of human fetal osteoblasts on PDLLA containing Bioglass® composite films in the absence of osteogenic supplements, Journal of Biomedical Materials Research 80A (2007) 837–851, https://doi.org/10.1002/jbm.a.30910.
[122] V. Maquet, A.R. Boccaccini, L. Pravata, I. Notingher, R. Jérôme, Porous poly(α-hydroxyacid)/Bioglass® composite scaffolds for bone tissue engineering. I: preparation and in vitro characterisation, Biomaterials 25 (2004) 4185–4194, https://doi.org/10.1016/j.biomaterials.2003.10.082.
[123] V. Maquet, A.R. Boccaccini, L. Pravata, I. Notingher, R. Jérôme, Preparation, characterization, and in vitro degradation of bioresorbable and bioactive composites based on Bioglass®-filled polylactide foams, Journal of Biomedical Materials Research 66A (2003) 335–346, https://doi.org/10.1002/jbm.a.10587.
[124] S. Verrier, J.J. Blaker, V. Maquet, L.L. Hench, A.R. Boccaccini, PDLLA/Bioglass® composites for soft-tissue and hard-tissue engineering: an in vitro cell biology assessment, Biomaterials 25 (2004) 3013–3021, https://doi.org/10.1016/j.biomaterials.2003.09.081.
[125] A.R. Boccaccini, V. Maquet, Bioresorbable and bioactive polymer/Bioglass® composites with tailored pore structure for tissue engineering applications, Composites Science and Technology 63 (2003) 2417–2429, https://doi.org/10.1016/S0266-3538(03)00275-6.
[126] H.H. Lu, S.F. El-Amin, K.D. Scott, C.T. Laurencin, Three-dimensional, bioactive, biodegradable, polymer–bioactive glass composite scaffolds with improved mechanical properties support collagen synthesis and mineralization of human osteoblast-like cells in vitro, Journal of Biomedical Materials Research 64A (2003) 465–474, https://doi.org/10.1002/jbm.a.10399.
[127] S.K. Misra, F. Ohashi, S.P. Valappil, J.C. Knowles, I. Roy, S.R.P. Silva, V. Salih, A.R. Boccaccini, Characterization of carbon nanotube (MWCNT) containing P(3HB)/bioactive glass composites for tissue engineering applications, Acta Biomaterialia 6 (2010) 735–742, https://doi.org/10.1016/j.actbio.2009.09.023.
[128] S.K. Misra, S.E. Philip, W. Chrzanowski, S.N. Nazhat, I. Roy, J.C. Knowles, V. Salih, A.R. Boccaccini, Incorporation of vitamin E in poly(3hydroxybutyrate)/Bioglass composite films: effect on surface properties and cell attachment, Journal of The Royal Society Interface 6 (2009) 401–409, https://doi.org/10.1098/rsif.2008.0278.
[129] S.K. Misra, T. Ansari, D. Mohn, S.P. Valappil, T.J. Brunner, W.J. Stark, I. Roy, J.C. Knowles, P.D. Sibbons, E.V. Jones, A.R. Boccaccini, V. Salih, Effect of nanoparticulate bioactive glass particles on bioactivity and cytocompatibility of poly(3-hydroxybutyrate) composites, Journal of The Royal Society Interface 7 (2010) 453–465, https://doi.org/10.1098/rsif.2009.0255.

[130] S.K. Misra, D. Mohn, T.J. Brunner, W.J. Stark, S.E. Philip, I. Roy, V. Salih, J.C. Knowles, A.R. Boccaccini, Comparison of nanoscale and microscale bioactive glass on the properties of P(3HB)/Bioglass® composites, Biomaterials 29 (2008) 1750–1761, https://doi.org/10.1016/j.biomaterials.2007.12.040.

[131] W. Helen, J.E. Gough, Cell viability, proliferation and extracellular matrix production of human annulus fibrosus cells cultured within PDLLA/Bioglass® composite foam scaffolds in vitro, Acta Biomaterialia 4 (2008) 230–243, https://doi.org/10.1016/j.actbio.2007.09.010.

[132] W. Helen, C.L.R. Merry, J.J. Blaker, J.E. Gough, Three-dimensional culture of annulus fibrosus cells within PDLLA/Bioglass® composite foam scaffolds: assessment of cell attachment, proliferation and extracellular matrix production, Biomaterials 28 (2007) 2010–2020, https://doi.org/10.1016/j.biomaterials.2007.01.011.

[133] X.B. Yang, D. Webb, J. Blaker, A.R. Boccaccini, V. Maquet, C. Cooper, R.O.C. Oreffo, Evaluation of human bone marrow stromal cell growth on biodegradable polymer/Bioglass® composites, Biochemical and Biophysical Research Communications 342 (2006) 1098–1107, https://doi.org/10.1016/j.bbrc.2006.02.021.

[134] N. Barroca, A.L. Daniel-da-Silva, P.M. Vilarinho, M.H.V. Fernandes, Tailoring the morphology of high molecular weight PLLA scaffolds through bioglass addition, Acta Biomaterialia 6 (2010) 3611–3620, https://doi.org/10.1016/j.actbio.2010.03.032.

[135] S. Deville, E. Saiz, A.P. Tomsia, Freeze casting of hydroxyapatite scaffolds for bone tissue engineering, Biomaterials 27 (2006) 5480–5489, https://doi.org/10.1016/j.biomaterials.2006.06.028.

[136] S.K. Swain, S. Bhattacharyya, D. Sarkar, Preparation of porous scaffold from hydroxyapatite powders, Materials Science and Engineering: C 31 (2011) 1240–1244, https://doi.org/10.1016/j.msec.2010.11.014.

[137] G. Tripathi, B. Basu, A porous hydroxyapatite scaffold for bone tissue engineering: physico-mechanical and biological evaluations, Ceramics International 38 (2012) 341–349, https://doi.org/10.1016/j.ceramint.2011.07.012.

[138] S. Kunjalukkal Padmanabhan, F. Gervaso, M. Carrozzo, F. Scalera, A. Sannino, A. Licciulli, Wollastonite/hydroxyapatite scaffolds with improved mechanical, bioactive and biodegradable properties for bone tissue engineering, Ceramics International 39 (2013) 619–627, https://doi.org/10.1016/j.ceramint.2012.06.073.

[139] P. Feng, P. Wei, P. Li, C. Gao, C. Shuai, S. Peng, Calcium silicate ceramic scaffolds toughened with hydroxyapatite whiskers for bone tissue engineering, Materials Characterization 97 (2014) 47–56, https://doi.org/10.1016/j.matchar.2014.08.017.

[140] M.B. Nair, S. Suresh Babu, H.K. Varma, A. John, A triphasic ceramic-coated porous hydroxyapatite for tissue engineering application, Acta Biomaterialia 4 (2008) 173–181, https://doi.org/10.1016/j.actbio.2007.07.004.

[141] Y. Zhang, L. Chen, J. Zeng, K. Zhou, D. Zhang, Aligned porous barium titanate/hydroxyapatite composites with high piezoelectric coefficients for bone tissue engineering, Materials Science and Engineering: C 39 (2014) 143–149, https://doi.org/10.1016/j.msec.2014.02.022.

[142] M.S. Islam, M. Todo, Effects of sintering temperature on the compressive mechanical properties of collagen/hydroxyapatite composite scaffolds for bone tissue engineering, Materials Letters 173 (2016) 231–234, https://doi.org/10.1016/j.matlet.2016.03.028.

[143] L. Stipniece, I. Narkevica, M. Sokolova, J. Locs, J. Ozolins, Novel scaffolds based on hydroxyapatite/poly(vinyl alcohol) nanocomposite coated porous TiO_2 ceramics for bone tissue engineering, Ceramics International 42 (2016) 1530–1537, https://doi.org/10.1016/j.ceramint.2015.09.101.

[144] C.-P. Jiang, Y.-Y. Chen, M.-F. Hsieh, Biofabrication and in vitro study of hydroxyapatite/mPEG–PCL–mPEG scaffolds for bone tissue engineering using air pressure-aided deposition technology, Materials Science and Engineering: C 33 (2013) 680–690, https://doi.org/10.1016/j.msec.2012.10.018.

[145] M. Rinaudo, Chitin and chitosan: properties and applications, Progress in Polymer Science 31 (2006) 603–632, https://doi.org/10.1016/j.progpolymsci.2006.06.001.

[146] J.M. Oliveira, M.T. Rodrigues, S.S. Silva, P.B. Malafaya, M.E. Gomes, C.A. Viegas, I.R. Dias, J.T. Azevedo, J.F. Mano, R.L. Reis, Novel hydroxyapatite/chitosan bilayered scaffold for osteochondral tissue-engineering applications: scaffold design and its performance when seeded with goat bone marrow stromal cells, Biomaterials 27 (2006) 6123–6137, https://doi.org/10.1016/j.biomaterials.2006.07.034.

[147] A. Shavandi, A.E.-D.A. Bekhit, M.A. Ali, Z. Sun, M. Gould, Development and characterization of hydroxyapatite/β-TCP/chitosan composites for tissue engineering applications, Materials Science and Engineering: C 56 (2015) 481–493, https://doi.org/10.1016/j.msec.2015.07.004.

[148] A. Shavandi, A.E.-D.A. Bekhit, Z. Sun, A. Ali, M. Gould, A novel squid pen chitosan/hydroxyapatite/β-tricalcium phosphate composite for bone tissue engineering, Materials Science and Engineering: C 55 (2015) 373–383, https://doi.org/10.1016/j.msec.2015.05.029.

[149] H.-H. Jin, D.-H. Kim, T.-W. Kim, K.-K. Shin, J.S. Jung, H.-C. Park, S.-Y. Yoon, In vivo evaluation of porous hydroxyapatite/chitosan–alginate composite scaffolds for bone tissue engineering, International Journal of Biological Macromolecules 51 (2012) 1079–1085, https://doi.org/10.1016/j.ijbiomac.2012.08.027.

[150] Z. Cui, B. Nelson, Y. Peng, K. Li, S. Pilla, W.-J. Li, L.-S. Turng, C. Shen, Fabrication and characterization of injection molded poly (ε-caprolactone) and poly (ε-caprolactone)/hydroxyapatite scaffolds for tissue engineering, Materials Science and Engineering: C 32 (2012) 1674–1681, https://doi.org/10.1016/j.msec.2012.04.064.

[151] L.J. Gibson, The mechanical behaviour of cancellous bone, Journal of Biomechanics 18 (1985) 317–328, https://doi.org/10.1016/0021-9290(85)90287-8.

[152] I. Sabree, J.E. Gough, B. Derby, Mechanical properties of porous ceramic scaffolds: influence of internal dimensions, Ceramics International 41 (2015) 8425–8432, https://doi.org/10.1016/j.ceramint.2015.03.044.

Recent research trends

6

A vast number of research trends are currently active in the field of bioceramics. However, in this book, the student has been shown the first steps in the rapid progress in bioceramics research and development. The content of this chapter is limited to aspects of nanotechnology in hard tissue engineering and drug delivery, including various materials and processes.

Nanotechnology is not merely using nanosized materials and the fabrication of nanostructures. Nanotechnology embraces the noticeable rise of properties quantitatively and/or qualitatively. The student will see that nanotechnology gives surprising flexibility in tailoring the microstructure and final properties of biomaterials. Apart from the alumina and zirconia implants fabricated from nanostarting powders, tissue hard engineering has benefited considerably from nanotechnology.

Well-controlled 3D pore architectures and high porosity (90% and above) scaffolds are achieved by utilizing nanohydroxyapatite (nHAP)/polymer composites dissolved in dioxane or benzene and applying the thermally induced phase separation technique, as detailed in Ref. [1]. Nanohydroxyapatite–poly(L-lactic acid) (nHAP/PLLA) with a dioxane/water mixture solvent system develops scaffolds of fibrous morphology, as seen in Fig. 6.1. The figure shows the difference in pore morphology between the pure PLLA scaffold, microhydroxyapatite (μHAP)/PLLA 50:50 scaffold and nHAP/PLLA 50:50 scaffold. The nHAP/PLLA scaffold shows a regular internal ladder-like pore structure, and the hydroxyapatite (HA) particles are uniformly distributed within the pore walls of the scaffolds and are free of large aggregates. On the other hand, HA particles in the μHAP/PLLA scaffold are randomly distributed in the PLLA matrix. The tubular pore architecture for the nHAP/PLLA scaffolds is obtained using benzene as a solvent and controlling the heat transfer direction.

When the PLLA of inherent viscosity of 1.4–1.8 dL/g is replaced with another copolymer (poly(lactic acid) [PLA] and poly(glycolic acid) copolymer [PLGA], LA:GA = 85:15), of inherent viscosity of 0.6 dL/g, an interconnected pore structure and leaf-like morphology results, as seen in Fig. 6.2. The regular ladder-like pore structure is replaced with smaller pores and random pore structure when small amounts of water are added to the solvent, as is obvious in Fig. 6.3. Fetal bovine serum/phosphate buffered saline (FBS/PBS) solution incubation of the scaffolds is used to investigate protein adsorption. The results show that the protein adsorption for the fibrous textured scaffolds is about four times greater than of that of the smooth pore walls, which indicates excellent cell attachment and migration in the fibrous textured scaffolds.

The aforementioned phase separation process starts by mixing the polymer with a proper solvent and heating up the mixture; then, the solution is cooled to achieve solidification of the solvent and phase separation takes place. Another process is called the phase inversion technique, in which the mixture is thermodynamically unstable

Bioceramics: For Materials Science and Engineering. https://doi.org/10.1016/B978-0-08-102233-7.00006-9

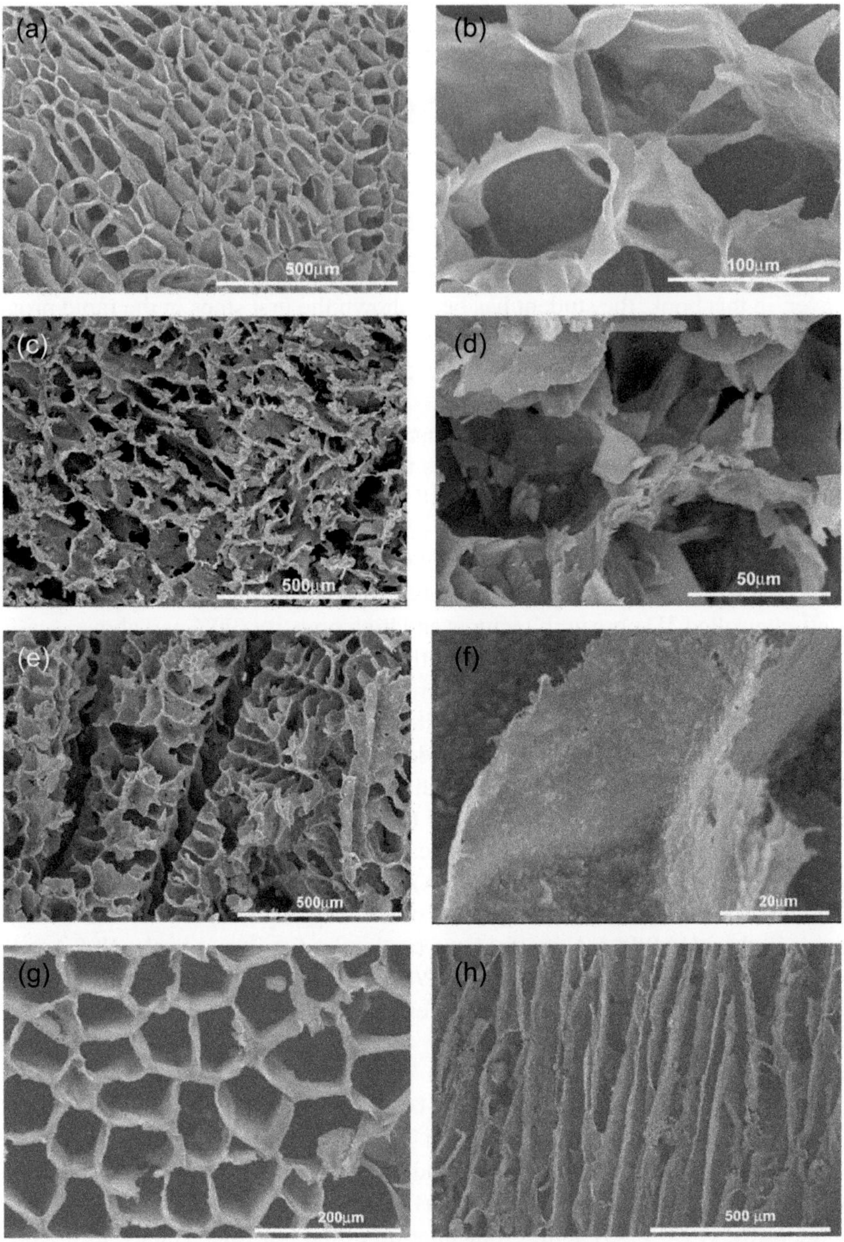

Figure 6.1 Scanning electron microscope micrographs of plain poly(L-lactic acid) PLLA, nanohydroxyapatite (nHAP)/PLLA, and microhydroxyapatite (μHAP)/PLLA scaffolds fabricated from 5% dioxane (a–e) and benzene (f and g) solution. (a and b) Pure PLLA scaffold, ×50, ×400; (c and d) μHAP/PLLA 50:50 scaffold, ×100, ×500; (e and f) nHAP/PLLA 50:50 scaffold, ×100, ×1000; (g) Tubular nHAP/PLLA scaffold, cross-section, ×200; (h) Tubular nHAP/PLLA scaffold, longitudinal section, ×100.
Reused from G. Wei, P.X. Ma, Structure and properties of nano-hydroxyapatite/polymer composite scaffolds for bone tissue engineering, Biomaterials 25 (2004) 4749–4757. https://doi.org/10.1016/j.biomaterials.2003.12.005 after license via (copyright.com) number 4275170434034.

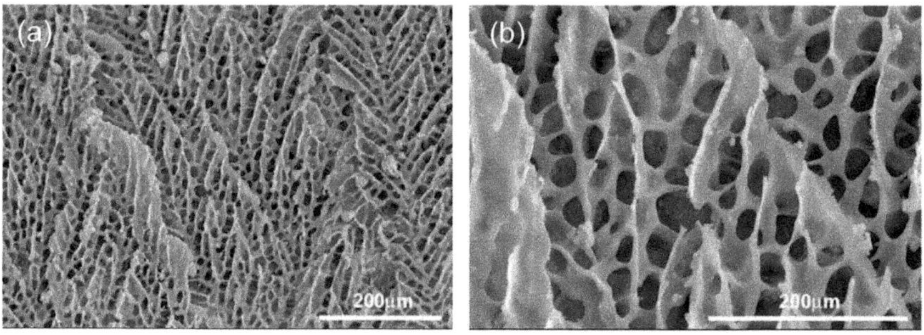

Figure 6.2 Scanning electron microscope micrographs of nanohydroxyapatite /poly(glycolic acid) copolymer 85 (30:70) scaffolds fabricated from 10% dioxane solution quenched at −70°C, (a) ×150 and (b) ×500.
Reused from G. Wei, P.X. Ma, Structure and properties of nano-hydroxyapatite/polymer composite scaffolds for bone tissue engineering, Biomaterials 25 (2004) 4749–4757. https://doi.org/10.1016/j.biomaterials.2003.12.005 after license via (copyright.com) number 4275170434034.

and a phase inversion of the solvent can be induced thermally, in some cases by cooling and in other cases by heating. The phase inversion technique is utilized with an nHAP/polyamide composite mixed with alcohol by heating the system to 80°C to let the phase inversion of the liquid alcohol to the gaseous phase take place [2]. The resultant microstructure is highly porous (70% porosity) and consists of micropores located on the pore walls of macropores. The resultant scaffolds show good biocompatibility and extensive osteoconductivity with the bone of rabbit mandibles. When the scaffolds are seeded with mesenchymal stem cells derived from bone marrow of neonatal rabbits, the mineralization and regeneration of bone are accelerated.

Almost the same methodology of Ref. [1] is followed by two separate studies [3,4] for the synthesis of rod-like or needle-like nHAP/PLLA composite scaffolds. Practically, equivalent conclusions are drawn concerning the resultant microstructure, in vitro cell attachment, and proliferation. In addition, it is shown that the compressive strength of the nanocomposite scaffolds is higher than that of the microcomposite scaffolds, and both of them are far higher than that of pure PLLA scaffolds. These two studies also add X-ray diffraction (XRD), Fourier transform infrared (FTIR), energy dispersive X-ray, and porosimetry analysis.

Once more, as the polymer ceramic composites are recurrently encountered in ceramic materials science and engineering, the development in polymer processing reflects directly on the processing of the polymer ceramic composites. Electrospinning of polymer solution emerged as a successful and tunable method for the formation of polymer nanofibers. In this method, the selected polymer solution is pumped to a metallic needle called the spinneret. The polymer jet is charged and collected on a rapidly rotating grounded collector. Controlling the process parameters fabricates a predesigned micro-/nanofiber mat. The details, advantages, and applications of the polymer electrospinning fabrication process can be found in these excellent reviews [5,6].

The electrospinning technique is utilized to fabricate PLGA and PLGA/collagen nanofibers before incorporating nHAP via a procedure detailed in Ref. [7].

Fig. 6.4 shows that the electrospun nanofibers are smooth and almost of uniform thickness, and the PLGA/collagen nanofibers are of smaller average diameter. nHAP is more uniformly distributed on PLGA/collagen nanofibers than that of PLGA nanofibers alone, as seen in Fig. 6.5. Cell culturing is studied using human fetal osteoblasts, which are an embryonic osteoblast cell line, i.e., nontumor cells. Fig. 6.6 shows that the cells adhere to the nanofibers in mineralized and nonmineralized regions. The

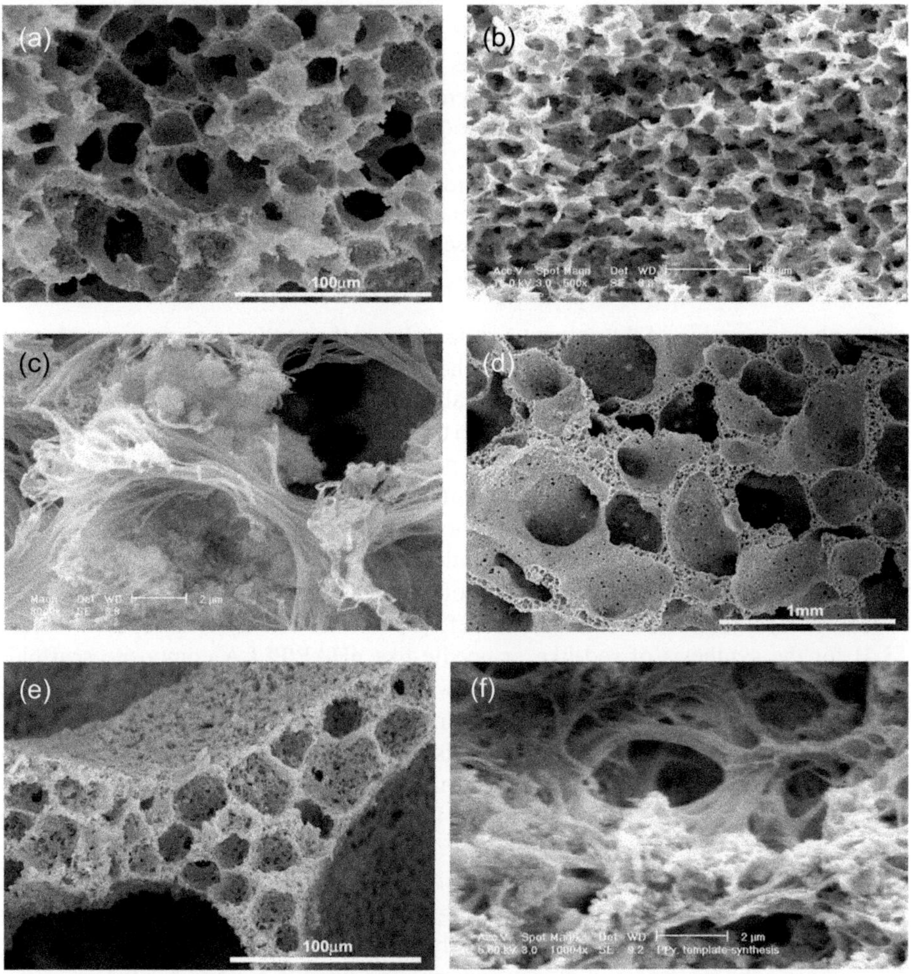

Figure 6.3 Scanning electron microscope micrographs of nanohydroxyapatite/poly(L-lactic acid)(30:70) scaffolds fabricated using dioxane/water mixture solvents. (a) Dioxane:water = 95:5, ×500. (b and c) Dioxane:water = 90:10, ×500, ×8000. (d–f) Dioxane:water = 87:13, ×45, ×500, ×10,000.
Reused from G. Wei, P.X. Ma, Structure and properties of nano-hydroxyapatite/polymer composite scaffolds for bone tissue engineering, Biomaterials 25 (2004) 4749–4757. https://doi.org/10.1016/j.biomaterials.2003.12.005 after license via (copyright.com) number 4275170434034.

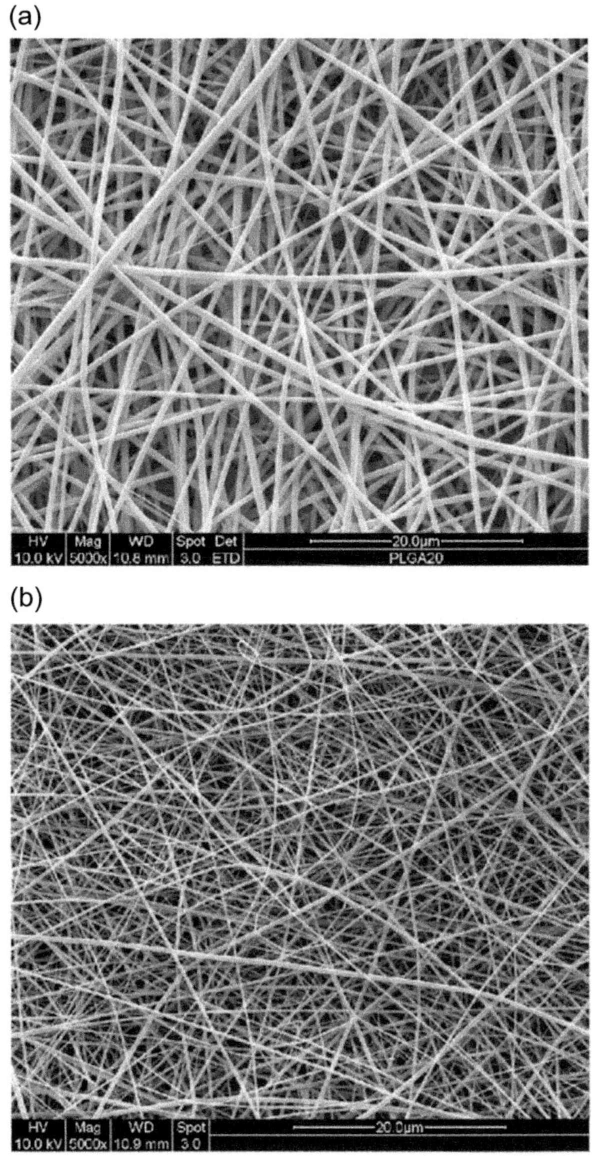

Figure 6.4 Morphology of electrospun (a) pure poly(glycolic acid) (PLGA) and (b) PLGA/collagen nanofibers.
Reused from M. Ngiam, S. Liao, A.J. Patil, Z. Cheng, C.K. Chan, S. Ramakrishna, The fabrication of nano-hydroxyapatite on PLGA and PLGA/collagen nanofibrous composite scaffolds and their effects in osteoblastic behavior for bone tissue engineering, Bone 45 (2009) 4–16. https://doi.org/10.1016/j.bone.2009.03.674 after license via (copyright.com) number 4276390071938.

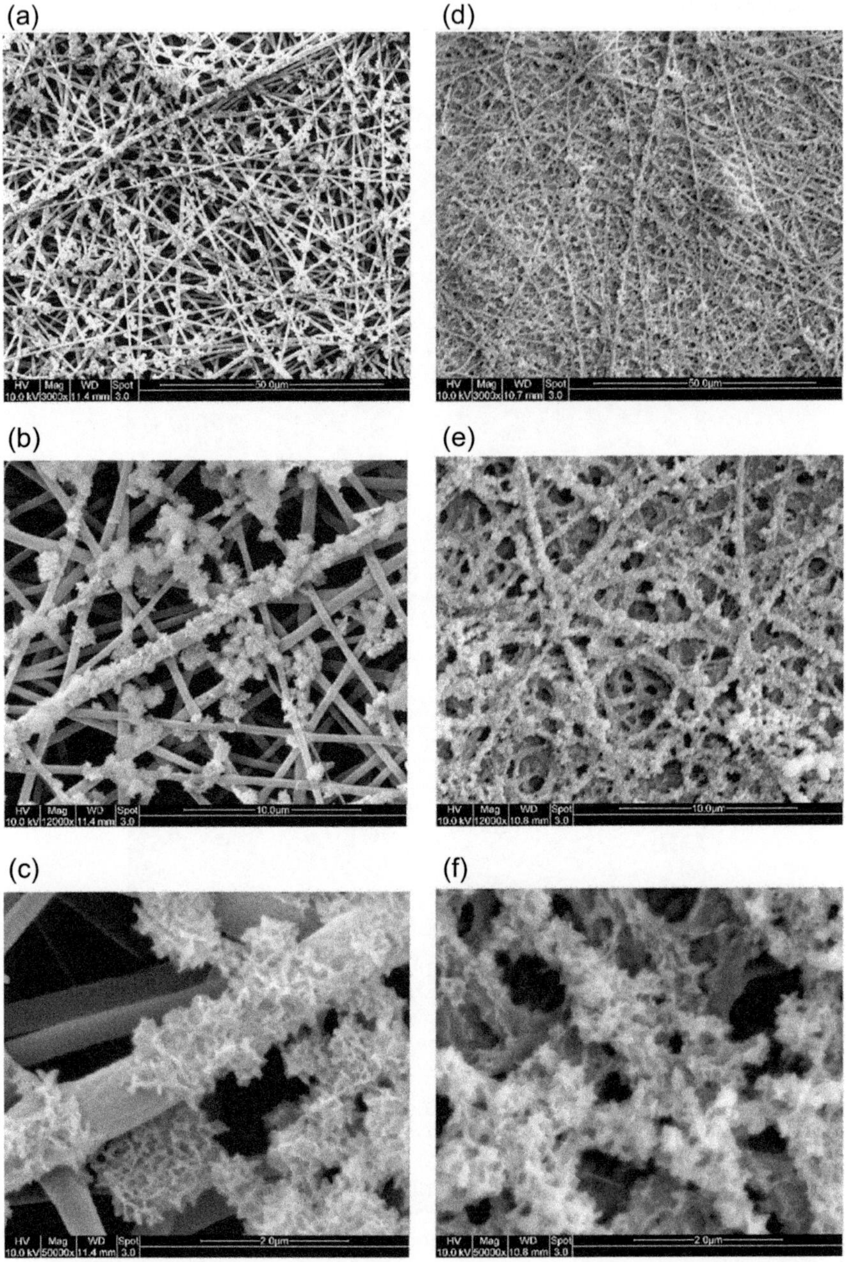

Figure 6.5 Distribution of nanohydroxyapatite (nHA) on nanofibers. (a–c) denote nHA deposition on poly(glycolic acid) (PLGA) nanofibers. (d–f) represent nHA deposition on PLGA/collagen nanofibers.
Reused from M. Ngiam, S. Liao, A.J. Patil, Z. Cheng, C.K. Chan, S. Ramakrishna, The fabrication of nano-hydroxyapatite on PLGA and PLGA/collagen nanofibrous composite scaffolds and their effects in osteoblastic behavior for bone tissue engineering, Bone 45 (2009) 4–16. https://doi.org/10.1016/j.bone.2009.03.674 after license via (copyright.com) number 4276390071938.

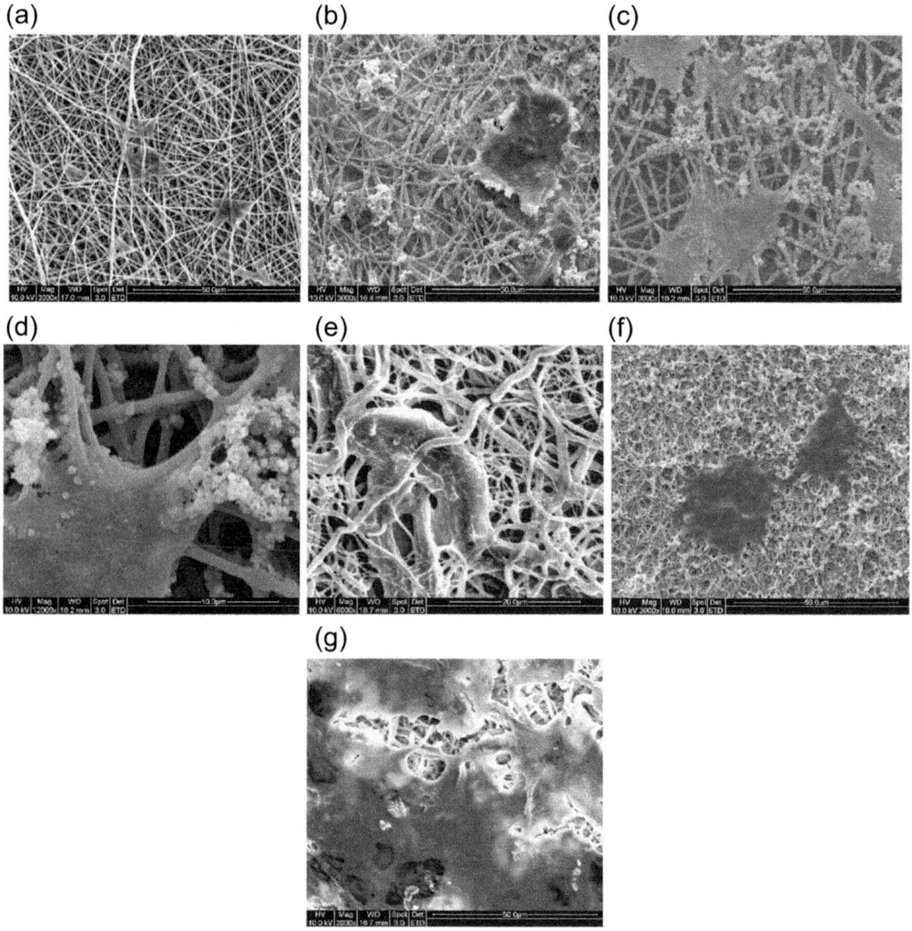

Figure 6.6 Osteoblasts on mineralized and nonmineralized nanofibers. (a) Poly(glycolic acid) (PLGA) (day 1), (b) PLGA + nanohydroxyapatite (nHA) (day 1), (c) PLGA + nHA (day 4), (d) is the enlargement of the central part of (c), (e) PLGA/collagen (day 1), (f) PLGA/collagen + nHA (day 1), (g) PLGA/collagen + nHA (day 4).
Reused from M. Ngiam, S. Liao, A.J. Patil, Z. Cheng, C.K. Chan, S. Ramakrishna, The fabrication of nano-hydroxyapatite on PLGA and PLGA/collagen nanofibrous composite scaffolds and their effects in osteoblastic behavior for bone tissue engineering, Bone 45 (2009) 4–16. https://doi.org/10.1016/j.bone.2009.03.674 after license via (copyright.com) number 4276390071938.

existence of nHAP enhances cell spreading. Also, cell spreading is encouraged in the case of PLGA/collagen nanofibers compared with PLGA nanofibers alone. Other details and a discussion in the same study should be found valuable for the reader. Also, an nHAP composite of a chitosan (CS)/poly(vinyl alcohol)(PVA) mixture matrix [8] may be found informative to students.

Before proceeding, it may be the right place for a short summary of the process of research and development study of bioactive ceramic–polymer composites to fabricate scaffolds for hard tissue engineering:

1. The selection of polymer, copolymer, or polymer blends and also the selection of synthetic or natural polymers. The type of polymer may contribute to the final properties of the scaffolds, as reviewed in Ref. [9].
2. The selection of the bioactive ceramic, such as HA or other calcium phosphate, ready-to-use bioceramics or their precursors, or micro-/nanobioceramics. A helpful review can be found in Ref. [10].
3. The selection of the fabrication process of the scaffold. A variety of suggested processes can be found in the literature and it is useful to start with this review [11].
4. Determination of the necessary characterizations needed to accomplish a complete study. Example characterizations are position-sensitive detector, XRD, FTIR, and scanning electron microscope (SEM). The references mentioned in Chapter 5 and and in this chapter contain a number of characterization examples.
5. Examination of cell proliferation and attachment, which is normally contained in research concerning engineering. More comprehensive studies also contain histology examination.

In situ precipitation, a distinguishable composite preparation process, is used to prepare a chitosan–polylactic acid/hydroxyapatite (CS–PLA/HA) nanocomposite scaffold [12]. The process starts with dissolved CS solution, dissolving the HA precursors in the CS solution, adding dissolved PLA solution, adding a cross-linker agent, and finally precipitation of the nHAP by soaking with ammonia solution. The chitosan/hydroxyapatite (CS/HA) nanocomposite scaffold is also prepared using the same steps without adding PLA. In this process, the polymer matrix acts as a template that controls the morphology of the inorganic phase. In this case, the resultant morphology is a rod-like shape composed of aligned spheres. The diameter of rods is about 50 nm, and the length is about 300 nm. The rod-like nHAP nanoparticles are homogeneously distributed in the polymer matrix. Compressive strength and elastic modulus are improved when PLA is incorporated. Fig. 6.7 shows the morphology of both CS–PLA/HA and CS/HA composites. The interconnected network of the HA rods can be visualized after calcination of the composite, as shown in Fig. 6.8. The polymer network is revealed by removing the inorganic phase by adding hydrochloric acid, as shown in Fig. 6.9. The figure shows that the polymer network is not interconnected. The porous scaffolds are then obtained after the freeze-drying process that yields scaffolds of 85% porosity. The scaffolds have a hierarchical porous morphology that also contains primary pores (100–200 μm) and subpores (2–10 μm).

In dental or maxillofacial surgery, the surgeon may encounter a situation where there is insufficient space for bone growth. Thus bioactive biodegradable membranes are used to direct the growth of the hard tissue, and the process is called guided bone regeneration (GBR). Guided tissue regeneration is also known for gingival esthetics or prosthetic restoration.

In a novel study, *N*-carboxyethylchitosan/nHAP nanocomposite films were fabricated for potential application in GBR [13]. Cell adhesion and growth were investigated, utilizing the rabbit tracheal cartilage cells. Carboxyethylchitosan (CECS) films

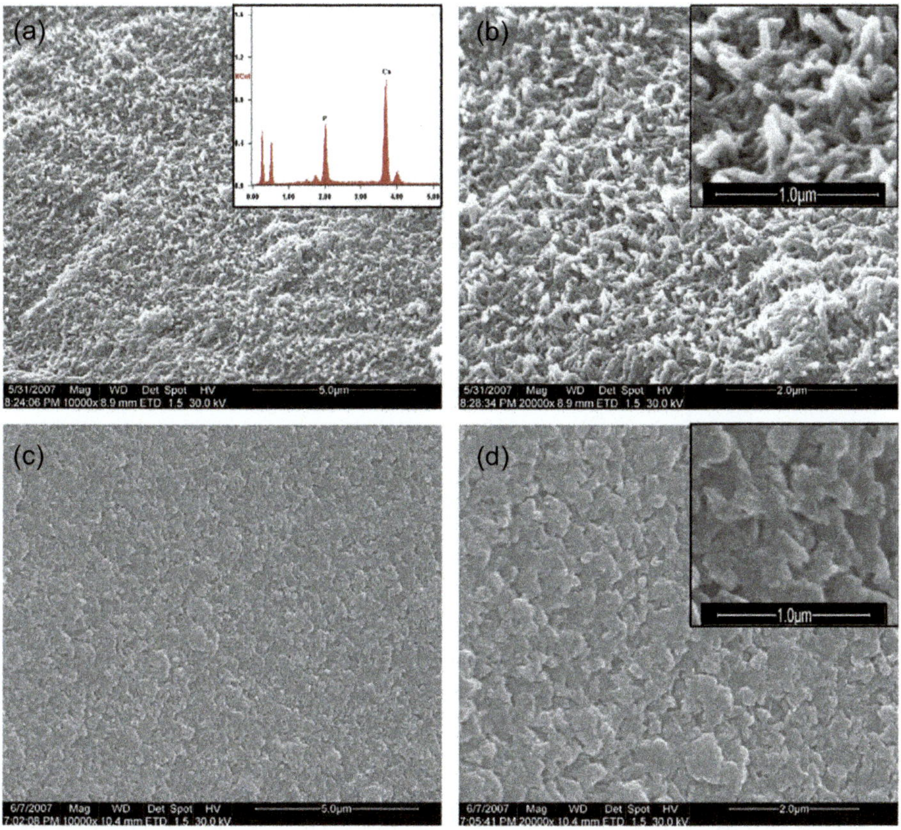

Figure 6.7 Scanning electron microscope (SEM) micrographs of (a) the chitosan–polylactic acid/hydroxyapatite (CS–PLA/HA) composite (the inset shows the calibrated energy dispersive X-ray area analysis of the composite); (b) a highly magnified SEM image of the CS–PLA/HA composite; (c) the CS/HA composite; and (d) a highly magnified SEM image of the CS/HA composite.

Reused from X. Cai, H. Tong, X. Shen, W. Chen, J. Yan, J. Hu, Preparation and characterization of homogeneous chitosan–polylactic acid/hydroxyapatite nanocomposite for bone tissue engineering and evaluation of its mechanical properties, Acta Biomaterialia 5 (2009) 2693–2703. https://doi.org/10.1016/j.actbio.2009.03.005 after license via (copyright.com) number 4276730600480.

have shown compatibility with cartilage cells and improved cell growth behavior was shown with the nanocomposite films. The addition of nHAP to the CECS improved both cell density and morphology.

A different attempt to fabricate films or membranes for GBR is done utilizing an nHAP/CS cross-linking composite [14]. The cross-linker was a natural water-soluble cross-linking agent called genipin. Genipin is usually used for the cross-linking of proteins, collagen, gelatin, and CS because it is much less toxic than other commonly used synthetic cross-linkers. In this study, the choice of genipin is to adjust the

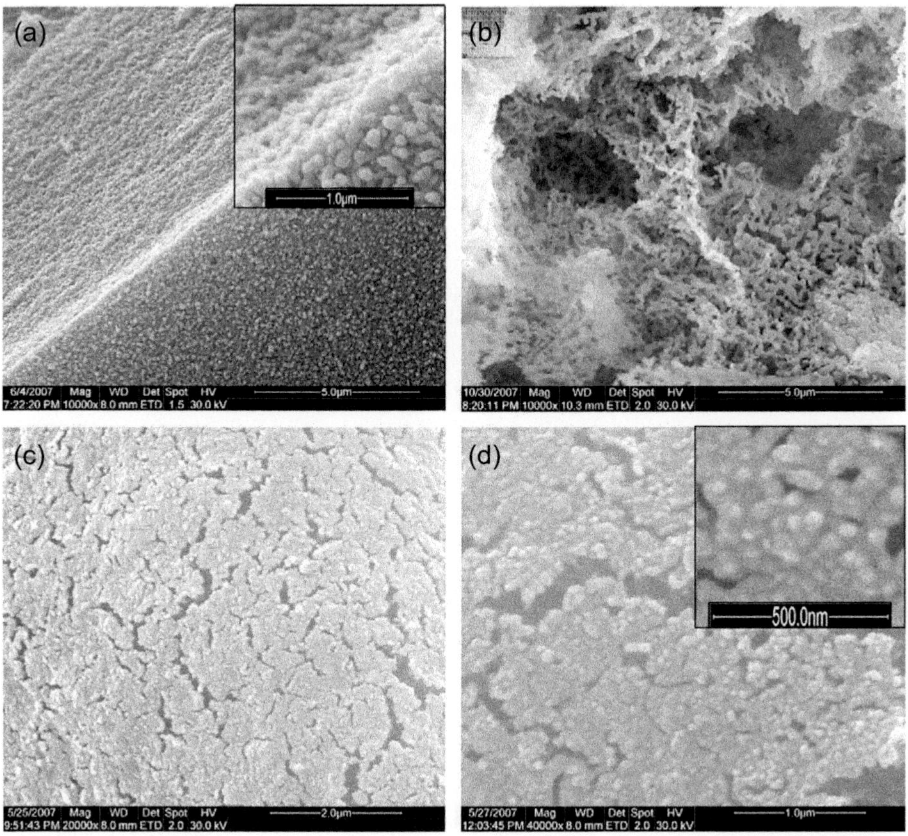

Figure 6.8 Scanning electron microscope (SEM) micrographs of (a) the profile morphology of the chitosan–polylactic acid/hydroxyapatite (CS–PLA/HA) composite; (b) the inner structure of the inorganic block after calcining; (c) the surface of the remaining CS–PLA matrix after removal of the inorganic phase; and (d) a highly magnified SEM image of the surface of the remaining CS–PLA matrix.
Reused from X. Cai, H. Tong, X. Shen, W. Chen, J. Yan, J. Hu, Preparation and characterization of homogeneous chitosan–polylactic acid/hydroxyapatite nanocomposite for bone tissue engineering and evaluation of its mechanical properties, Acta Biomaterialia 5 (2009) 2693–2703. https://doi.org/10.1016/j.actbio.2009.03.005 after license via (copyright.com) number 4276730600480.

hydrophobic properties of CS that only dissolve in acidic solution and activate the cross-linking to improve its mechanical properties.

nHAP was synthesized by a hydrothermal precipitation process, and the resultant particle morphology was needle-like rods (or nanorods) of dimensions of about 20 nm × 100 nm, as shown in Fig. 6.10. The composite membranes were made with different amounts of nHAP content, as shown in Table 6.1, and the resultant morphology of the upper and lower surfaces is shown in Fig. 6.11 for each composition listed

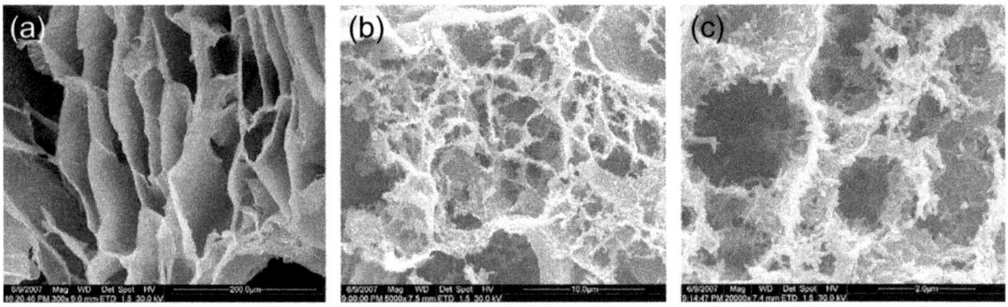

Figure 6.9 Scanning electron microscope micrographs of freeze-drying chitosan–polylactic acid/hydroxyapatite composite: (a) primary pores; (b) subpores; (c) nanocomposites of subpore walls.
Reused from X. Cai, H. Tong, X. Shen, W. Chen, J. Yan, J. Hu, Preparation and characterization of homogeneous chitosan–polylactic acid/hydroxyapatite nanocomposite for bone tissue engineering and evaluation of its mechanical properties, Acta Biomaterialia 5 (2009) 2693–2703. https://doi.org/10.1016/j.actbio.2009.03.005 after license via (copyright.com) number 4276730600480.

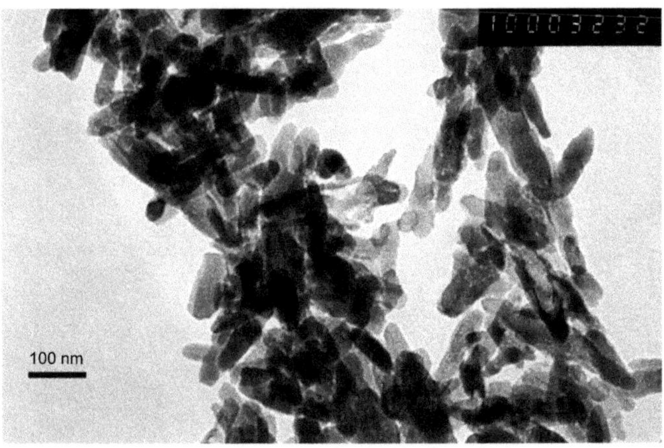

Figure 6.10 Transmission electron microscopy photograph of the nanohydroxyapatite.
Reused from X. Li, K. Nan, S. Shi, H. Chen, Preparation and characterization of nano-hydroxyapatite/chitosan cross-linking composite membrane intended for tissue engineering, International Journal of Biological Macromolecules 50 (2012) 43–49. https://doi.org/10.1016/j.ijbiomac.2011.09.021 after license via (copyright.com) number 4278671343254.

in Table 6.1. The figure shows that increasing nHAP leads to an increase in roughness of both surfaces, especially the lower surface because of the settlement of the nHaP particles. When the nHAP content exceeds 15%, cracks start to appear at the lower surfaces. These results encourage future attempts to improve the fabrication process.

The HA nanorods were again synthesized via the hydrothermal process but this time with the assistance of a triblock copolymer P123, also called pluronic. A simple

Table 6.1 Nanohydroxyapatite (nHAP)/chitosan cross-linking composite membrane made from various HA contents

Samples	Chitosan concentration (mg/mL)	nHAP content (%)	Genipin concentration (mM)
S-1	20	0	0.5
S-2	20	5	0.5
S-3	20	10	0.5
S-4	20	15	0.5
S-5	20	20	0.5
S-6	20	30	0.5

Reused from X. Li, K. Nan, S. Shi, H. Chen, Preparation and characterization of nanohydroxyapatite/chitosan cross-linking composite membrane intended for tissue engineering, International Journal of Biological Macromolecules 50 (2012) 43–49. https://doi.org/10.1016/j.ijbiomac.2011.09.021 after license via (copyright.com) number 4278671343254.

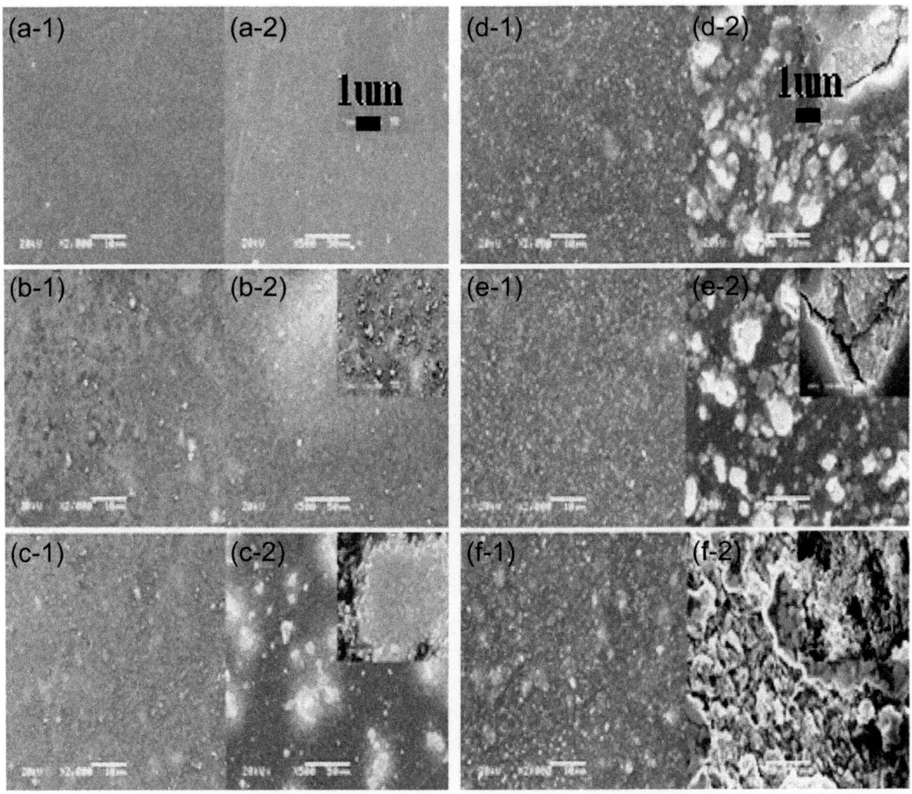

Figure 6.11 Scanning electron microscope micrographs: (a-1) upper surfaces of S1; (b-1) upper surfaces of S2; (c-1) upper surfaces of S3; (d-1) upper surfaces of S4; (e-1) upper surfaces of S5; (f-1) upper surfaces of S6. (a-2) Bottom surfaces of S1; (b-2) bottom surfaces of S2; (c-2) bottom surfaces of S3; (d-2) bottom surfaces of S4; (e-2) bottom surfaces of S5; (f-2) bottom surfaces of S6.

Reused from X. Li, K. Nan, S. Shi, H. Chen, Preparation and characterization of nano-hydroxy-apatite/chitosan cross-linking composite membrane intended for tissue engineering, International Journal of Biological Macromolecules 50 (2012) 43–49. https://doi.org/10.1016/j.ijbiomac.2011.09.021 after license via (copyright.com) number 4278671343254.

Table 6.2 Characteristics of representative hydroxyapatite nanorod samples

Sample codes	Mean diameter ±SD (nm)	Mean length ± SD (nm)	Aspect ratios	Ca/P	Morphology
0P123	103 ± 26	585 ± 315	5.68	1.55	Rod-like shape
1P123	74 ± 25	383 ± 152	5.18	1.61	Rod-like shape
2P123	28 ± 5	120 ± 32	4.29	1.66	Rod-like shape

description of P123 is a central ethylene oxide chain (hydrophobic) surrounded by two ethylene oxide chains (hydrophilic). The mean diameter and length of the synthesized HA nanorods is reduced by increasing the addition of P123 (0, 1, 2 g) to the recipe, as shown in Table 6.2 and Fig. 6.12. The detailed methodology and chemistry are described in the source article [15]. The authors show that the N_2 adsorption–desorption isotherms of the HA nanorods exhibit a type III isotherm with an H_3 hysteresis loop, as shown in Fig. 6.13. These results signify primary large pores and secondary slit-shaped pores within the aggregates of nanoparticles. The reader is referred to the review article [16] for self-learning of porosimetry and interpretation of the results. Finally, composite films of poly(D,L) lactic acid (PDLLA)–HA nanorods were prepared. SEM micrographs of the composite film of 2P123, after incubation in simulated body fluid (SBF) (7 days), show early formation of flower-like apatite composed of tiny needle-like crystallites, which is typical in bone-like apatite.

In addition, an innovative process is introduced and called the salt leaching–phase inverse process to fabricate porous scaffolds. It is a delicate process and is described in Refs. [17,18]. In short, controlled polymer transformation from a liquid phase to a solid phase, called phase inversion, creates micropores, while subsequent salt leaching is the dissolving of a type of salt, called the porogen, from the set molded polymer to create larger pores.

The salt leaching–phase inverse technique has been utilized to fabricate nanohydroxyapatite/poly(ester-urethane) (nHAP/PU) composite scaffolds [19]. The produced scaffolds with this method, Figs. 6.14 and 6.15, have interconnected micropores, and the macropores are not interconnected (Fig. 6.16).

Other than phase inversion, solvent casting is also used to synthesize polymeric scaffolds. In solvent casting, the polymer is dissolved via a suitable solvent and then the solution is cast in a mold. Various preparation processes for polymeric scaffolds are described in an informative article [20]. A combined solvent-casting–salt-leaching method is utilized for the synthesis of HA nanorod/PDLLA scaffolds [21]. The HA nanorods were prepared using the same methodology described earlier. The produced scaffolds mimic the structure of natural bone because of the macropore networks (117–183 μm), high porosity (80%–84%), and high HA content (30%). Yet again, a rapid formation of flower-like apatite takes place after 7 days of incubation in SBF.

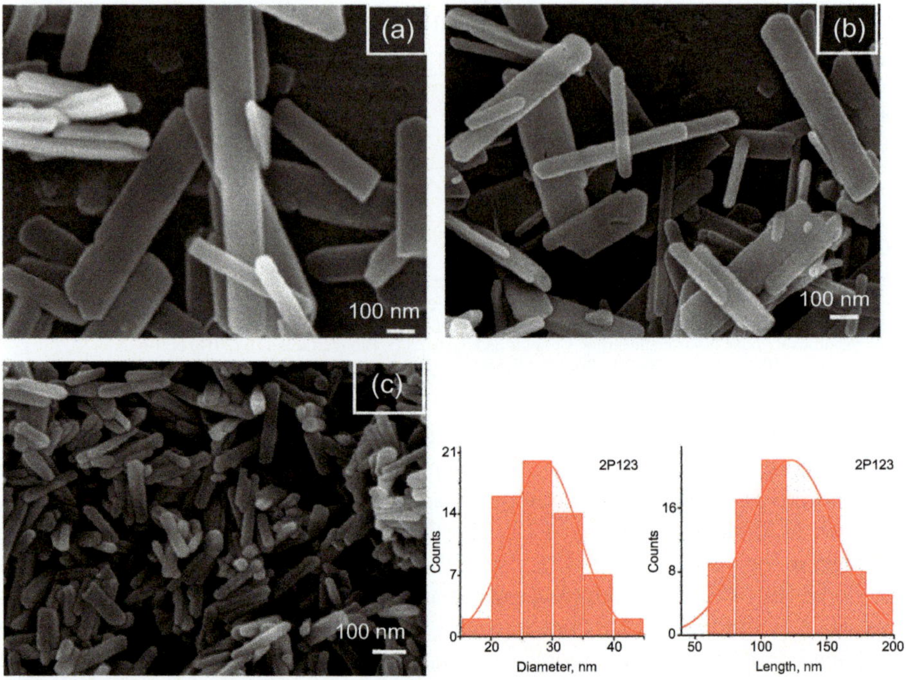

Figure 6.12 Field-emission scanning electron microscope images of representative hydroxyapatite samples synthesized at different concentrations of P123: (a) 0P123, (b) 1P123, and (c) 2P123 calcinated at 500°C for 1 h. The inset shows the particle size distribution of 2P123. Reused from N.K. Nga, L.T. Giang, T.Q. Huy, P.H. Viet, C. Migliaresi, Surfactant-assisted size control of hydroxyapatite nanorods for bone tissue engineering, Colloids and Surfaces B: Biointerfaces 116 (2014) 666–673. https://doi.org/10.1016/j.colsurfb.2013.11.001 after license via (copyright.com) number 4278951234804.

In most nanoceramic/polymer scaffold studies, different types of solvents are added that depend on the type of polymer. Polymer dilution is necessary in most cases to create pores and/or to decrease the polymer viscosity to encourage homogeneous distribution of the ceramic nanoparticles within the polymer matrix. However, incorporating solvents has negative effects such as reducing the mechanical properties of the composite and the harmful effects of residual solvents to cells and tissues, as claimed by some authors. Fabrication of nHAP/poly(3-hydroxybutyrate) composite scaffolds has been successfully performed without the use of organic solvents [22]. The incorporation of nHAP was successful to produce interconnected porosity, high porosities, and optimized pore size range for 10% and 15% content of nHAP; nevertheless, agglomerates are formed at a content of 20%. Improved mechanical properties have been reported, which are in the range of those of cancellous bone.

Another promising method for creating an interconnected pore network in the body of bioceramic scaffolds is the space holder technique. In this method, a bioceramic–porogen powder mixture is compacted via, e.g., uniaxial pressing. The porogen is

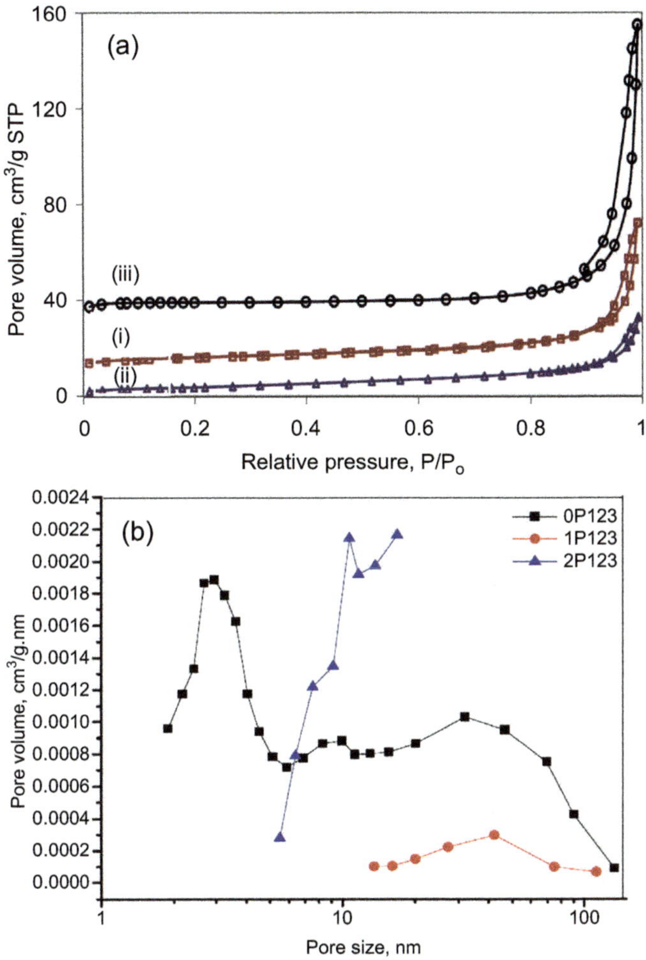

Figure 6.13 (a) Nitrogen adsorption–desorption isotherms of hydroxyapatite (HA) samples synthesized at different concentrations of P123: (i) 0P123, (ii) 1P123, and (iii) 2P123. (b) Pore size distributions of HA samples.
Reused from Reused from N.K. Nga, L.T. Giang, T.Q. Huy, P.H. Viet, C. Migliaresi, Surfactant-assisted size control of hydroxyapatite nanorods for bone tissue engineering, Colloids and Surfaces B: Biointerfaces 116 (2014) 666–673. https://doi.org/10.1016/j.colsurfb.2013.11.001 after license via (copyright.com) number 4278951234804.

not dissolved but withdrawn by heat treatment of the compact to leave pores behind. The space holder technique allows better control of the resultant pore network and because of this the pore size and distribution represent, to a high degree, a replica of the particle size and distribution of the porogen. HA–bredigite ($Ca_7MgSi_4O_{16}$) scaffolds have been fabricated using the space holder technique [23]. Fig. 6.17 shows that the scaffolds contain interconnected pores with suitable pore sizes for tissue ingrowth

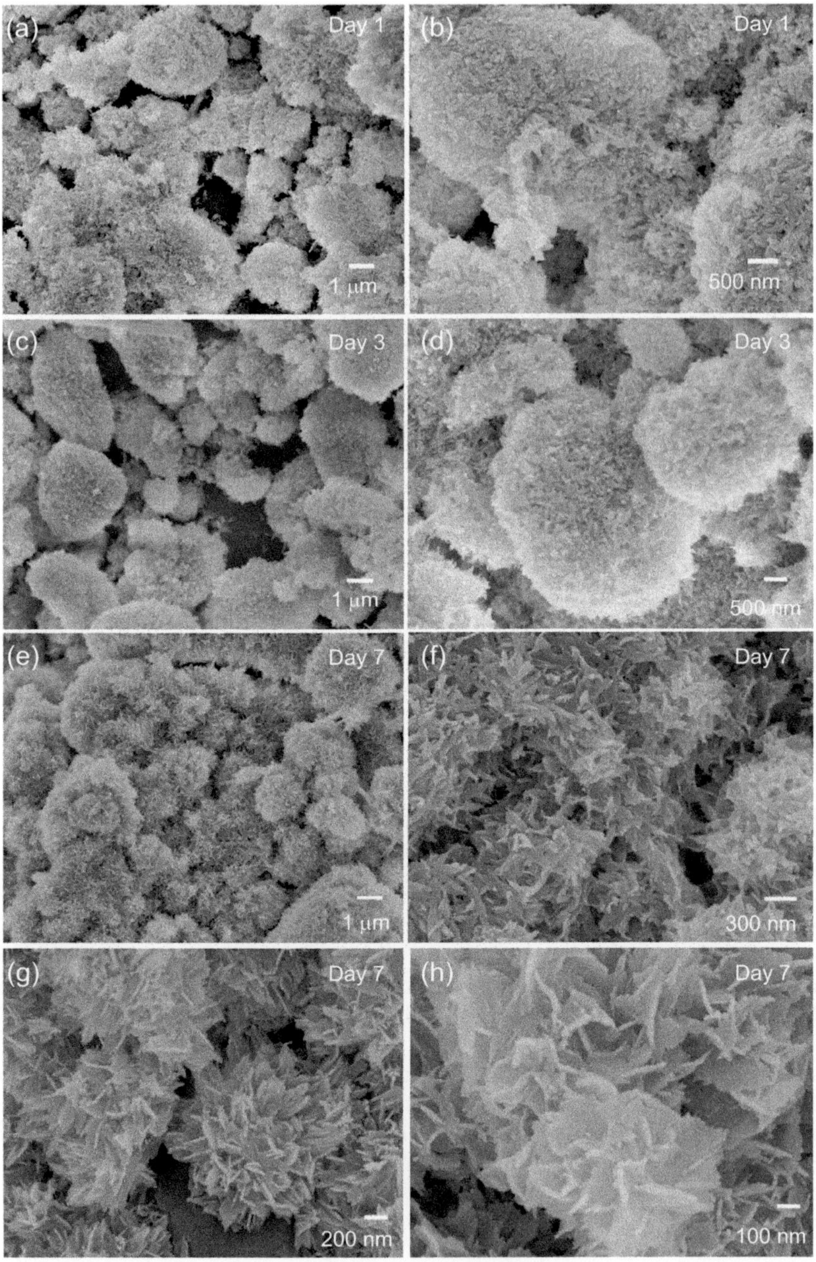

Figure 6.14 Field-emission scanning electron microscope micrographs of poly(D,L) lactic acid/hydroxyapatite composite film of 2P123 after soaking in simulated body fluid for (a and b) 1 day, (c and d) 3 days, and (e–h) 7 days.
Reused from Reused from N.K. Nga, L.T. Giang, T.Q. Huy, P.H. Viet, C. Migliaresi, Surfactant-assisted size control of hydroxyapatite nanorods for bone tissue engineering, Colloids and Surfaces B: Biointerfaces 116 (2014) 666–673. https://doi.org/10.1016/j.colsurfb.2013.11.001 after license via (copyright.com) number 4278951234804.

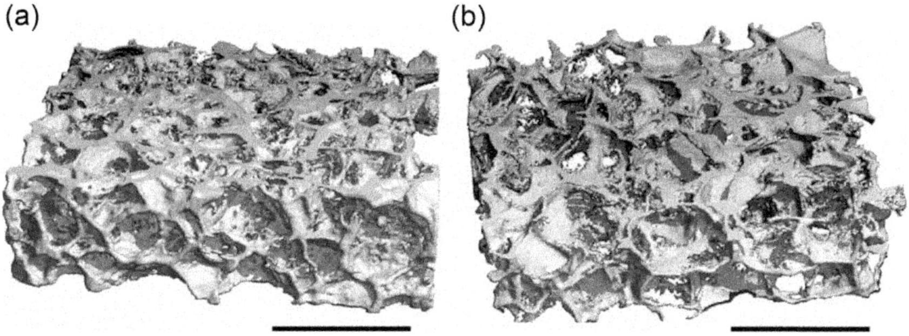

Figure 6.15 Representative 3D microcomputed X-ray tomography reconstructions of (a) a nanohydroxyapatite/poly(ester-urethane) and (b) poly(ester-urethane) scaffold. Note that both scaffold types exhibit a comparable porous macrostructure. Scale bars: 1 mm.
Reused from M.W. Laschke, A. Strohe, M.D. Menger, M. Alini, D. Eglin, In vitro and in vivo evaluation of a novel nanosize hydroxyapatite particles/poly(ester-urethane) composite scaffold for bone tissue engineering, Acta Biomaterialia 6 (2010) 2020–2027. https://doi.org/10.1016/j.actbio.2009.12.004 after license via (copyright.com) number 4278370323931.

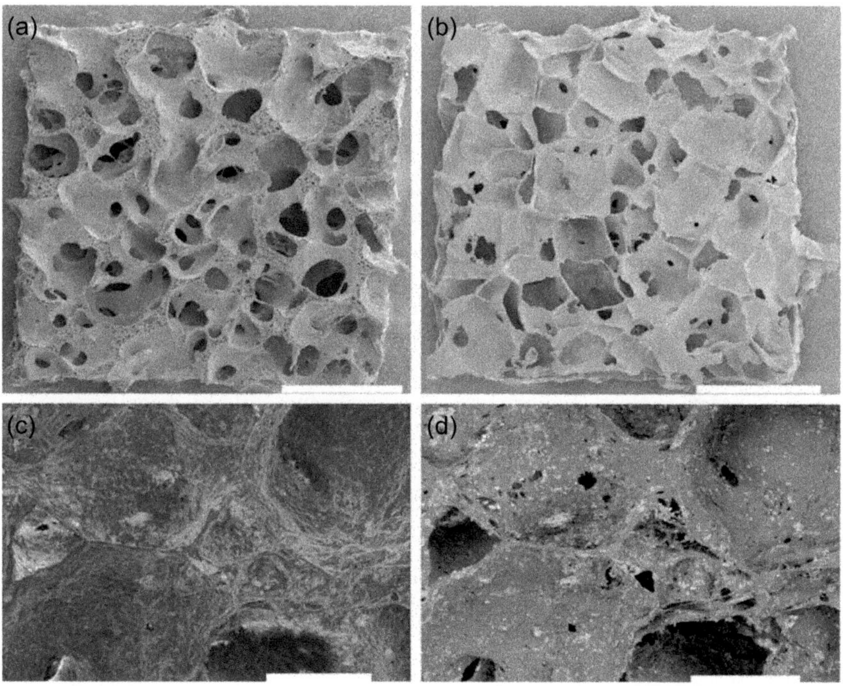

Figure 6.16 Representative scanning electron microscope micrographs of (a) a poly(ester-urethane) (PU) and (b) a nanohydroxyapatite/poly(ester-urethane) (nHAP/PU) scaffold. Note that the nHAP/PU scaffold exhibits a decreased microporosity when compared with the PU scaffold. Scale bars: 1 mm. (c and d) Higher magnification of the nHAP/PU scaffold imaged in (c) SE and (d) BSE mode indicates the presence of nHAP particle aggregates (*light gray*) distributed within and on the PU matrix. Scale bars: 100 μm.
Reused from M.W. Laschke, A. Strohe, M.D. Menger, M. Alini, D. Eglin, In vitro and in vivo evaluation of a novel nanosize hydroxyapatite particles/poly(ester-urethane) composite scaffold for bone tissue engineering, Acta Biomaterialia 6 (2010) 2020–2027. https://doi.org/10.1016/j.actbio.2009.12.004 after license via (copyright.com) number 4278370323931.

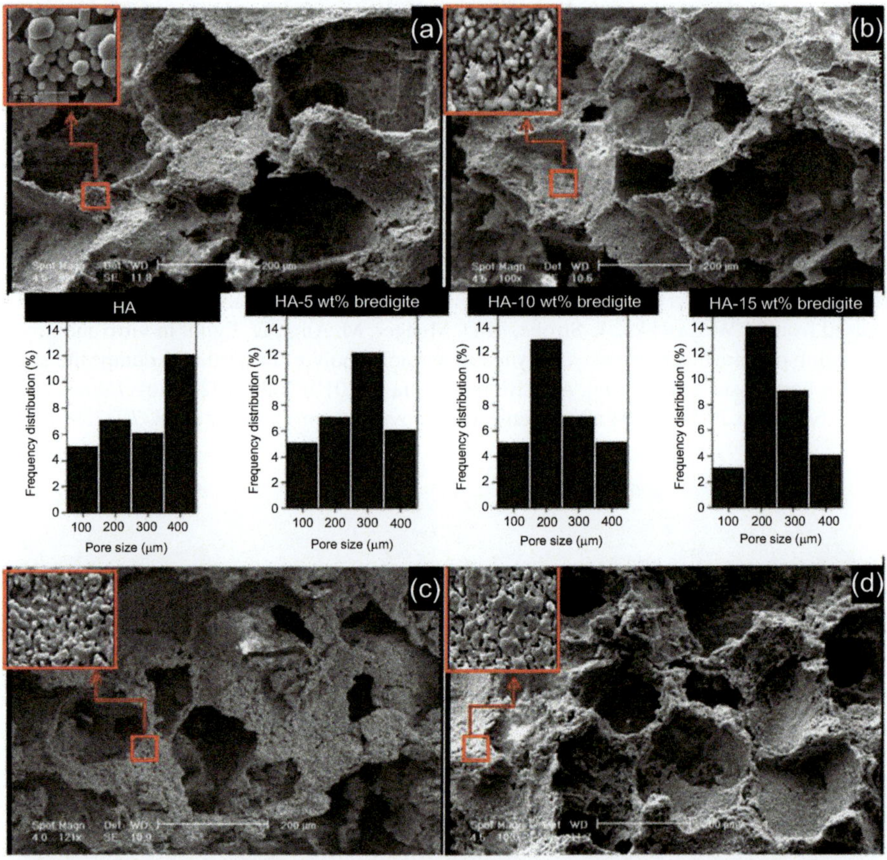

Figure 6.17 Scanning electron microscope micrographs (two different magnifications) of fractured surfaces of hydroxyapatite (HA) (a), HA-5 wt% bredigite (b), HA-10 wt% bredigite (c), and HA-15 wt% bredigite (d) scaffolds, as well as their macropore size distribution histograms. The average sizes are 311.1 ± 8.7, 256.7 ± 18.7, 232.8 ± 17.1, and 227.5 ± 20.2 µm, respectively.
Reused from M. Eilbagi, R. Emadi, K. Raeissi, M. Kharaziha, A. Valiani, Mechanical and cytotoxicity evaluation of nanostructured hydroxyapatite-bredigite scaffolds for bone regeneration, Materials Science and Engineering: C 68 (2016) 603–612. https://doi.org/10.1016/j.msec.2016.06.030 after license via (copyright.com) number 4283570758472.

and exchanging body fluid. Macropore sizes, according to the attached histograms, were decreased with the increase in bredigite in the composite. In addition, micropore sizes were also decreased with the increase in bredigite nanopowder, as seen in Fig. 6.18. The compressive strength, shown in Fig. 6.19, of HA and the composite was in the range 1–1.7 MPa. The moduli were in the range 150–215 MPa. These results are close to those reported for cancellous bone in Ref. [24]. HA–bredigite composites also show improved bioactivity with the increase in bredigite content via soaking in SBF solution and culturing in SaOS2 cells.

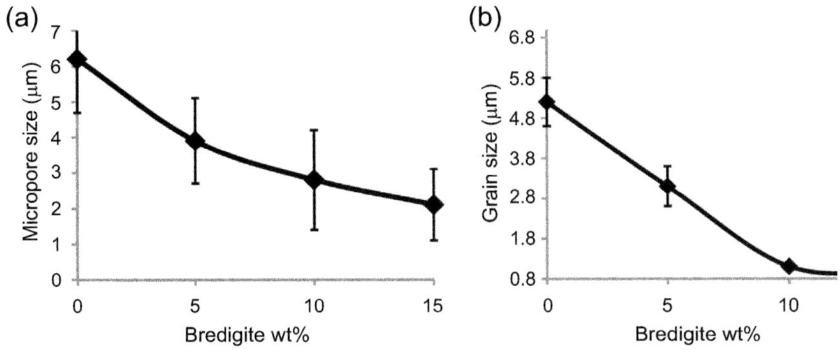

Figure 6.18 The average micropore size (a) and grain size (b) of the sintered scaffolds versus bredigite content.
Reused from M. Eilbagi, R. Emadi, K. Raeissi, M. Kharaziha, A. Valiani, Mechanical and cytotoxicity evaluation of nanostructured hydroxyapatite-bredigite scaffolds for bone regeneration, Materials Science and Engineering: C 68 (2016) 603–612. https://doi.org/10.1016/j.msec.2016.06.030 after license via (copyright.com) number 4283570758472.

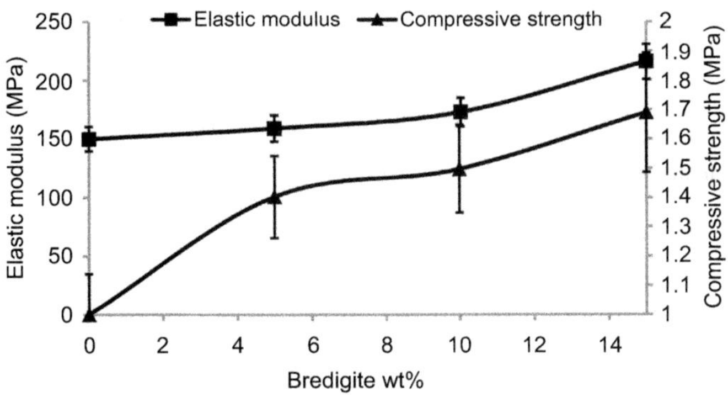

Figure 6.19 Compressive modulus and strength of scaffolds as a function of bredigite content.
Reused from M. Eilbagi, R. Emadi, K. Raeissi, M. Kharaziha, A. Valiani, Mechanical and cytotoxicity evaluation of nanostructured hydroxyapatite-bredigite scaffolds for bone regeneration, Materials Science and Engineering: C 68 (2016) 603–612. https://doi.org/10.1016/j.msec.2016.06.030 after license via (copyright.com) number 4283570758472.

The space holder method is also used in subsequent studies to prepare composite scaffolds and reach nearly equivalent results in the case of diopside/biphasic calcium phosphate nanocomposite scaffolds [25] and diopside/forsterite nanocomposite scaffolds [26].

One of the recent research trends is the incorporation of graphene oxide (GO) and the study of its effect on the final properties of the scaffolds. Graphene is a 2D carbon nanosheet and can be visualized as an opened carbon nanotube. However, there are versatile procedures to prepare graphene directly or GO as an intermediate stage. Graphene, particularly of high purity, is preferred for electronic material applications, whereas the cheaper GO gives better mechanical properties when incorporated in a composite, mainly of polymer matrix.

Scaffolds of PVA/GO have been prepared incorporating GO in the polymer precursor of the electrospinning process [27]. Scaffolds of nanofibers have been loaded with GO that improves the mechanical properties up to 1% content. MC3T3-E1 cells are successfully spread on these scaffolds. Another incorporation of graphene is that performed via the chemical precipitation method [28]. Functionalized graphene was prepared via the reduction of GO in the presence of biocompatible ethylenediamine. The results show successful grafting of exfoliated graphene nanosheets (GNS) on HA without destroying their structure.

An outstanding work is the synthesis of GNS/HA composite via spark plasma sintering (SPS) [29]. SPS involves the application of pressure and electrical current at the same time. Densification is accomplished in a few minutes; thus there is not enough time for grain growth and the mechanical properties are improved. GNS survive under these conditions, as seen in Fig. 6.20(a). An improvement in fracture toughness (80%) as compared with pure HA was attained with the incorporation of 1% in the composite. The major toughening mechanisms may include crack deflection caused by sheet-like reinforcement [30], grain bridging by GNS, as shown in Fig. 6.20(b), GNS pullout from the interface between GNS ridge and matrix grain, as illustrated by Fig. 6.21, and crack bridging, as seen in Fig. 6.22. The results also show that osteoblast spreading is preserved during incorporation of GNS. However, incubation in SBF for 7 days yields a thicker apatite layer in the case of the composite compared with that of HA alone. In addition, the needle-like-shaped apatite morphology found on the incubated HA surface is changed to curled sheet-shaped apatite in the case of the incubated composite.

Coating with a bioactive ceramic may represent a solution in cases such as unsatisfied mechanical strength of the bulk bioceramic or the lack of bioactivity of e.g.

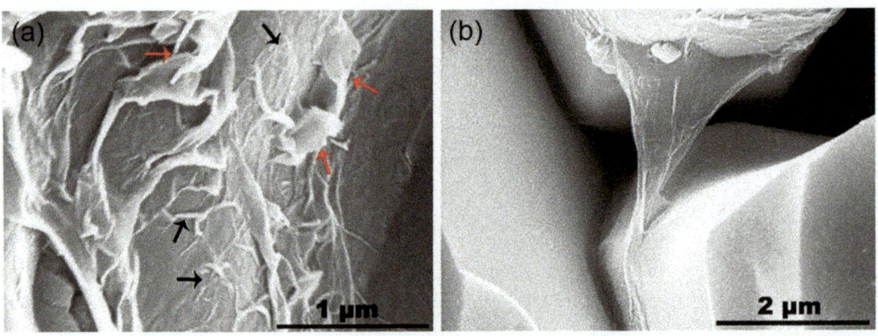

Figure 6.20 Scanning electron microscope micrographs showing (a) wrinkled surface texture of a graphene nanosheet (GNS) wrapped around the hydroxyapatite (HA) grain (wrinkles are pointed out by *black arrows* and ridges are pointed out by *red arrows* [*gray in print version*]) and (b) grain bridging by GNS on the fracture surface of 1.0 wt% GNS/HA composite. Reused from L. Zhang, W. Liu, C. Yue, T. Zhang, P. Li, Z. Xing, Y. Chen, A tough graphene nanosheet/hydroxyapatite composite with improved in vitro biocompatibility, Carbon 61 (2013) 105–115. https://doi.org/10.1016/j.carbon.2013.04.074 after license via (copyright.com) number 4284681227882.

titanium alloy implant. $CaO–SiO_2$-based ceramics are usually used for bone bioactivity and high bonding strength to titanium alloys. Thus a plasma-sprayed coating of wollastonite, dicalcium silicate, and diopside is usually found in the literature and reviewed in this work [31]. The bioactivity of $CaO–SiO_2$ ceramics in the body fluid environment is explained in [32]. In short, the dissolution of $CaO–SiO_2$ in the body fluid provides calcium ions needed for the formation of the apatite that found favorable sites on the hydrated silica on the surfaces of $CaO–SiO_2$ ceramics.

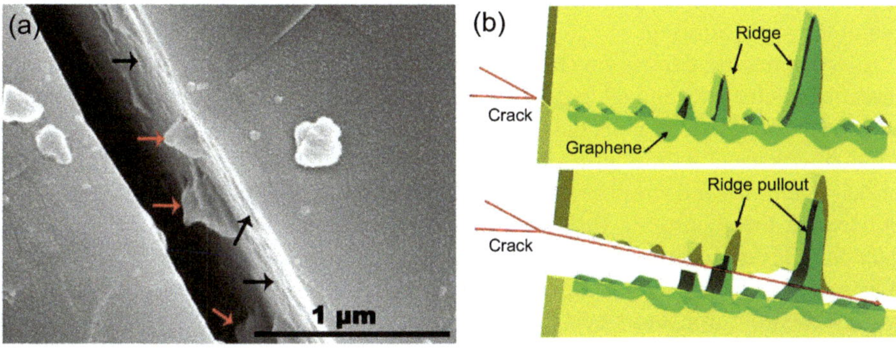

Figure 6.21 (a) Scanning electron microscope micrographs showing Vickers indentation-induced radial crack of 0.5 wt% graphene nanosheet/hydroxyapatite (GNS/HA) composite, in which wrinkled texture (pointed out by *black arrows*) and GNS pullout (pointed out by *red arrows*) are visible on the crack surface. (b) Schematic illustration of GNS pullout in the GNS/HA composite.
Reused from L. Zhang, W. Liu, C. Yue, T. Zhang, P. Li, Z. Xing, Y. Chen, A tough graphene nanosheet/hydroxyapatite composite with improved in vitro biocompatibility, Carbon 61 (2013) 105–115. https://doi.org/10.1016/j.carbon.2013.04.074 after license via (copyright.com) number 4284681227882.

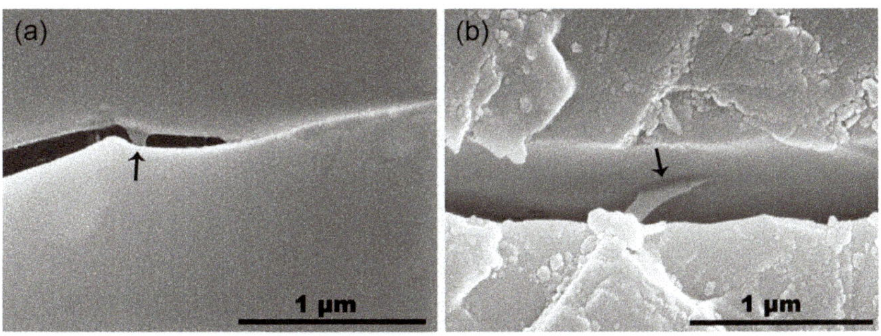

Figure 6.22 Scanning electron microscope micrographs of (a) inhibition of the Vickers indentation-induced crack by a graphene nanosheet (GNS) and (b) crack bridging by GNS.
Reused from L. Zhang, W. Liu, C. Yue, T. Zhang, P. Li, Z. Xing, Y. Chen, A tough graphene nanosheet/hydroxyapatite composite with improved in vitro biocompatibility, Carbon 61 (2013) 105–115. https://doi.org/10.1016/j.carbon.2013.04.074 after license via (copyright.com) number 4284681227882.

A GO/HA nanorod composite coat was synthesized by the one-pot hydrothermal process, as described in Ref. [33]. The coating was deposited on glass slides by the method of spin coating. Nanoindentation was utilized for mechanical characterization of the coat. The technique of nanoindentation utilized a special set of nanoindenters, actuators, and sensors that can obtain the load displacement curve, hardness, and Young's modulus. Fig. 6.23 compares the results of the nanoindentation measurement for the HA coat and the GNS/HA composite. The figure clearly shows enhanced mechanical properties of the composite coat compared with those of HA alone. In addition, bioactivity is confirmed via incubation in SBF solution and MC3T3-E1 osteoblast cell culturing.

Electrophoretic deposition (EPD) is also used as a technique for coating. It is different from electrochemical deposition or electrodeposition in that it does not include ionic species (salts). EPD includes ceramic particles that are charged in a suspension; then, an electrical field is utilized to force migration of the charged particles to one of the electrodes (electrophoresis) to perform coating. The cathodic EPD process is utilized for the coating of Ti substrate by GO/HA. The resultant coat represents HA nanoparticles uniformly decorated on GO sheets [34]. The EPD process in this work is illustrated in Fig. 6.24. The weight versus deposition time for the coatings is increased with deposition time and reaches almost a plateau for pure HA, 2% GO/HA, and 5% GO/HA, as seen in Fig. 6.25(a). Increasing the deposition voltage also increases the coating weight and reaches almost saturation plateaus.

The results also show that the coating adhesion strength is increased from about 1.55 MPa for pure HA to 2.75 MPa for 2% GO/HA and 3.3 MPa for 5% GO/HA. Cell proliferation is improved with the incorporation of GO, and it is optimum at 2% GO/HA composite coat, as seen in Fig. 6.26, with two types of cell lines. In this figure, the notation "positive" means the "positive control." The positive control is a type of

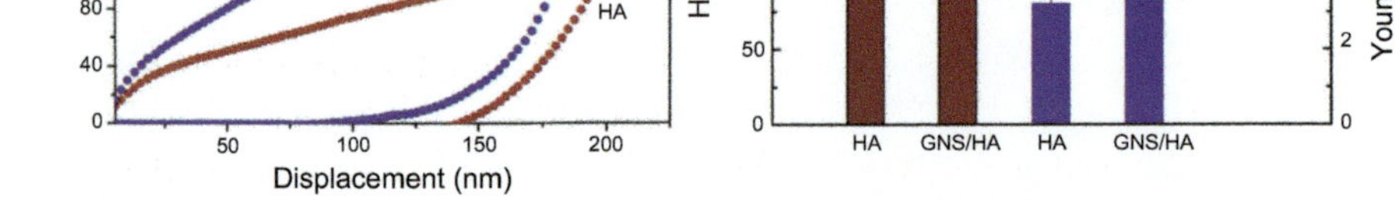

Figure 6.23 (a) Typical load–displacement curves of hydroxyapatite (HA) and graphene nanosheet/hydroxyapatite (GNS/HA) coatings obtained by nanoindentation at a fixed displacement of 200 nm. (b) The values of hardness and Young's modulus of HA and GNS/HA coatings, respectively. HA and GNS/HA labels are added to part (a) of the figure for clarity. Reused from Z. Fan, J. Wang, Z. Wang, H. Ran, Y. Li, L. Niu, P. Gong, B. Liu, S. Yang, One-pot synthesis of graphene/hydroxyapatite nanorod composite for tissue engineering, Carbon 66 (2014) 407–416. https://doi.org/10.1016/j.carbon.2013.09.016 after license via (copyright.com) number 4284990666443.

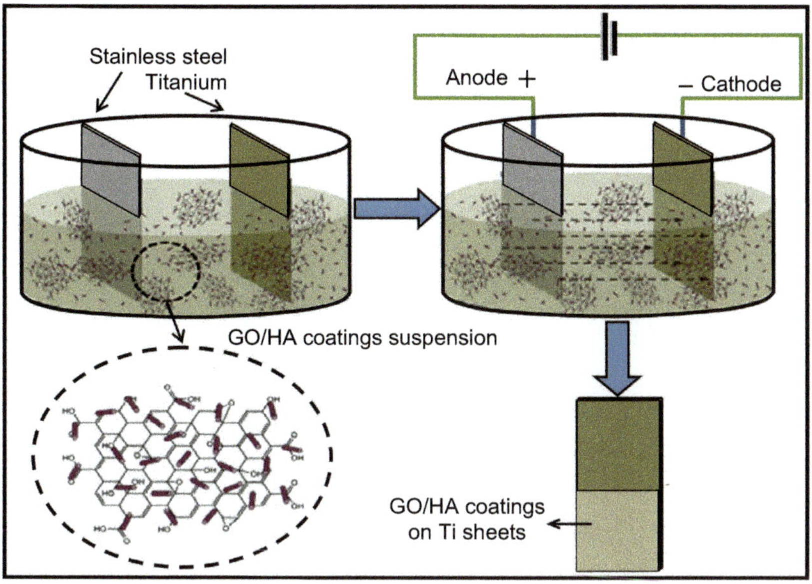

Figure 6.24 Schematic illustration of the electrophoretic deposition process.
Reused from M. Li, Q. Liu, Z. Jia, X. Xu, Y. Cheng, Y. Zheng, T. Xi, S. Wei, Graphene oxide/hydroxyapatite composite coatings fabricated by electrophoretic nanotechnology for biological applications, Carbon 67 (2014) 185–197. https://doi.org/10.1016/j.carbon.2013.09.080 after license via (copyright.com) number 4285281406018.

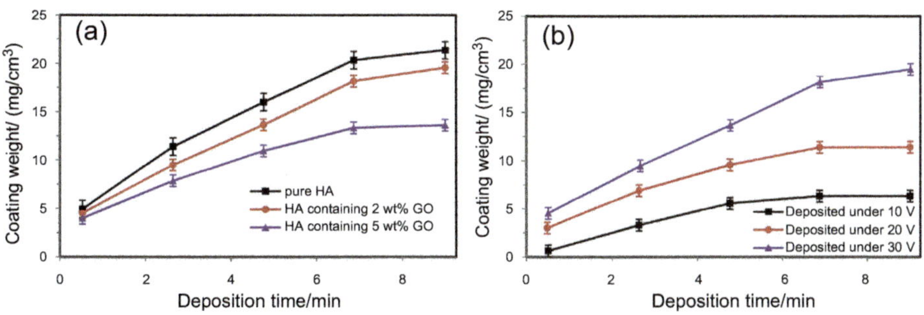

Figure 6.25 The weight versus deposition time for the coatings prepared from 5 mg/mL GO/HA suspension with different GO contents at a deposition voltage of 30 V (a) and with 2 wt% GO at a different deposition voltage (b). *GO*, graphene oxide; *HA*, hydroxyapatite.
Reused from M. Li, Q. Liu, Z. Jia, X. Xu, Y. Cheng, Y. Zheng, T. Xi, S. Wei, Graphene oxide/hydroxyapatite composite coatings fabricated by electrophoretic nanotechnology for biological applications, Carbon 67 (2014) 185–197. https://doi.org/10.1016/j.carbon.2013.09.080 after license via (copyright.com) number 4285281406018.

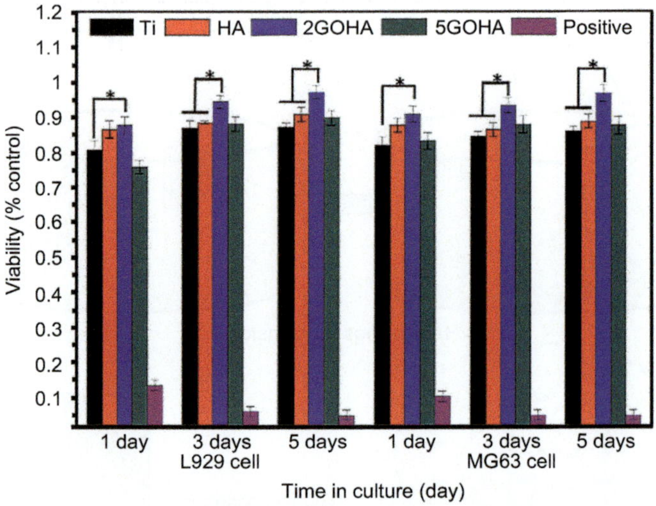

Figure 6.26 The cell proliferation rates of L929 cell lines and MG63 cell lines cultured in media for 1, 3, and 5 days with prepared samples. * represents $P < .05$.
Reused from M. Li, Q. Liu, Z. Jia, X. Xu, Y. Cheng, Y. Zheng, T. Xi, S. Wei, Graphene oxide/hydroxyapatite composite coatings fabricated by electrophoretic nanotechnology for biological applications, Carbon 67 (2014) 185–197. https://doi.org/10.1016/j.carbon.2013.09.080 after license via (copyright.com) number 4285281406018.

material that receives the same treatment with known response. Thus the response of the positive control can be compared with that of the material under test. Also, a "negative control" is the response that is expected with it. It is used in complicated experiments for certain purposes, e.g., the detection of contamination.

The frequently encountered problem where Ti or its alloys are coated with HA is the mismatch of the coefficient of thermal expansion between the coat and the substrate. In an attempt to overcome this problem, a graded coating of Ti6Al4V substrates by TiO_2 and HA is performed by atmospheric plasma spraying (APS) [35]. The process parameters of APS are versatile, and the interested reader is referred to the original work for details of obtaining the optimum process parameters. Here, we point to graded coating, especially via APS, which continues as an active field of research and development. The microstructure of the graded coating before heat treatment is shown in Fig. 6.27. The TiO_2 layer is directly deposited on the Ti alloy and appears as light gray. HA is included within the TiO_2 layer and its content is increased gradually away from the substrate. Then, a mere HA layer appears at the outermost of the coat. This configuration greatly reduces the stresses accompanied by mismatch of the thermal expansion. Fig. 6.28 (scale bar = 100 μm) shows the microstructure of the coat at different annealing temperatures. The residual porosity at the HA layer appears to be increased at an annealing temperature of 850°C. Residual porosity is caused by the melting and recrystallization of HA at this annealing temperature. However, the higher magnification micrograph of Fig. 6.29 (scale bar = 20 μm) shows that the cracks start

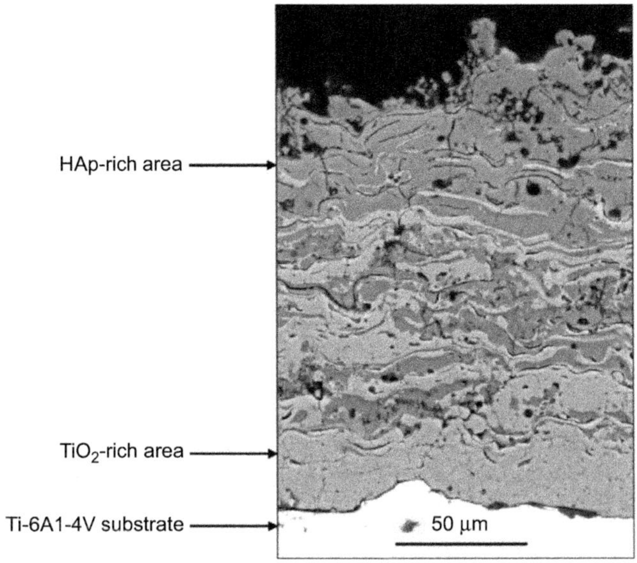

Figure 6.27 Cross-section of the TiO_2–hydroxyapatite-graded coating.
Reused from V. Cannillo, L. Lusvarghi, A. Sola, Production and characterization of plasma-sprayed TiO_2–hydroxyapatite functionally graded coatings, Journal of the European Ceramic Society 28 (2008) 2161–2169. https://doi.org/10.1016/j.jeurceramsoc.2008.02.026 after license via (copyright.com) number 4285560238619.

to initiate at an annealing temperature of 750°C. Thus the optimum annealing temperature for this type of graded coat is 650°C, which gives an optimal microstructure.

The concept of functionally graded materials is not limited to coating applications. A bulk HA–alumina-stabilized zirconia functionally graded material (FGM) biocomposite has been synthesized to combine bulk properties, strength, toughness, and hardness with the known bioactivity of the HA surface [36]. The fracture toughness of the utilized HA–Al_2O_3– yttria-stabilized zirconia FGM materials is around 1.5–3.5–6.2 MPa·$m^{1/2}$, respectively. Accordingly, Al_2O_3 represents a transition layer to reduce the gradient of the mechanical properties. SPS is utilized for the fabrication of FGM. SPS is performed at 1200°C under a vacuum of 6 Pa to drive out any possible CO_2. The sintering duration is 5 min. Obtaining an optimum hardness profile guided the choice of sintering parameters. The hardness and toughness profiles are shown in Figs. 6.30 and 6.31, respectively. It can be seen that the stepwise variation of toughness of the prepared FGM may help to reduce the probability of crack propagation along the interfaces. In addition, Fig. 6.32 shows that the interfaces are free of cracking even with the polished samples. In addition, the fracture surfaces elucidate that an integrated microstructure is obtained with the utilized parameters of SPS. This work also contains an in vitro cytocompatibilty examination of the prepared FGM using L929 fibroblast cells and SaOS2 osteoblast cells that proves their adhesion and growth.

The aforementioned work, as far as the author knows, may be the best bio-FGM report. The nanostructured HA–biphasic calcium phosphate [37] FGM is also

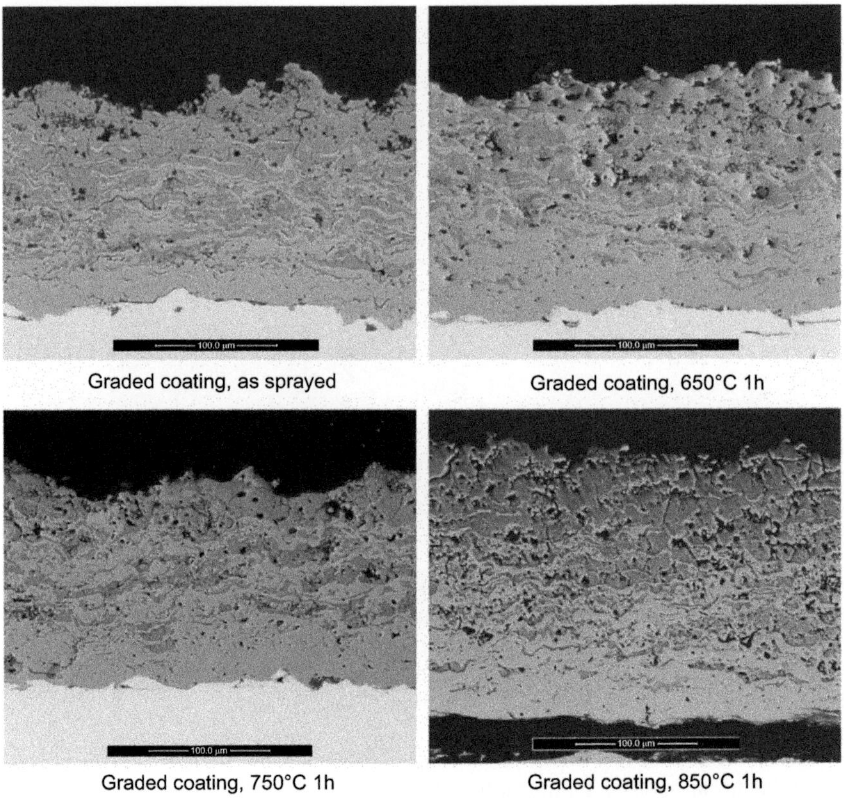

Figure 6.28 Effect of different heat treatments on the graded coating.

illuminating and educating because the starting materials are the stoichiometric HA and the calcium-deficient HA that are converted to biphasic calcium phosphate (HA + β-tricalcium phospate [β-TCP]) after sintering to the final FGM. However, a great deal of FGM work can be found in the literature and the review paper [38] is comprehensive and useful.

Calcium phosphate cements (CPCs) have known applications as bioceramics because of their biocompatibility, osteoconductivity, and in situ setting capability. However, research work always attempts to improve their performance. Thus incorporation of Bioglass (BG), with or without PLGA, has shown advantages in in vitro physicochemical studies. In addition, biological performance studies [39] showed improved in vivo performance for bone regeneration. The prepared CPCs and their composites are shown in Table 6.3. The morphology of the starting materials, CPCs,

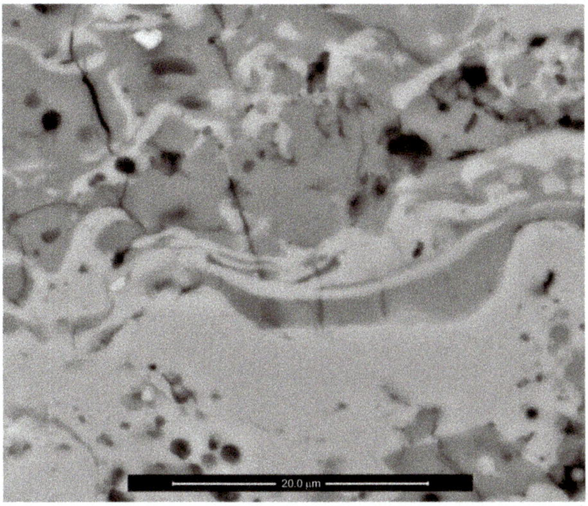

Figure 6.29 Cracks induced by hydroxyapatite recrystallization in the sample heat treated at 750°C for 1 h.
Reused from V. Cannillo, L. Lusvarghi, A. Sola, Production and characterization of plasma-sprayed TiO_2–hydroxyapatite functionally graded coatings, Journal of the European Ceramic Society 28 (2008) 2161–2169. https://doi.org/10.1016/j.jeurceramsoc.2008.02.026 after license via (copyright.com) number 4285560238619.

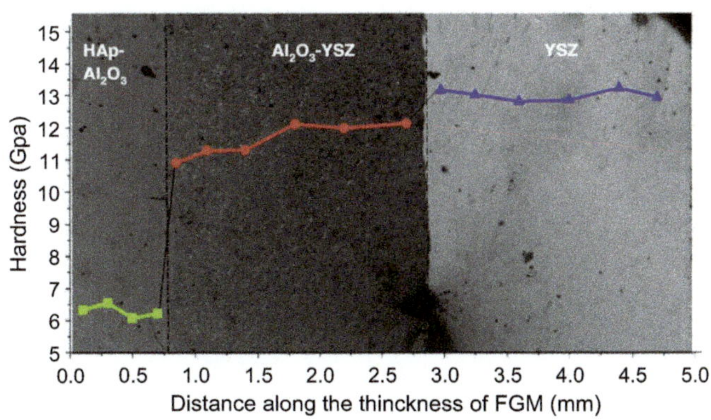

Figure 6.30 Hardness profile of functionally graded materials across the cross-section.
Reused from M.A.F. Afzal, P. Kesarwani, K.M. Reddy, S. Kalmodia, B. Basu, K. Balani, Functionally graded hydroxyapatite-alumina-zirconia biocomposite: synergy of toughness and biocompatibility, Materials Science and Engineering: C 32 (2012) 1164–1173. https://doi.org/10.1016/j.msec.2012.03.003 after license via (copyright.com) number 4285890235235.

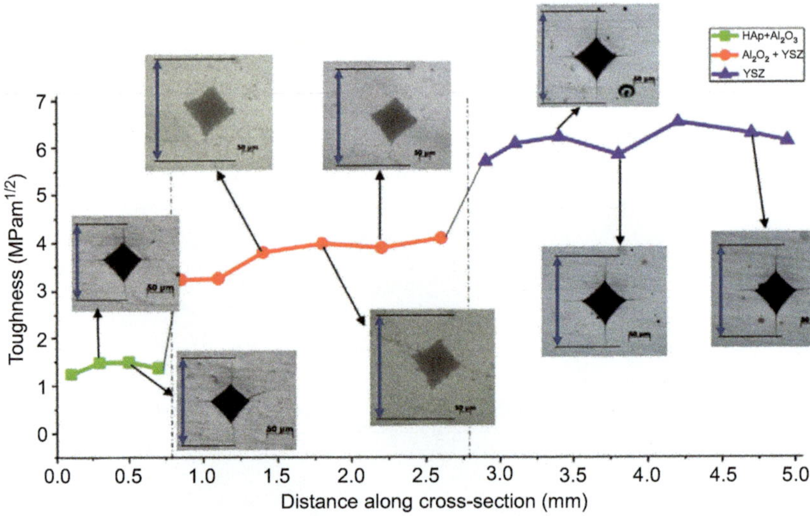

Figure 6.31 Toughness profile of functionally graded materials across the cross-section. A load of 500 g was applied on hydroxyapatite–Al_2O_3 and a 2 kg load on Al_2O_3–yttria-stabilized zirconia (YSZ) layer and YSZ layer.
Reused from M.A.F. Afzal, P. Kesarwani, K.M. Reddy, S. Kalmodia, B. Basu, K. Balani, Functionally graded hydroxyapatite-alumina-zirconia biocomposite: synergy of toughness and biocompatibility, Materials Science and Engineering: C 32 (2012) 1164–1173. https://doi.org/10.1016/j.msec.2012.03.003 after license via (copyright.com) number 4285890235235.

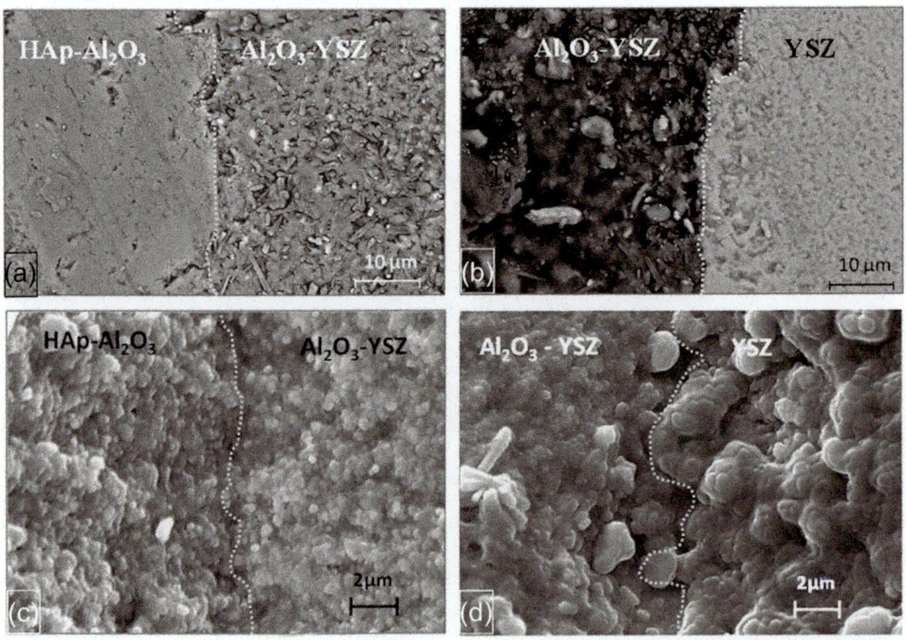

Figure 6.32 (a) and (b) show the polished surfaces of functionally graded materials (FGM) cross-section depicting the two interfaces. (c) and (d) show the fractured surfaces of FGM cross-section.
Reused from M.A.F. Afzal, P. Kesarwani, K.M. Reddy, S. Kalmodia, B. Basu, K. Balani, Functionally graded hydroxyapatite-alumina-zirconia biocomposite: synergy of toughness and biocompatibility, Materials Science and Engineering: C 32 (2012) 1164–1173. https://doi.org/10.1016/j.msec.2012.03.003 after license via (copyright.com) number 4285890235235.

Table 6.3 Composition and porosity values of preset composite materials

Groups	Ca/P wt%	BG wt%	PLGA wt%	Macroporosity	Total porosity
CPC	100	0	0	–	40.6±0.7
CPC/BG	70	30	0	–	41.6±0.8
CPC/PLGA	70	0	30	40.5±1.2	55.7±0.9
CPC/PLGA/BG	40	30	30	41.2±0.8	56.5±1.5

BG, Bioglass; *CPC*, calcium phosphate cements; *PLGA*, poly(glycolic acid) copolymer.
Reused from A.C.M. Renno, F.C.J. van de Watering, M.R. Nejadnik, M.C. Crovace, E.D. Zanotto, J.G.C. Wolke, J.A. Jansen, J.J.J.P. van den Beucken, Incorporation of bioactive glass in calcium phosphate cement: an evaluation, Acta Biomaterialia 9 (2013) 5728–5739. https://doi.org/10.1016/j.actbio.2012.11.009 after license via (copyright.com) number 4286900390737.

and their composites is shown in Fig. 6.33. The figure shows the BG and PLA particles are uniformly distributed in the CPC matrix. The incorporation of BG into CPCs and CPC/PLGA shows higher degradation and bone formation, as indicated in Fig. 6.34.

Biphasic dicalcium phosphate-rich cement is fabricated from tetracalcium phosphate (TTCP) and surface-modified dicalcium phosphate anhydrous (DCPA). The surface modification of DCPA is performed via deposition of TTCP nanocrystals of the particle surfaces of the DCPA by a method described in Ref. [40]. An injectable bone graft substitute is produced with adequate mechanical strength, nondispersibility, and biocompatibility, as shown in the original article. It is claimed that the TTCP nanocrystals help in stabilizing the Ca ion concentration. In addition, the nanocrystals encourage the nondispersive behavior that leads to the rapid growth and interlocking of particles, as illustrated in the graphical abstract of the article (Fig. 6.35).

Brushite ($CaHPO_4{\cdot}2H_2O$) cement is modified by the incorporation of Mg^{2+} ions by introducing magnesium phosphate 3-hydrate ($MgHPO_4{\cdot}3H_2O$), as described in Ref. [41]. The aim of the study is to increase the bioactivity of the brushite scaffolds. The addition of Mg seems to accelerate the degradation of the CPC cements that improve osteoblast proliferation and provide higher new bone formation. Thus the employment of magnesium ions assists controllable biodegradable properties and improved bone regeneration.

In another study, brushite-forming CPCs based on β-TCP/phosphoric acid were developed with PLGA fiber reinforcement [42]. The fibers were of small diameter (25 μm) and different lengths (0.25, 1, or 2 mm). The cements contain different weight ratios (2.5%, 5%, or 7.5%). The aim of the study is to develop cement with better mechanical properties. The PLGA fiber reinforcement increased the diametrical tensile strength, biaxial flexural strength, and flexural strength by up to 25%. Concurrently, the injectability and biocompatibility of the cements are preserved.

The injectability of CPCs is the core of various studies. For example, it is found that the partially aggregated particles enhance injectability [43]. High-energy ball milling improves injectability, bioactivity, and strength because of smaller powder particle size

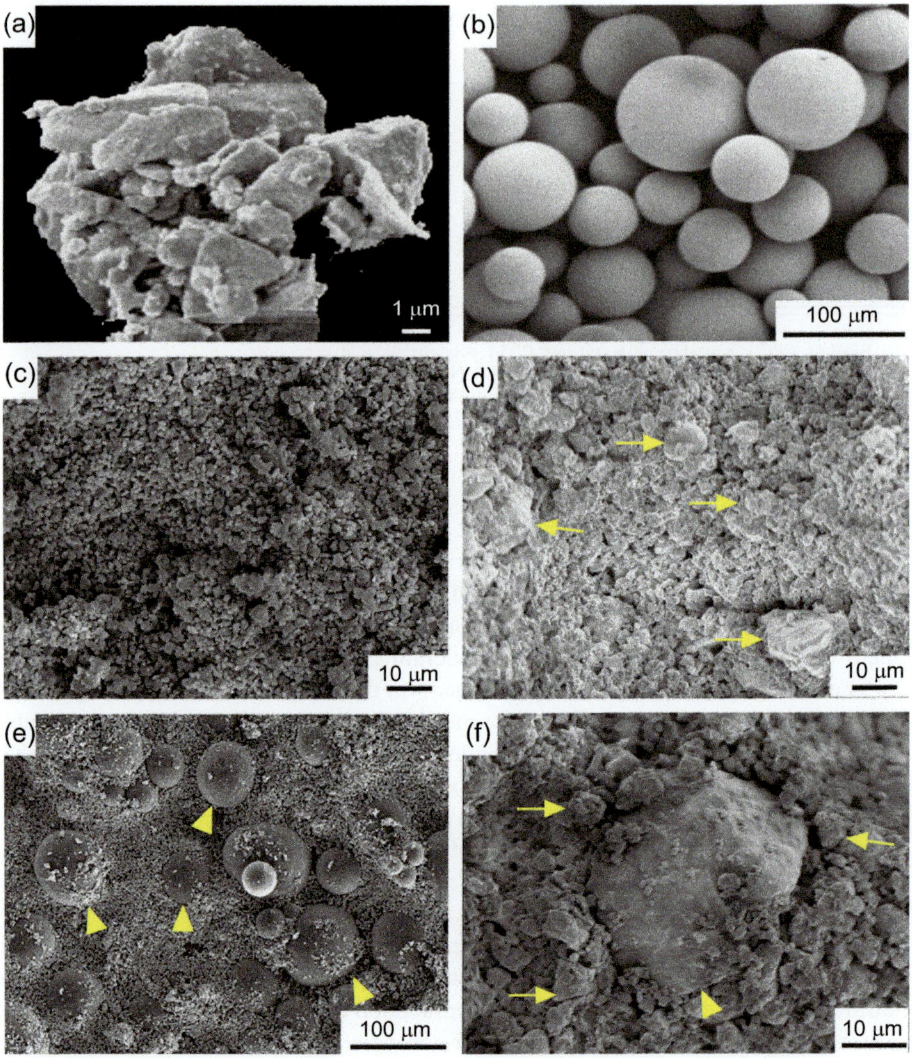

Figure 6.33 Scanning electron microscope (SEM) micrographs of (a) Bioglass (BG) particles, (b) dense poly(glycolic acid) (PLGA) microparticles, (c) calcium phosphate cement (CPC), (d) CPC/BG, (e) CPC/PLGA, and (f) CPC/PLGA/BG. BG (*arrow*) and PLGA microparticles (*arrowheads*) are indicated in the SEM micrographs. Bar represents 1, 10, or 100 μm. Reused from A.C.M. Renno, F.C.J. van de Watering, M.R. Nejadnik, M.C. Crovace, E.D. Zanotto, J.G.C. Wolke, J.A. Jansen, J.J.J.P. van den Beucken, Incorporation of bioactive glass in calcium phosphate cement: an evaluation, Acta Biomaterialia 9 (2013) 5728–5739. https://doi.org/10.1016/j.actbio.2012.11.009 after license via (copyright.com) number 4286900390737.

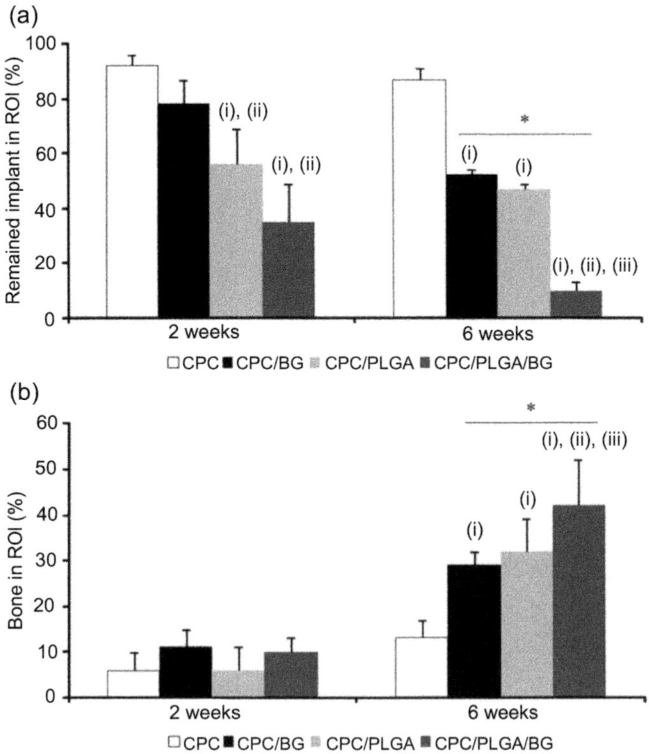

Figure 6.34 Results of histomorphometrical evaluation of different formulations, i.e., CPC, CPC/BG, CPC/PLGA, and CPC/PLGA/BG. (a) The amount of remaining implant and (b) the amount of newly formed bone after 2 and 6 weeks are expressed as a percentage of the region of interest (i.e., a standardized region of interest with similar dimensions as a created defect). Error bars represent means ± standard deviation. (i) $P<.05$ compared to CPC; (ii) $P<.05$ compared to CPC/BG; (iii) $P<.05$ compared to CPC/PLGA; (*) $P<.05$ compared to 2-week equivalent. *BG*, Bioglass; *CPC*, calcium phosphate cement; *PLGA*, poly(glycolic acid); *ROI*, region of interest.
Reused from A.C.M. Renno, F.C.J. van de Watering, M.R. Nejadnik, M.C. Crovace, E.D. Zanotto, J.G.C. Wolke, J.A. Jansen, J.J.J.P. van den Beucken, Incorporation of bioactive glass in calcium phosphate cement: an evaluation, Acta Biomaterialia 9 (2013) 5728–5739. https://doi.org/10.1016/j.actbio.2012.11.009 after license via (copyright.com) number 4286900390737.

and crystal size that lead to higher dissolution rate [44]. From materials science we have learned that high-energy ball milling, blast milling, and similar milling techniques lead to higher concentrations of defects within solid particles, which are responsible for higher chemical reactivity, i.e., higher bioactivity. Apart from this, the high concentration of defects enhances active diffusion coefficient during the sintering of powder compacts. Syringe foaming via hydrophilic viscous polymeric solution (silanized-hydroxypropyl methylcellulose) has also been used to improve injectability [45].

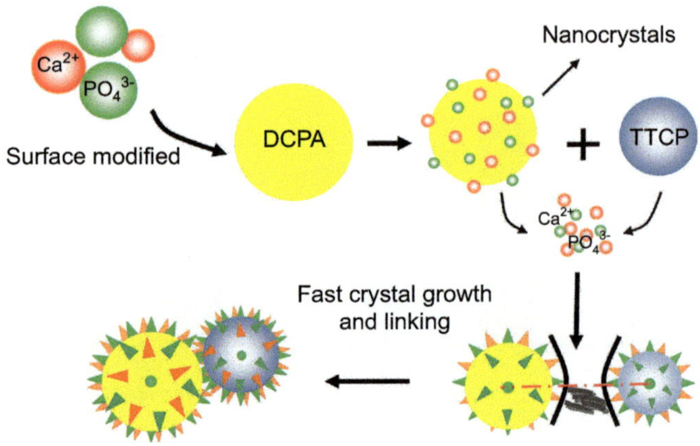

Figure 6.35 Graphical abstract illustrating the function of the TTCP nanocrystals incorporated in the CPC. *CPC*, calcium phosphate cement; *DCPA*, dicalcium phosphate anhydrous; *TTCP*, tetracalcium phosphate.
Reused from C.-L. Ko, J.-C. Chen, C.-C. Hung, J.-C. Wang, Y.-C. Tien, W.-C. Chen, Biphasic products of dicalcium phosphate-rich cement with injectability and nondispersibility, Materials Science and Engineering: C 39 (2014) 40–46. https://doi.org/10.1016/j.msec.2014.02.033 after license via (copyright.com) number 4286991461263.

The study shows the adequate initial mechanical properties. In addition, a preliminary in vivo study shows that there is evidence of new bone growth in the central zone of the implantation site.

The composition of CPCs is also subjected to various studies. In an innovative study, the Ca/P ratio and solubility of calcium silicate phosphate cement are tailored to improve the setting properties, biocompatibility, and bioactivity [46]. The cement is a mixture of brushite with amorphous hydrated calcium silicate phosphate or annealed calcium silicate phosphate. The final setting times of the composite cements decreased by 50% from 25 to 17 min with the incorporation of the amorphous hydrated calcium silicate phosphate. On the other hand, reducing the content of the amorphous phase to 10% results in a rougher microstructure because of coarser particles of plate-like morphology, which encourage better in vitro cell adherence and proliferation. In a different study [47], bioactive glass is reacted with milled $Ca(H_2PO_4)_2$ powder obtaining a Ca/P ratio of 1.33, which is the stoichiometry of octacalcium phosphate ($Ca_8(HPO_4)_2(PO_4)_4{\cdot}5H_2O$) and 2.5% Na_2HPO_4 solution with a liquid-to-powder ratio of 0.70 mL/g. It is shown that a minimum of 4 mol% of P_2O_5 is necessary for the bioactive glass to produce cement. The authors of this study claimed that this procedure to produce cement has the advantages of flexibility of the starting glass composition (but maintaining the Ca/P ratio of 1.33), tailorable dissolution rate and reactivity based on the bioactive glass composition, and the possibility of the incorporation of a wide variety of therapeutic ions into the glass.

Wollastonite has been incorporated into CPCs, and various properties have been studied, as detailed in Ref. [48]. It is found that the setting time is shortened with the

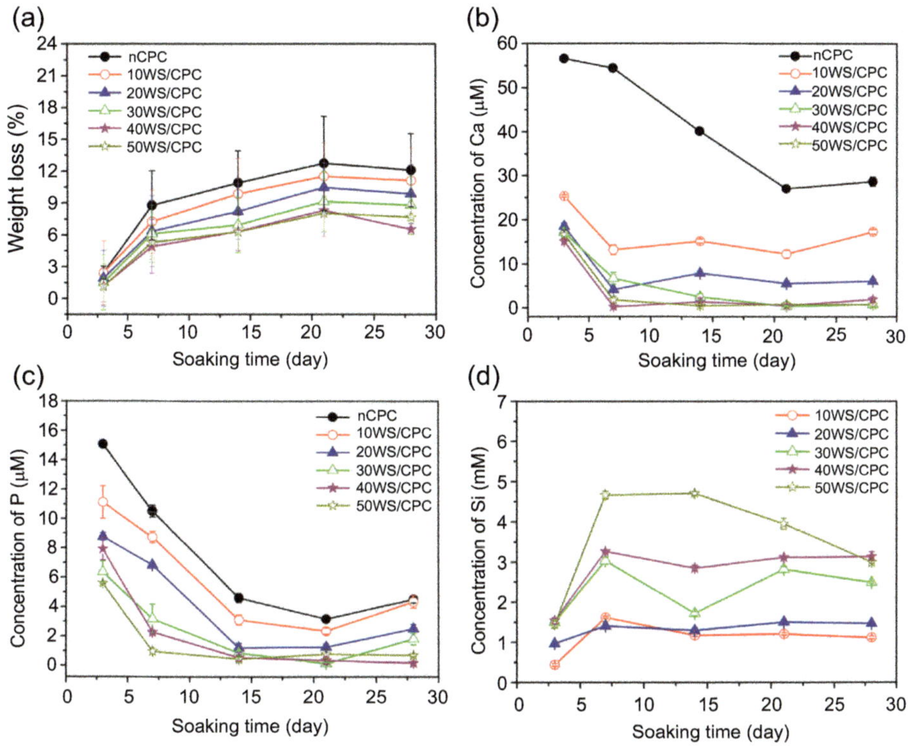

Figure 6.36 Influence of wollastonite amount on (a) the weight loss of the cements during in vitro degradation and variation of the concentrations of (b) Ca, (c) P, and (d) Si ions released from the cements immersed in phosphate buffered saline solution with the soaking time.

Reused from J. Liu, J. Li, J. Ye, F. He, Setting behavior, mechanical property and biocompatibility of anti-washout wollastonite/calcium phosphate composite cement, Ceramics International 42 (2016) 13670–13681. https://doi.org/10.1016/j.ceramint.2016.05.165 after license via (copyright.com) number 4287520017320.

incorporation of wollastonite. In addition, better antiwashout property, more compact microstructure, compressive strength, slowing down of the degradation of the cement (Fig. 6.36), and favorable attachment, proliferation, and differentiation are obtained. On the other hand, injectability was rapidly reduced for wollastonite in excess of 20%.

Another alternative to CPC is biphasic cement composed of carbonate apatite and β-TCP [49]. Carbonate apatite is known to have a faster dissolving rate in the body fluid. A mixture of α-TCP/β-TCP powder (ratio 40%) is treated with 1.0 M $NaHCO_3$ solution to obtain the biphasic cement. The mechanical property and composition ratio of carbonate apatite are tailorable by varying the treatment time with 1.0 M $NaHCO_3$ solution. These cements were examined for in vitro bioactivity using MC3T3-E1 cell lines [50]. It is found that cell proliferation could be enhanced via increasing the β-TCP content. PLLA microfillers are incorporated in CPCs for mechanical reinforcement [51].

The initial setting time is reduced but there is no observed improvement in the mechanical properties.

To promote surface degradation of an injectable CPC, the porosity of the cement should be increased. Incorporation of fast-dissolving glucose porogen is one of the strategies to increase porosity [52]. The introduced porosity and distribution can be tailored according to the selection of the porogen properties. The initial setting time is decreased, but the compressive strength is also decreased, which suggests further research on the use of porogen materials with cement. The use of porogens is more successful when associated with sintered ceramics, as mentioned earlier in this chapter. In conclusion, research trends in the development of CPCs are improving the current strategies or developing new methodologies to improve the injectability, biodegradation, bioactivity, and final mechanical properties of bone regeneration.

The story of cements does not end here; bone cements can be loaded with drugs and become a medium for drug delivery in addition to their original function in bone regeneration. Much of the literature includes the drug delivery capabilities of various cements. However, for education purposes, the distinguishing work that appears in Ref. [53] is quite useful and it is advised to read the full article. Among the important points that are highlighted in this article are the following:

1. There are two major types of CPCs; for details, see Ref. [54]. The first is the HA-forming cements, which consume little or no water during setting reaction. The second type is the brushite-forming cements, which consume a lot of water during setting.
2. The second type has fast-setting reaction that needs to include a retardant, normally citric acid. On the other hand, it can produce reduced porosity after setting, which would depress the burst release profile of incorporated drugs.
3. Accordingly, adjusting the final porosity via particle size, particle size distribution, powder-to-liquid ratio (PLR), and citric acid concentration can minimize drug release rates. The solubility of the incorporated drugs also contributes to drug release rates.

The brushite cement system in this study was composed of sintered and crushed β-TCP and monocalcium phosphate monohydrate (MCPM) powder. Equimolar amounts of β-TCP and MCPM powders are mixed to prepare cements, as shown in Table 6.4. The table also shows the measured physical and mechanical properties of the fabricated cements. An obtained relation between the compressive strength and the relative density is shown in Fig. 6.37. Vancomycin or ciprofloxacin (2 wt%) is included to study the drug release of these cements as detailed in the original article. Vancomycin and ciprofloxacin are antibiotics that are used to treat a number of bacterial infections, including bone and joint infections. The results for cumulative release of these antibiotics, with two different PLRs, are shown in Fig. 6.38.

A nonsteroidal (contains no hormone) antiinflammatory drug, indomethacin (IM), is loaded to both CPC and a composite of 50 wt% calcium sulfate + 50 wt% nanocrystalline apatite [55]. It was found that IM release reached 97% after 48 h in the case of loaded CPC. On the other hand, only 80% of IM is released in the case of the loaded composite over a longer time (144 h).

Controlling the porosity of α-TCP (HA-forming) cements by modifying the processing parameters is the subject of another study [56]. The prepared cements were of different open porosities (35%–55%) because of different PLRs and of different

Table 6.4 Properties of brushite cements produced with unfractioned monocalcium phosphate monohydrate (MCPM) and different particle size fractions after hand mixing and pressureless setting at different powder-to-liquid ratios (PLRs) (n≥5)

Cement made with	Molarity of retardant liquid (mM)	PLR (g/mL)	Compressive strength (MPa)	Initial setting time (min)	Apparent dry density (g/cm³)	Strut density (g/cm³)	Relative porosity (%)
Unfractioned MCPM (d_{50}=62 μm)	500	2.5	18.5±2.4	4.5±0.5	1.57±0.03	2.39±0.02	34±1
	500	3.3	22.8±2.7	2.5±0.5	1.72±0.03	2.42±0.02	29±1
	800	3.3	21.4±2.4	6.5±0.5	1.73±0.03	2.37±0.02	27±1
	800	4.0	36.4±3.6	3.5±0.5	1.97±0.03	2.35±0.02	16±1
Sieved <45 μm (d_{50}=32 μm)	800	4.0	46.7±6.6	3.0±0.5	2.01±0.03	2.33±0.02	14±1
Sieved <63 μm (d_{50}=42 μm)	500	4.0	45.7±9.8	3.5±0.5	2.00±0.03	2.28±0.02	12±1
	800	4.0	51.6±6.9	4.5±0.5	2.02±0.03	2.26±0.02	11±1
Sieved 45–63 μm (d_{50}=54 μm)	800	4.0	37.7±8.9	5.0±0.5	1.95±0.03	2.33±0.02	16±1
Sieved >63 μm (d_{50}=99 μm)	800	4.0	20.0±2.3	4.5±0.5	1.89±0.03	2.41±0.02	22±1

Reused from M.P. Hofmann, A.R. Mohammed, Y. Perrie, U. Gbureck, J.E. Barralet, High-strength resorbable brushite bone cement with controlled drug-releasing capabilities, Acta Biomaterialia 5 (2009) 43–49. https://doi.org/10.1016/j.actbio.2008.08.005 after license via (copyright.com) number 4290620751714.

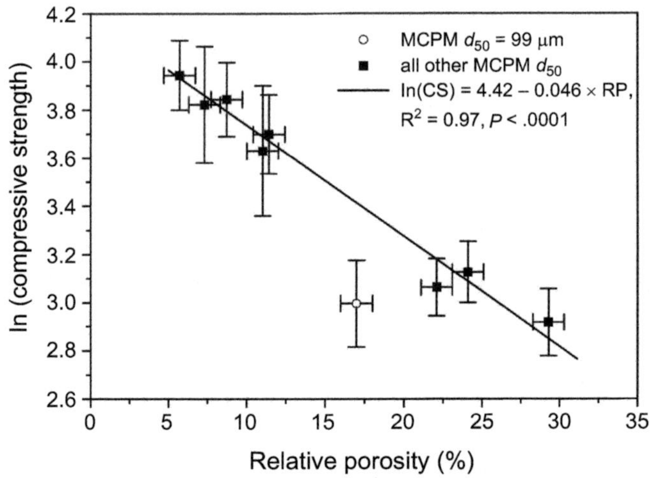

Figure 6.37 Correlation between the porosity of brushite cement formulations and the natural logarithm of wet compressive strength. *MCPM*, monocalcium phosphate monohydrate. Reused from M.P. Hofmann, A.R. Mohammed, Y. Perrie, U. Gbureck, J.E. Barralet, High-strength resorbable brushite bone cement with controlled drug-releasing capabilities, Acta Biomaterialia 5 (2009) 43–49. https://doi.org/10.1016/j.actbio.2008.08.005 after license via (copyright.com) number 4290620751714.

specific surface areas (~20 and ~37 m^2/g) because of different starting particle sizes. It was found that, e.g., protein-based drugs and high-intrinsic porosity are not sufficient. An adequate pore size distribution is necessary for protein macromolecule penetration.

Biodegradable polymer microspheres, loaded with a selected drug, in the cement are one of the strategies for drug delivery. The synthetic polymer PLGA is usually used for this purpose [57–60]. The polymer–bioceramic composite as a scaffold for drug delivery is reviewed in depth in Ref. [61].

However, the use of pectin, a water-soluble fiber that becomes gel-like when mixed with water and found in a variety of fruits and vegetables, is attractive because of its biocompatibility (nontoxic) and biodegradability. Low-methoxy amidated pectin (LMAP) is used as a drug envelope because it can gel with an "egg-box" configuration in certain chemical environments, as described in Ref. [62]. LMAP is loaded with ibuprofen (an analgesic and antiinflammatory drug) and incorporated in CPC in three ratios: 2, 4, and 6 wt%. Fig. 6.39 shows the morphology of the unloaded and loaded LMAP with ibuprofen. The composition of the used CPC was not stated in the original article, but the results seem applicable for most known compositions. Encapsulation of the drug in LMAP was found to control drug release rates, as seen in Figs. 6.40 and 6.41.

Paclitaxel is a chemotherapy medication used to treat a number of types of cancer. Including paclitaxel in calcium cement has been performed in an injectable formula of the cement [63]. The cement composition was 85% α-TCP, 10% DCPA, and 5 wt% precipitated HA. The paclitaxel was loaded in a drop of 100 mL Dulbecco's Modified Eagle Medium solution on the CPC discs and allowed to adsorb for 30 min; then, the CPC discs were freeze dried. The cell viability tests indicated that the paclitaxel

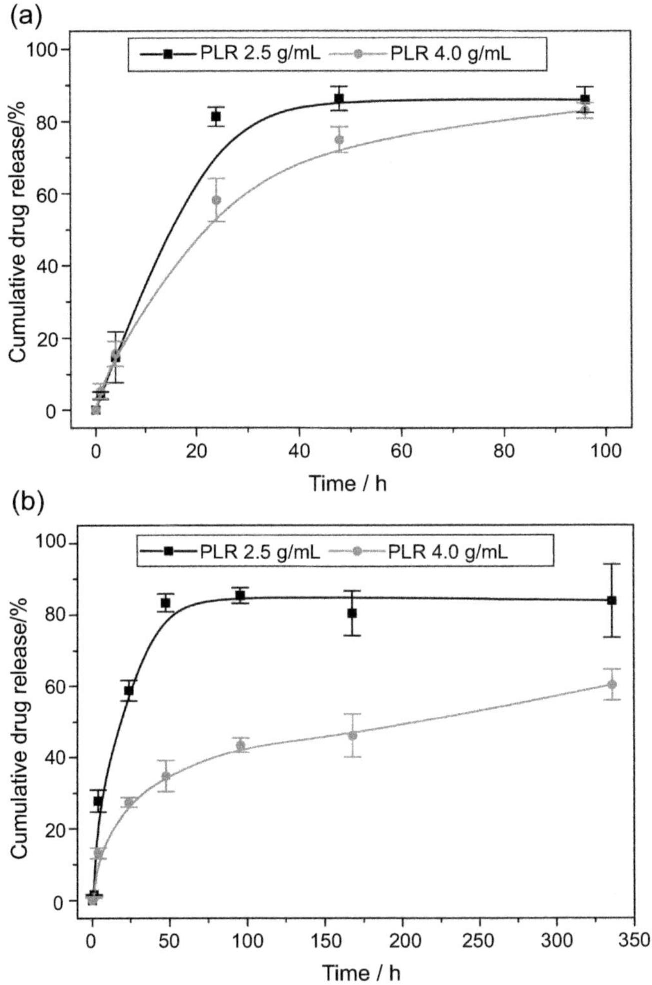

Figure 6.38 (a) Cumulative release of vancomycin (2 wt% addition to the paste) for up to 96 h from brushite cement for two different powder-to-liquid ratios. (b) Release of ciprofloxacin (2 wt% addition) for up to 14 days (336 h). B-Spline fits are included to illustrate the overall trend in drug release.

Reused from M.P. Hofmann, A.R. Mohammed, Y. Perrie, U. Gbureck, J.E. Barralet, High-strength resorbable brushite bone cement with controlled drug-releasing capabilities, Acta Biomaterialia 5 (2009) 43–49. https://doi.org/10.1016/j.actbio.2008.08.005 after license via (copyright.com) number 4290620751714.

minimal lethal dose is 90 μg/mL. One of the outcomes of this research is that paclitaxel did arrest breast cancer MDA-MB-231 cell proliferation completely.

Mesoporous material contains pores with a size range of 2–50 nm. If the pore size is below the lower bound, the material is called microporous; and if the pore size is above the upper bound, the material is called macroporous. Mesoporous silica is

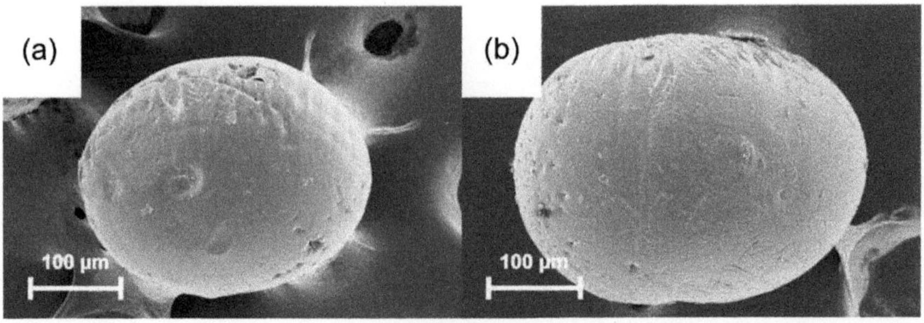

Figure 6.39 Scanning electron microscope photographs of low-methoxy amidated pectin (LMAP) microspheres: (a) LMAP microspheres; (b) LMAP microspheres loaded with ibuprofen–LMAP.
Reused from S. Girod Fullana, H. Ternet, M. Freche, J.L. Lacout, F. Rodriguez, Controlled release properties and final macroporosity of a pectin microspheres–calcium phosphate composite bone cement, Acta Biomaterialia 6 (2010) 2294–2300. https://doi.org/10.1016/j.actbio.2009.11.019 after license via (copyright.com) number 4291041118795.

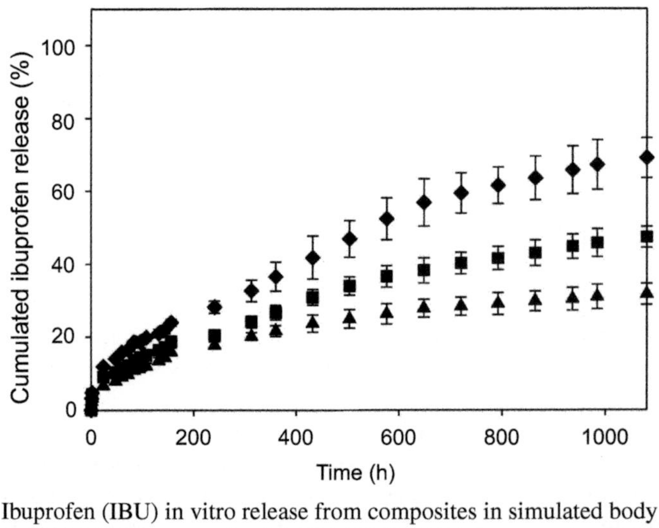

Figure 6.40 Ibuprofen (IBU) in vitro release from composites in simulated body fluid, pH 7.25 (▲, CP/IBU–LMAP6% composite; ■, CP/IBU–LMAP4% composite; ◆, CP/IBU–LMAP2% composite). *CP*, calcium phosphate; *LMAP*, low-methoxy amidated pectins.
Reused from S. Girod Fullana, H. Ternet, M. Freche, J.L. Lacout, F. Rodriguez, Controlled release properties and final macroporosity of a pectin microspheres–calcium phosphate composite bone cement, Acta Biomaterialia 6 (2010) 2294–2300. https://doi.org/10.1016/j.actbio.2009.11.019 after license via (copyright.com) number 4291041118795.

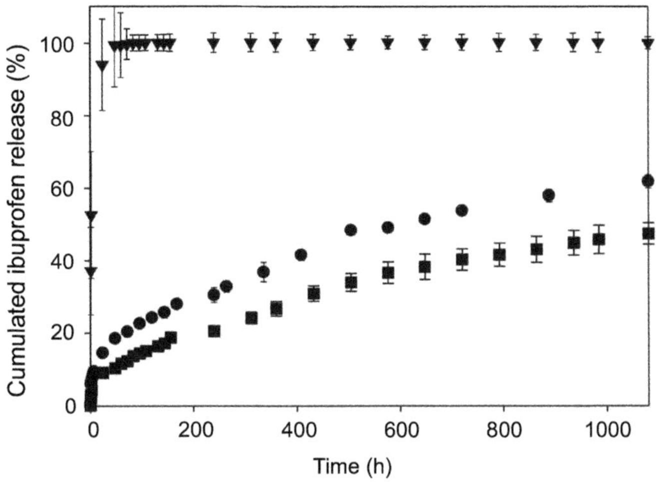

Figure 6.41 Ibuprofen (IBU) in vitro release from composites in simulated body fluid, pH 7.25, comparison with the same quantity of IBU (4 mg) encapsulated into LMAP microspheres or directly incorporated into CPC reference (●, IBU–LMAP microspheres; ■, CP/IBU–LMAP4% composite; ▼, IBU–CPC). *CP*, calcium phosphate; *CPC*, calcium phosphate cement; *LMAP*, low-methoxy amidated pectins.
Reused from S. Girod Fullana, H. Ternet, M. Freche, J.L. Lacout, F. Rodriguez, Controlled release properties and final macroporosity of a pectin microspheres–calcium phosphate composite bone cement, Acta Biomaterialia 6 (2010) 2294–2300. https://doi.org/10.1016/j.actbio.2009.11.019 after license via (copyright.com) number 4291041118795.

widely included in tissue engineering and drug delivery. It allows the regulation of drug release via a variety of stimuli such as temperature and magnetic field. The reader is referred to the informative articles in Refs. [64,65] for calcium phosphate–based cements. Mesoporous silica also proves superior to HA nanorods and carbon nanotubes in PMMA-based bone cements [66].

In hard or bone tissue engineering, the loaded drug in the implanted biomaterials becomes wider to promote osteoinductivity, the healing process, and to treat various musculoskeletal disorders. Accordingly, the concept of the drug is extended to include growth factors. Growth factors are biomaterials capable of stimulating cellular growth, proliferation, healing, and cellular differentiation such as proteins or certain hormones. The drug can also include bioactive proteins, enzymes, and nonviral genes (DNAs, RNAs). This revelation of loaded drugs makes tissue engineering a rapidly growing field of research. A well-organized review that appears in Ref. [67] describes that revelation in calcium phosphate ceramics. In addition, the article that appears in Ref. [68] reviews different aspects of calcium phosphates as cements and drug carriers for the three drug groups: low-molecular weight drugs, high-molecular weight biomolecules, and ions. This review is excellent for self-study.

As is usual in materials science and engineering, the evolved microstructure affects the final properties. In the case of CPCs, the microstructure is developed during the setting reaction and thus determines its drug release properties. The evolution of the microstructure may also be affected by the liquid part of the cement; accordingly, including the drug within the liquid phase may affect the final microstructure and drug release. These effects are studied with the incorporation of doxycycline hyclate in the α-TCP CPC [69]. Doxycycline hyclate, of the family of tetracyclines, is a broad-spectrum antibiotic commonly used in the treatment of bone infections. It is found that the drug acts as a nucleating agent for the heterogeneous precipitation of HA crystals modifying the final microstructure to be nanoporous rather than macroporous, as seen in Fig. 6.42. This situation moderates the burst release of the drug in the case of fresh CPCs (1 h incubation at 37°C in 100% relative humidity in the setting media) and the preset CPCs (7 days of incubation), as shown in Fig. 6.43. This work is further improved by tailoring the macroporosity of the prepared self-setting CPCs [70]. These cements were prepared by foaming the liquid phase at 6000 rpm for 30 s followed by mixing with the solid phase. It is shown that macroporosity enhances osteoconduction and material resorption in addition to the tuning of drug delivery rates.

A novel cement paste formulation is formulated by including a water-immiscible carrier liquid combined with suitable surfactants to control the water supply to the CPC and perform better cement-setting reaction, as detailed in Ref. [71]. The newly formulated set cement has controlled release of antibiotics (gentamicin, vancomycin). The highly developed methodology of this study is well described in the original article.

Another strategy for drug delivery is to include the drug in porous granules. Methotrexate (a chemotherapy agent of multiple uses, including the treatment of cancer) is successfully loaded in octacalcium phosphate–HA composite spherical porous granules [72]. The composite porous granules are prepared via immersing α-TCP spherical granules in a pH 5.0 buffered solution at 60°C. It is shown that the prepared porous granules release the drugs continuously.

Silver-containing bioactive glass powders in a PMMA matrix is another trend in the synthesis of scaffolds with drug delivery functionality [73]. In vitro testing with SBF is successful but further cell culturing and/or in vivo tests are necessary to validate the usefulness of such a drug delivery system.

It seems that there is no limit to the number of alternatives for CPC compositions for drug delivery. A brushite-forming cement is loaded with novel PLA/vancomycin microcapsules [74]. The microcapsules are coated with nanosized HA. Vancomycin release is slowed down with this composition, and only $85.3 \pm 3.1\%$ of the incorporated vancomycin is released within 43 days. To conclude regarding drug delivery, an all-inclusive review on the design of calcium phosphate ceramics for drug delivery appears in Ref. [75] and it is a must read in the field of drug delivery.

The last topic in this chapter is a brief description of a manufacturing process called "additive manufacturing" (AM). The ASTM definition of AM is "a process of joining materials to make objects from 3D model data, usually layer upon layer, as opposed to subtractive manufacturing methodologies" [76]. The same reference states the following synonyms for AM: additive fabrication, additive processes, additive techniques, additive layer manufacturing, layer manufacturing, and freeform fabrication. As far as hard tissue engineering is concerned, AM is a process for the production of freeform

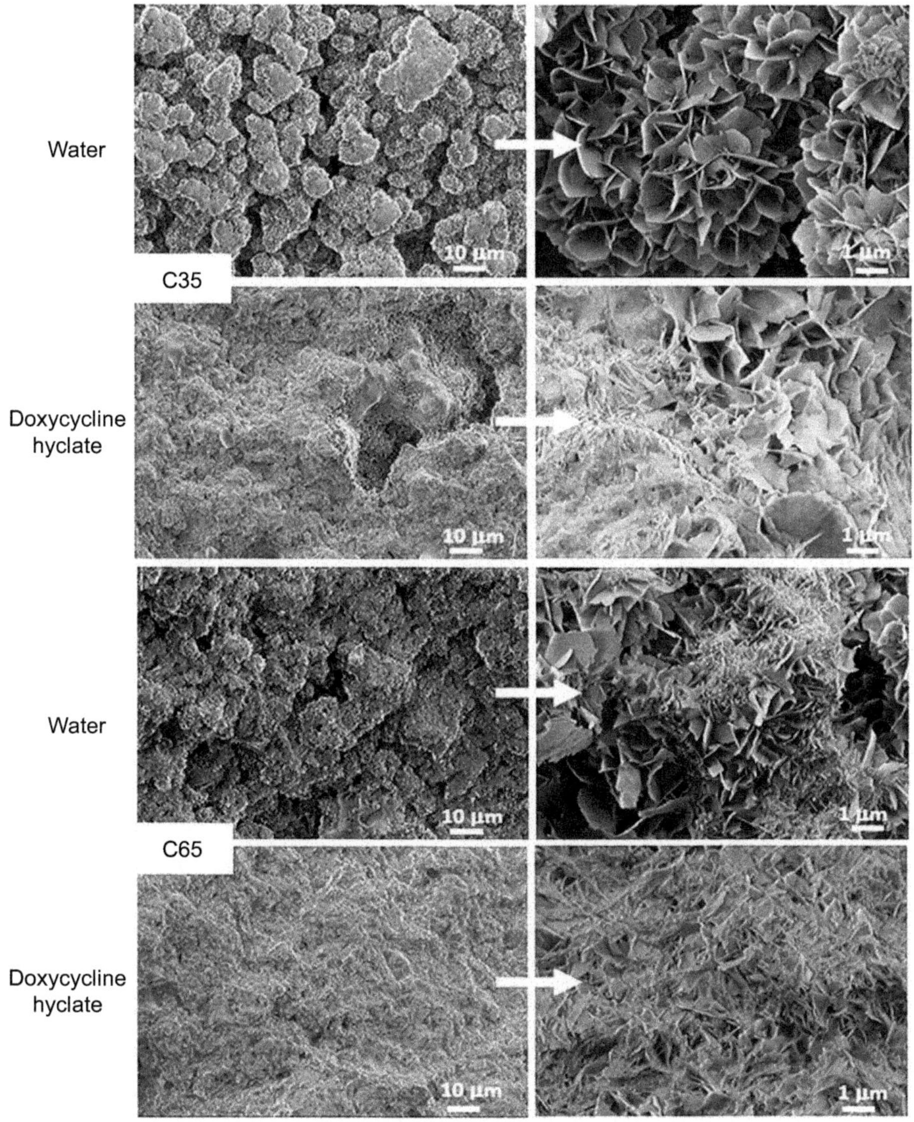

Figure 6.42 Field-emission scanning electron microscope micrographs of the fracture surfaces of cements prepared with different liquid-to-powder ratios (C35 or C65), using either water or a doxycycline hyclate solution as liquid phase. Low magnification in the left column and higher magnification in the right column.
Reused from C. Canal, D. Pastorino, G. Mestres, P. Schuler, M-P. Ginebra, Relevance of microstructure for the early antibiotic release of fresh and pre-set calcium phosphate cements, Acta Biomaterialia 9 (2013) 8403–8412. https://doi.org/10.1016/j.actbio.2013.05.016 after license via (copyright.com) number 4292070453184.

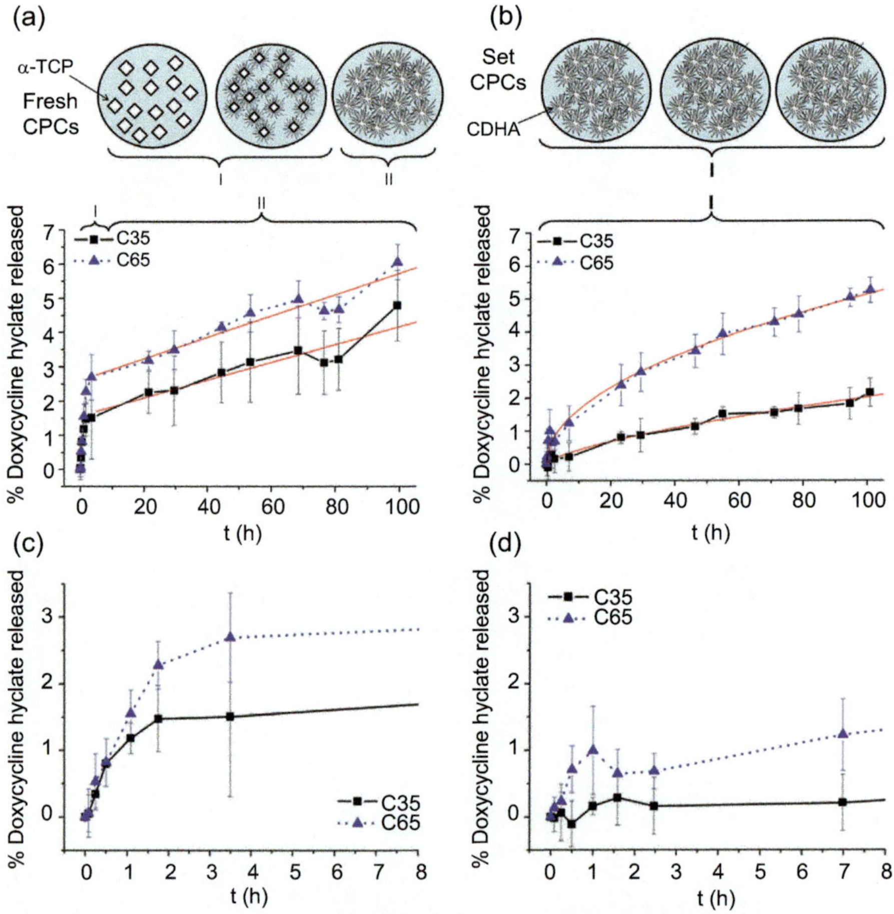

Figure 6.43 Accumulated doxycycline release (%) from calcium phosphate cements (CPCs) prepared with liquid phase (L/P) containing antibiotic at L/P ratios of 0.35 and 0.65. Release curves of the (a) fresh CPCs, (b) preset CPCs with the corresponding fitting (*red lines* [*gray in print version*]) and zoom of the first 8 h for (c) fresh and (d) preset CPCs. A schematic representation of the evolution of the microstructure of fresh and preset CPCs with time is included. *α-TCP*, α-tricalcium phosphate; *CDHA*, calcium-deficient hydroxyapatites.
Reused from C. Canal, D. Pastorino, G. Mestres, P. Schuler, M-P. Ginebra, Relevance of microstructure for the early antibiotic release of fresh and pre-set calcium phosphate cements, Acta Biomaterialia 9 (2013) 8403–8412. https://doi.org/10.1016/j.actbio.2013.05.016 after license via (copyright.com) number 4292070453184.

porous scaffolds with custom-tailored architectures. A simple image of the AM is the printing, layer by layer, of a 3D object using biomaterial composite ink. This is why the term "3D printing" is frequently found in publications. However, AM may start with 3D CAD design followed by a type of rapid prototyping that utilizes a 3D printer. Note that the rapid prototyping represents a collection of techniques, including 3D

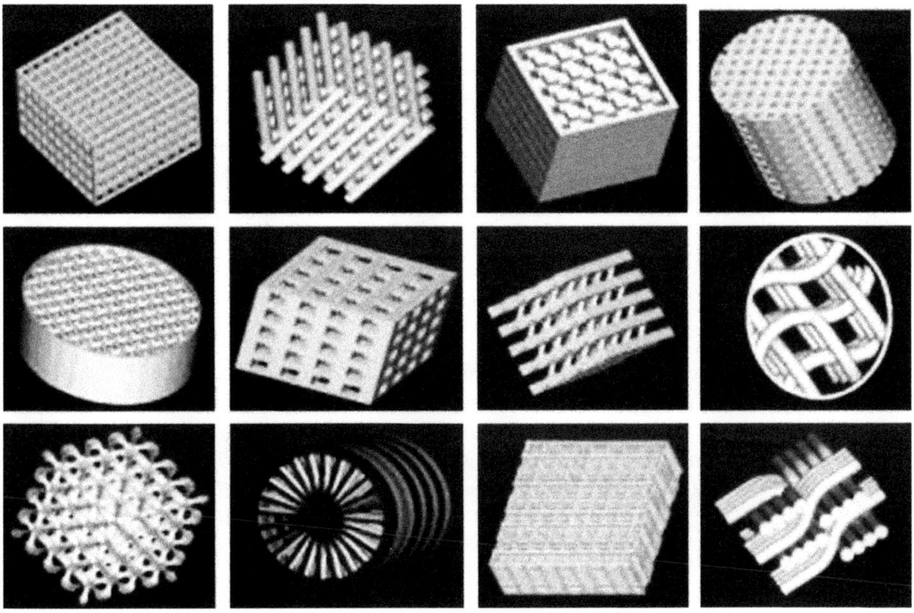

Figure 6.44 A library of designed scaffold unit cells based on different feature primitives. Reused from W. Sun, B. Starly, J. Nam, A. Darling, Bio-CAD modeling and its applications in computer-aided tissue engineering, Computer-Aided Design 37 (2005) 1097–1114. https://doi.org/10.1016/j.cad.2005.02.002 after license via (copyright.com) number 4292631251448.

printing, that builds 3D objects. These techniques are fully described in a comprehensive book [77]. Definitions found in the literature are not necessarily consistent, thus the above ASTM definition is a good start for AM.

CAD design takes into account the model microstructure (architecture) of the printed object and the desired final mechanical properties. Thus there are various architectures based on a selected "unit cell," as seen in Fig. 6.44. Each unit cell in the figure has its particular pore size and shape. Thus the choice of unit cell is reflected in the final mechanical properties. In addition, the choice of unit cell material and porosity also affects the resultant mechanical properties, as seen in Fig. 6.45. The figure compares the effective Young's modulus between the unit cell materials of HA, poly(L-glutamic acid), and PLLA at different porosities [78].

AM is largely applicable via printing molten polymers and metals. On the other hand, ceramics and glasses are difficult to melt. Therefore robocasting has emerged as an alternative AM process that is based on extruding a filament of paste/ink via a 3D printer nozzle [79]. The process of robocasting is successfully applied in fabrication of biphasic calcium phosphate scaffolds (HA/β-TCP ≈ 1.5) [80]. Codoped composite scaffolds with Sr and Ag improve the mechanical strength, provide antimicrobial activity, and induce cellular proliferation. The reader is referred to the extensive review in Ref. [81] for current trends in AM utilizing bioceramics. This review

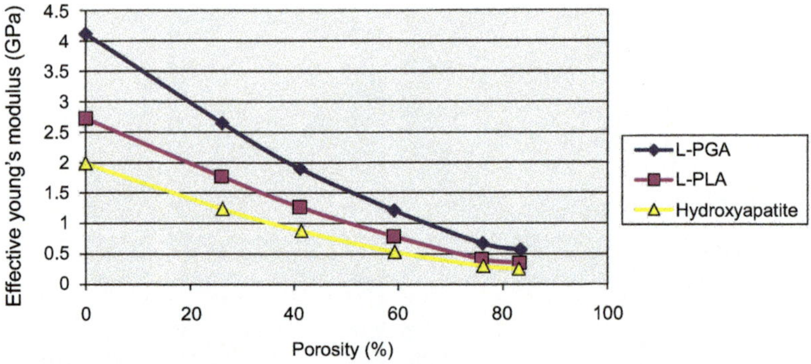

Figure 6.45 Effect of unit cell material and porosity on the effective Young's modulus. *L-PGA*, L-Poly(glycolic acid); *L-PLA*, L-poly(lactic acid).
Reused from W. Sun, B. Starly, J. Nam, A. Darling, Bio-CAD modeling and its applications in computer-aided tissue engineering, Computer-Aided Design 37 (2005) 1097–1114. https://doi.org/10.1016/j.cad.2005.02.002 after license via (copyright.com) number 4292631251448.

provides excellent classification of the methodologies and discusses the optimization strategies to compromise between mechanical and biological properties. However, the door is wide open for new innovations in this field and it is expected that the field of AM for ceramic biomaterials will be the subject of extensive research activity for a long time.

Review questions

1. Prepare a report that contains brief descriptions of the processes mentioned in this chapter for the fabrication of scaffolds. Add extra methods from the literature if necessary.
2. Prepare a report that classifies the materials used for the scaffolds as ceramic–ceramic composites and polymer–ceramic composites.
3. Prepare another report that discusses the materials and process selection of the scaffolds and their effects on the final pore size and shape.
4. Discuss the characterization methods that are utilized to evaluate the fabricated scaffolds and the benefit of each characterization technique.
5. How does nanotechnology improve cell proliferation and growth of the scaffolds? Write a complete report.
6. Discuss the differences in the utilization of sintered bioceramics and cement bioceramics.
7. Discuss the differences between the two major types of CPCs and their applicability.
8. Tabulate the loaded drugs mentioned in this chapter as a core of a new report that contains a brief description, the method of loading, and the resultant release rate.
9. Discuss the learned strategies in this chapter to control drug release. Refer to additional literature if required to write a self-contained report.
10. Discuss the relations between these concepts: 3D printing, rapid prototyping, AM, and robocasting.

References

[1] G. Wei, P.X. Ma, Structure and properties of nano-hydroxyapatite/polymer composite scaffolds for bone tissue engineering, Biomaterials 25 (2004) 4749–4757, https://doi.org/10.1016/j.biomaterials.2003.12.005.

[2] H. Wang, Y. Li, Y. Zuo, J. Li, S. Ma, L. Cheng, Biocompatibility and osteogenesis of biomimetic nano-hydroxyapatite/polyamide composite scaffolds for bone tissue engineering, Biomaterials 28 (2007) 3338–3348, https://doi.org/10.1016/j.biomaterials.2007.04.014.

[3] E. Nejati, H. Mirzadeh, M. Zandi, Synthesis and characterization of nano-hydroxyapatite rods/poly(l-lactide acid) composite scaffolds for bone tissue engineering, Composites Part A: Applied Science and Manufacturing 39 (2008) 1589–1596, https://doi.org/10.1016/j.compositesa.2008.05.018.

[4] E. Nejati, V. Firouzdor, M.B. Eslaminejad, F. Bagheri, Needle-like nano hydroxyapatite/poly(l-lactide acid) composite scaffold for bone tissue engineering application, Materials Science and Engineering: C 29 (2009) 942–949, https://doi.org/10.1016/j.msec.2008.07.038.

[5] Z.-M. Huang, Y.-Z. Zhang, M. Kotaki, S. Ramakrishna, A review on polymer nanofibers by electrospinning and their applications in nanocomposites, Composites Science and Technology 63 (2003) 2223–2253, https://doi.org/10.1016/S0266-3538(03)00178-7.

[6] N. Bhardwaj, S.C. Kundu, Electrospinning: a fascinating fiber fabrication technique, Biotechnology Advances 28 (2010) 325–347, https://doi.org/10.1016/j.biotechadv.2010.01.004.

[7] M. Ngiam, S. Liao, A.J. Patil, Z. Cheng, C.K. Chan, S. Ramakrishna, The fabrication of nano-hydroxyapatite on PLGA and PLGA/collagen nanofibrous composite scaffolds and their effects in osteoblastic behavior for bone tissue engineering, Bone 45 (2009) 4–16, https://doi.org/10.1016/j.bone.2009.03.674.

[8] D. Yang, Y. Jin, G. Ma, X. Chen, F. Lu, J. Nie, Fabrication and characterization of chitosan/PVA with hydroxyapatite biocomposite nanoscaffolds, Journal of Applied Polymer Science 110 (2008) 3328–3335, https://doi.org/10.1002/app.28829.

[9] M. Swetha, K. Sahithi, A. Moorthi, N. Srinivasan, K. Ramasamy, N. Selvamurugan, Biocomposites containing natural polymers and hydroxyapatite for bone tissue engineering, International Journal of Biological Macromolecules 47 (2010) 1–4, https://doi.org/10.1016/j.ijbiomac.2010.03.015.

[10] H. Zhou, J. Lee, Nanoscale hydroxyapatite particles for bone tissue engineering, Acta Biomaterialia 7 (2011) 2769–2781, https://doi.org/10.1016/j.actbio.2011.03.019.

[11] F. Sun, H. Zhou, J. Lee, Various preparation methods of highly porous hydroxyapatite/polymer nanoscale biocomposites for bone regeneration, Acta Biomaterialia 7 (2011) 3813–3828, https://doi.org/10.1016/j.actbio.2011.07.002.

[12] X. Cai, H. Tong, X. Shen, W. Chen, J. Yan, J. Hu, Preparation and characterization of homogeneous chitosan–polylactic acid/hydroxyapatite nanocomposite for bone tissue engineering and evaluation of its mechanical properties, Acta Biomaterialia 5 (2009) 2693–2703, https://doi.org/10.1016/j.actbio.2009.03.005.

[13] Y. Lu, A. Zhu, W. Wang, H. Shi, New bioactive hybrid material of nano-hydroxyapatite based on N-carboxyethylchitosan for bone tissue engineering, Applied Surface Science 256 (2010) 7228–7233, https://doi.org/10.1016/j.apsusc.2010.05.056.

[14] X. Li, K. Nan, S. Shi, H. Chen, Preparation and characterization of nano-hydroxyapatite/chitosan cross-linking composite membrane intended for tissue engineering, International Journal of Biological Macromolecules 50 (2012) 43–49, https://doi.org/10.1016/j.ijbiomac.2011.09.021.

[15] N.K. Nga, L.T. Giang, T.Q. Huy, P.H. Viet, C. Migliaresi, Surfactant-assisted size control of hydroxyapatite nanorods for bone tissue engineering, Colloids and Surfaces B: Biointerfaces 116 (2014) 666–673, https://doi.org/10.1016/j.colsurfb.2013.11.001.
[16] K.S.W. Sing, R.T. Williams, Physisorption hysteresis loops and the characterization of nanoporous materials, Adsorption Science and Technology 22 (2004) 773–782, https://doi.org/10.1260/0263617053499032.
[17] K. Gorna, S. Gogolewski, Biodegradable porous polyurethane scaffolds for tissue repair and regeneration, Journal of Biomedical Materials Research 79A (2006) 128–138, https://doi.org/10.1002/jbm.a.30708.
[18] C.I.R. Boissard, P.-E. Bourban, A.E. Tami, M. Alini, D. Eglin, Nanohydroxyapatite/poly(ester urethane) scaffold for bone tissue engineering, Acta Biomaterialia 5 (2009) 3316–3327, https://doi.org/10.1016/j.actbio.2009.05.001.
[19] M.W. Laschke, A. Strohe, M.D. Menger, M. Alini, D. Eglin, In vitro and in vivo evaluation of a novel nanosize hydroxyapatite particles/poly(ester-urethane) composite scaffold for bone tissue engineering, Acta Biomaterialia 6 (2010) 2020–2027, https://doi.org/10.1016/j.actbio.2009.12.004.
[20] D. Puppi, F. Chiellini, A.M. Piras, E. Chiellini, Polymeric materials for bone and cartilage repair, Progress in Polymer Science 35 (2010) 403–440, https://doi.org/10.1016/j.progpolymsci.2010.01.006.
[21] N.K. Nga, T.T. Hoai, P.H. Viet, Biomimetic scaffolds based on hydroxyapatite nanorod/poly(d,l) lactic acid with their corresponding apatite-forming capability and biocompatibility for bone-tissue engineering, Colloids and Surfaces B: Biointerfaces 128 (2015) 506–514, https://doi.org/10.1016/j.colsurfb.2015.03.001.
[22] A. Nemati Hayati, S.M. Hosseinalipour, H.R. Rezaie, M.A. Shokrgozar, Characterization of poly(3-hydroxybutyrate)/nano-hydroxyapatite composite scaffolds fabricated without the use of organic solvents for bone tissue engineering applications, Materials Science and Engineering: C 32 (2012) 416–422, https://doi.org/10.1016/j.msec.2011.11.013.
[23] M. Eilbagi, R. Emadi, K. Raeissi, M. Kharaziha, A. Valiani, Mechanical and cytotoxicity evaluation of nanostructured hydroxyapatite-bredigite scaffolds for bone regeneration, Materials Science and Engineering: C 68 (2016) 603–612, https://doi.org/10.1016/j.msec.2016.06.030.
[24] H. Follet, G. Boivin, C. Rumelhart, P.J. Meunier, The degree of mineralization is a determinant of bone strength: a study on human calcanei, Bone 34 (2004) 783–789, https://doi.org/10.1016/j.bone.2003.12.012.
[25] S. Ramezani, R. Emadi, M. Kharaziha, F. Tavangarian, Synthesis, characterization and in vitro behavior of nanostructured diopside/biphasic calcium phosphate scaffolds, Materials Chemistry and Physics 186 (2017) 415–425, https://doi.org/10.1016/j.matchemphys.2016.11.013.
[26] S. Sadeghzade, R. Emadi, F. Tavangarian, M. Naderi, Fabrication and evaluation of silica-based ceramic scaffolds for hard tissue engineering applications, Materials Science and Engineering: C 71 (2017) 431–438, https://doi.org/10.1016/j.msec.2016.10.042.
[27] Y.Y. Qi, Z.X. Tai, D.F. Sun, J.T. Chen, H.B. Ma, X.B. Yan, B. Liu, Q.J. Xue, Fabrication and characterization of poly(vinyl alcohol)/graphene oxide nanofibrous biocomposite scaffolds, Journal of Applied Polymer Science 127 (2013) 1885–1894, https://doi.org/10.1002/app.37924.
[28] G.M. Neelgund, A. Oki, Z. Luo, In situ deposition of hydroxyapatite on graphene nanosheets, Materials Research Bulletin 48 (2013) 175–179, https://doi.org/10.1016/j.materresbull.2012.08.077.

[29] L. Zhang, W. Liu, C. Yue, T. Zhang, P. Li, Z. Xing, Y. Chen, A tough graphene nanosheet/hydroxyapatite composite with improved in vitro biocompatibility, Carbon 61 (2013) 105–115, https://doi.org/10.1016/j.carbon.2013.04.074.
[30] M.A. Rafiee, J. Rafiee, I. Srivastava, Z. Wang, H. Song, Z.-Z. Yu, N. Koratkar, Fracture and fatigue in graphene nanocomposites, Small 6 (2010) 179–183, https://doi.org/10.1002/smll.200901480.
[31] X.Liu,M.Morra,A.Carpi,B.Li,Bioactivecalciumsilicateceramicsandcoatings,Biomedicine and Pharmacotherapy 62 (2008) 526–529, https://doi.org/10.1016/j.biopha.2008.07.051.
[32] X. Liu, C. Ding, P.K. Chu, Mechanism of apatite formation on wollastonite coatings in simulated body fluids, Biomaterials 25 (2004) 1755–1761, https://doi.org/10.1016/j.biomaterials.2003.08.024.
[33] Z. Fan, J. Wang, Z. Wang, H. Ran, Y. Li, L. Niu, P. Gong, B. Liu, S. Yang, One-pot synthesis of graphene/hydroxyapatite nanorod composite for tissue engineering, Carbon 66 (2014) 407–416, https://doi.org/10.1016/j.carbon.2013.09.016.
[34] M. Li, Q. Liu, Z. Jia, X. Xu, Y. Cheng, Y. Zheng, T. Xi, S. Wei, Graphene oxide/hydroxyapatite composite coatings fabricated by electrophoretic nanotechnology for biological applications, Carbon 67 (2014) 185–197, https://doi.org/10.1016/j.carbon.2013.09.080.
[35] V. Cannillo, L. Lusvarghi, A. Sola, Production and characterization of plasma-sprayed TiO_2–hydroxyapatite functionally graded coatings, Journal of the European Ceramic Society 28 (2008) 2161–2169, https://doi.org/10.1016/j.jeurceramsoc.2008.02.026.
[36] M.A.F. Afzal, P. Kesarwani, K.M. Reddy, S. Kalmodia, B. Basu, K. Balani, Functionally graded hydroxyapatite-alumina-zirconia biocomposite: synergy of toughness and biocompatibility, Materials Science and Engineering: C 32 (2012) 1164–1173, https://doi.org/10.1016/j.msec.2012.03.003.
[37] S. Marković, M.J. Lukić, S.D. Škapin, B. Stojanović, D. Uskoković, Designing, fabrication and characterization of nanostructured functionally graded HAp/BCP ceramics, Ceramics International 41 (2015) 2654–2667, https://doi.org/10.1016/j.ceramint.2014.10.079.
[38] M. Naebe, K. Shirvanimoghaddam, Functionally graded materials: a review of fabrication and properties, Applied Materials Today 5 (2016) 223–245, https://doi.org/10.1016/j.apmt.2016.10.001.
[39] A.C.M. Renno, F.C.J. van de Watering, M.R. Nejadnik, M.C. Crovace, E.D. Zanotto, J.G.C. Wolke, J.A. Jansen, J.J.J.P. van den Beucken, Incorporation of bioactive glass in calcium phosphate cement: an evaluation, Acta Biomaterialia 9 (2013) 5728–5739, https://doi.org/10.1016/j.actbio.2012.11.009.
[40] C.-L. Ko, J.-C. Chen, C.-C. Hung, J.-C. Wang, Y.-C. Tien, W.-C. Chen, Biphasic products of dicalcium phosphate-rich cement with injectability and nondispersibility, Materials Science and Engineering: C 39 (2014) 40–46, https://doi.org/10.1016/j.msec.2014.02.033.
[41] J. Cabrejos-Azama, M.H. Alkhraisat, C. Rueda, J. Torres, L. Blanco, E. López-Cabarcos, Magnesium substitution in brushite cements for enhanced bone tissue regeneration, Materials Science and Engineering: C 43 (2014) 403–410, https://doi.org/10.1016/j.msec.2014.06.036.
[42] S. Maenz, E. Kunisch, M. Mühlstädt, A. Böhm, V. Kopsch, J. Bossert, R.W. Kinne, K.D. Jandt, Enhanced mechanical properties of a novel, injectable, fiber-reinforced brushite cement, Journal of the Mechanical Behavior of Biomedical Materials 39 (2014) 328–338, https://doi.org/10.1016/j.jmbbm.2014.07.028.
[43] P.M.C. Torres, S. Gouveia, S. Olhero, A. Kaushal, J.M.F. Ferreira, Injectability of calcium phosphate pastes: effects of particle size and state of aggregation of β-tricalcium phosphate powders, Acta Biomaterialia 21 (2015) 204–216, https://doi.org/10.1016/j.actbio.2015.04.006.

[44] J. Bae, Y. Ida, K. Sekine, F. Kawano, K. Hamada, Effects of high-energy ball-milling on injectability and strength of β-tricalcium-phosphate cement, Journal of the Mechanical Behavior of Biomedical Materials 47 (2015) 77–86, https://doi.org/10.1016/j.jmbbm.2015.03.005.
[45] J. Zhang, W. Liu, O. Gauthier, S. Sourice, P. Pilet, G. Rethore, K. Khairoun, J.-M. Bouler, F. Tancret, P. Weiss, A simple and effective approach to prepare injectable macroporous calcium phosphate cement for bone repair: syringe-foaming using a viscous hydrophilic polymeric solution, Acta Biomaterialia 31 (2016) 326–338, https://doi.org/10.1016/j.actbio.2015.11.055.
[46] T. Sopcak, L. Medvecky, M. Giretova, R. Stulajterova, J. Durisin, V. Girman, M. Faberova, Effect of phase composition of calcium silicate phosphate component on properties of brushite based composite cements, Materials Characterization 117 (2016) 17–29, https://doi.org/10.1016/j.matchar.2016.04.011.
[47] N.W. Kent, R.G. Hill, N. Karpukhina, A new way of forming a calcium phosphate cement using bioactive glasses as a reactive precursor, Materials Letters 162 (2016) 32–36, https://doi.org/10.1016/j.matlet.2015.09.099.
[48] J. Liu, J. Li, J. Ye, F. He, Setting behavior, mechanical property and biocompatibility of anti-washout wollastonite/calcium phosphate composite cement, Ceramics International 42 (2016) 13670–13681, https://doi.org/10.1016/j.ceramint.2016.05.165.
[49] T. Arahira, M. Maruta, S. Matsuya, Development and characterization of carbonate apatite/β-tricalcium phosphate biphasic cement, Materials Letters 194 (2017) 205–208, https://doi.org/10.1016/j.matlet.2017.02.071.
[50] T. Arahira, M. Maruta, S. Matsuya, Characterization and in vitro evaluation of biphasic α-tricalcium phosphate/β-tricalcium phosphate cement, Materials Science and Engineering: C 74 (2017) 478–484, https://doi.org/10.1016/j.msec.2016.12.049.
[51] A.G.B. Castro, A. Polini, Z. Azami, S.C.G. Leeuwenburgh, J.A. Jansen, F. Yang, J.J.J.P. van den Beucken, Incorporation of PLLA micro-fillers for mechanical reinforcement of calcium-phosphate cement, Journal of the Mechanical Behavior of Biomedical Materials 71 (2017) 286–294, https://doi.org/10.1016/j.jmbbm.2017.03.027.
[52] B.T. Smith, M. Santoro, E.C. Grosfeld, S.R. Shah, J.J.J.P. van den Beucken, J.A. Jansen, A.G. Mikos, Incorporation of fast dissolving glucose porogens into an injectable calcium phosphate cement for bone tissue engineering, Acta Biomaterialia 50 (2017) 68–77, https://doi.org/10.1016/j.actbio.2016.12.024.
[53] M.P. Hofmann, A.R. Mohammed, Y. Perrie, U. Gbureck, J.E. Barralet, High-strength resorbable brushite bone cement with controlled drug-releasing capabilities, Acta Biomaterialia 5 (2009) 43–49, https://doi.org/10.1016/j.actbio.2008.08.005.
[54] K. Ishikawa, Calcium phosphate cement, in: Advances in Calcium Phosphate Biomaterials, Springer, Berlin, Heidelberg, 2014, pp. 199–227, https://doi.org/10.1007/978-3-642-53980-0_7.
[55] S. Hesaraki, F. Moztarzadeh, N. Nezafati, Evaluation of a bioceramic-based nanocomposite material for controlled delivery of a non-steroidal anti-inflammatory drug, Medical Engineering and Physics 31 (2009) 1205–1213, https://doi.org/10.1016/j.medengphy.2009.07.019.
[56] M. Espanol, R.A. Perez, E.B. Montufar, C. Marichal, A. Sacco, M.P. Ginebra, Intrinsic porosity of calcium phosphate cements and its significance for drug delivery and tissue engineering applications, Acta Biomaterialia 5 (2009) 2752–2762, https://doi.org/10.1016/j.actbio.2009.03.011.
[57] Q.P. Ruhe, E.L. Hedberg, N.T. Padron, P.H.M. Spauwen, J.A. Jansen, A.G. Mikos, RHBMP-2 release from injectable poly(dl-lactic-co-glycolic acid)/calcium-phosphate cement composites, Journal of Bone and Joint Surgery 85 (2003) 75.

[58] P.Q. Ruhé, O.C. Boerman, F.G.M. Russel, P.H.M. Spauwen, A.G. Mikos, J.A. Jansen, Controlled release of rhBMP-2 loaded poly(dl-lactic-co-glycolic acid)/calcium phosphate cement composites in vivo, Journal of Controlled Release 106 (2005) 162–171, https://doi.org/10.1016/j.jconrel.2005.04.018.
[59] J. Schnieders, U. Gbureck, R. Thull, T. Kissel, Controlled release of gentamicin from calcium phosphate—poly(lactic acid-co-glycolic acid) composite bone cement, Biomaterials 27 (2006) 4239–4249, https://doi.org/10.1016/j.biomaterials.2006.03.032.
[60] Z. Fei, Y. Hu, D. Wu, H. Wu, R. Lu, J. Bai, H. Song, Preparation and property of a novel bone graft composite consisting of rhBMP-2 loaded PLGA microspheres and calcium phosphate cement, Journal of Materials Science: Materials in Medicine 19 (2008) 1109–1116, https://doi.org/10.1007/s10856-007-3050-5.
[61] V. Mouriño, J.P. Cattalini, J.A. Roether, P. Dubey, I. Roy, A.R. Boccaccini, Composite polymer-bioceramic scaffolds with drug delivery capability for bone tissue engineering, Expert Opinion on Drug Delivery 10 (2013) 1353–1365, https://doi.org/10.1517/17425247.2013.808183.
[62] S. Girod Fullana, H. Ternet, M. Freche, J.L. Lacout, F. Rodriguez, Controlled release properties and final macroporosity of a pectin microspheres–calcium phosphate composite bone cement, Acta Biomaterialia 6 (2010) 2294–2300, https://doi.org/10.1016/j.actbio.2009.11.019.
[63] M.A. Lopez-Heredia, G.J. Bernard Kamphuis, P.C. Thüne, F. Cumhur Öner, J.A. Jansen, X. Frank Walboomers, An injectable calcium phosphate cement for the local delivery of paclitaxel to bone, Biomaterials 32 (2011) 5411–5416, https://doi.org/10.1016/j.biomaterials.2011.04.010.
[64] M. Manzano, M. Vallet-Regí, Revisiting bioceramics: bone regenerative and local drug delivery systems, Progress in Solid State Chemistry 40 (2012) 17–30, https://doi.org/10.1016/j.progsolidstchem.2012.05.001.
[65] D. Arcos, M. Vallet-Regí, Bioceramics for drug delivery, Acta Materialia 61 (2013) 890–911, https://doi.org/10.1016/j.actamat.2012.10.039.
[66] S.-C. Shen, W.K. Ng, Y.-C. Dong, J. Ng, R.B.H. Tan, Nanostructured material formulated acrylic bone cements with enhanced drug release, Materials Science and Engineering: C 58 (2016) 233–241, https://doi.org/10.1016/j.msec.2015.08.011.
[67] S. Bose, S. Tarafder, Calcium phosphate ceramic systems in growth factor and drug delivery for bone tissue engineering: a review, Acta Biomaterialia 8 (2012) 1401–1421, https://doi.org/10.1016/j.actbio.2011.11.017.
[68] M.-P. Ginebra, C. Canal, M. Espanol, D. Pastorino, E.B. Montufar, Calcium phosphate cements as drug delivery materials, Advanced Drug Delivery Reviews 64 (2012) 1090–1110, https://doi.org/10.1016/j.addr.2012.01.008.
[69] C. Canal, D. Pastorino, G. Mestres, P. Schuler, M.-P. Ginebra, Relevance of microstructure for the early antibiotic release of fresh and pre-set calcium phosphate cements, Acta Biomaterialia 9 (2013) 8403–8412, https://doi.org/10.1016/j.actbio.2013.05.016.
[70] D. Pastorino, C. Canal, M.-P. Ginebra, Drug delivery from injectable calcium phosphate foams by tailoring the macroporosity–drug interaction, Acta Biomaterialia 12 (2015) 250–259, https://doi.org/10.1016/j.actbio.2014.10.031.
[71] E. Vorndran, M. Geffers, A. Ewald, M. Lemm, B. Nies, U. Gbureck, Ready-to-use injectable calcium phosphate bone cement paste as drug carrier, Acta Biomaterialia 9 (2013) 9558–9567, https://doi.org/10.1016/j.actbio.2013.08.009.
[72] N. Ito, M. Kamitakahara, K. Ioku, Preparation and evaluation of spherical porous granules of octacalcium phosphate/hydroxyapatite as drug carriers in bone cancer treatment, Materials Letters 120 (2014) 94–96, https://doi.org/10.1016/j.matlet.2014.01.040.

[73] M. Miola, M. Bruno, G. Maina, G. Fucale, G. Lucchetta, E. Vernè, Antibiotic-free composite bone cements with antibacterial and bioactive properties. A preliminary study, Materials Science and Engineering: C 43 (2014) 65–75, https://doi.org/10.1016/j.msec.2014.06.026.
[74] D. Loca, M. Sokolova, J. Locs, A. Smirnova, Z. Irbe, Calcium phosphate bone cements for local vancomycin delivery, Materials Science and Engineering: C 49 (2015) 106–113, https://doi.org/10.1016/j.msec.2014.12.075.
[75] M. Parent, H. Baradari, E. Champion, C. Damia, M. Viana-Trecant, Design of calcium phosphate ceramics for drug delivery applications in bone diseases: a review of the parameters affecting the loading and release of the therapeutic substance, Journal of Controlled Release 252 (2017) 1–17, https://doi.org/10.1016/j.jconrel.2017.02.012.
[76] ASTM F2792–12a, Standard Terminology for Additive Manufacturing Technologies. Astm.Org, https://doi.org/10.1520/f2792-12a.
[77] R. Narayan (Ed.), Rapid Prototyping of Biomaterials, Woodhead Publishing, 2014. https://www.sciencedirect.com/science/article/pii/B978085709599250012X.
[78] W. Sun, B. Starly, J. Nam, A. Darling, Bio-CAD modeling and its applications in computer-aided tissue engineering, Computer-Aided Design 37 (2005) 1097–1114, https://doi.org/10.1016/j.cad.2005.02.002.
[79] E. Feilden, C. Ferraro, Q. Zhang, E. García-Tuñón, E. D'Elia, F. Giuliani, L. Vandeperre, E. Saiz, 3D printing bioinspired ceramic composites, Scientific Reports 7 (2017) 13759, https://doi.org/10.1038/s41598-017-14236-9.
[80] C.F. Marques, F.H. Perera, A. Marote, S. Ferreira, S.I. Vieira, S. Olhero, P. Miranda, J.M.F. Ferreira, Biphasic calcium phosphate scaffolds fabricated by direct write assembly: mechanical, anti-microbial and osteoblastic properties, Journal of the European Ceramic Society 37 (2017) 359–368, https://doi.org/10.1016/j.jeurceramsoc.2016.08.018.
[81] S.M. Giannitelli, D. Accoto, M. Trombetta, A. Rainer, Current trends in the design of scaffolds for computer-aided tissue engineering, Acta Biomaterialia 10 (2014) 580–594, https://doi.org/10.1016/j.actbio.2013.10.024.

Index

Note: 'Page numbers followed by "f" indicate figures and "t" indicate tables.'

I

CPI Antony Rowe
Chippenham, UK
2018-10-11 20:14